ALL ABOUT
HEALTH AND BEAUTY
FOR THE
BLACK WOMAN

ALL ABOUT
HEALTH AND BEAUTY
FOR THE
BLACK WOMAN

by Naomi Sims

Illustrated by Harvey Boyd

Doubleday & Company, Inc., Garden City, New York   1976

Library of Congress Cataloging in Publication Data

Sims, Naomi, 1949–
    All about health and beauty for the Black woman.

    Includes index.
        1. Afro-American women—Health and hygiene.
2. Beauty, Personal. I. Title.
RA778.S585   613'.04'244
                ISBN 0-385-00389-7
Library of Congress Catalog Card Number 73–9047

For my mother,
the late
ELIZABETH SIMS
and my grandmother,
PRISCILLA PARHAM

CONTENTS

Foreword by Dr. Norma Goodwin, New York City Health and Hospital
  Corporation   *ix*

Preface   *xv*

Chapter   I OUR SKIN   *1*

Chapter   II OUR FACE   *13*

Chapter   III OUR HAIR   *53*

Chapter   IV OUR HANDS AND NAILS   *97*

Chapter   V OUR FEET AND LEGS   *107*

Chapter   VI THE VISIBLE BODY   *123*

Chapter   VII THE INVISIBLE BODY   *149*

Chapter VIII THE REPRODUCTIVE SYSTEM   *183*

Chapter   IX MENTAL HEALTH   *233*

Chapter   X BEAUTY AND BEHAVIOR   *241*

Chapter   XI FASHION: MYTH AND REALITY   *253*

Chapter   XII HOSPITALS AND HEALTH AGENCIES   *273*

Appendix   *285*

Index   *287*

FOREWORD

———————◆———————

In writing ALL ABOUT HEALTH AND BEAUTY FOR THE BLACK WOMAN, Naomi Sims has combined her own extensive and highly successful experience in portraying the beauty of the Black woman with four years of personal consultations with health-care and beauty experts and many women. The result for you, the reader, is a readable, comprehensive, very personal, and uniquely practical guide to a better understanding of those ingredients that contribute to the realization of health and beauty in the Black woman. The highly informative consultations alone afford the reader the benefit of years of experience by dermatologists, obstetrician/gynaecologists, internists, plastic surgeons, nutritionists, dentists, and other health-care specialists, plus numerous beauty specialists, all gained from their individual and collective efforts to enhance the lives of Black women.

From the title through the last chapter, the book consistently makes two points: 1) the varied and often unique physical needs and attributes of Black women, and 2) the inevitable interrelationships of health and beauty. In fact, Ms. Sims makes clear early in the book the importance of a mental state of well-being, as well as a bodily one, in bringing out the potential beauty intrinsic in every Black woman, regardless of her specific physical characteristics.

Another impression that emerges as one reads the book is that any Black woman who is willing to make an objective assessment of her assets and liabilities—in both appearance and health—can proceed to remove obstacles and maximize assets through both knowledge and understanding of self and a willingness to work toward this goal. While the book does not tell how to become a model, it contains much valuable information for the Black woman who wishes to project beauty for herself or for, and to, others.

Throughout the book, Ms. Sims shares many of her personal approaches to physical beauty, points out the fallacies of certain methods and products that have been promoted in the past for Black women, and gives guidelines that are general enough to be applicable to the broad variety of needs of Black women. Although Ms. Sims emphasizes that there is no one formula for make-up or dress that is applicable for all women of a particular color, size, or shape, she gives guidelines related to these considerations. Her viewpoint, most would acknowledge, is an informed one.

In fact, I consider this book a personalized encyclopedia on health and beauty for the Black woman because of its comprehensiveness. For example, in the chapter on skin, one is told what it is, what causes its color, its special conditions and problems such as dark patches, ashiness, keloids, acne, allergies, and the changes sometimes associated with pregnancy or the use of birth control pills. The effect of the sun on black skin, the when and how of skin care, and the aging process are also covered. The chapter on the face, in part an extension of that on skin, tells when and how to use moisturizers, cleansing creams and lotions, astringents, facial masks, and even soap and water. Further, the basis of how to select and use foundations, powders, eye shadow, mascara, and a variety of other products exemplifies the array of detailed information covered on caring for various parts of the body. The chapter on hair should be of particular interest, given the fact that Black women today, on the basis of personal preference and convenience, select from hairstyles encompassing the Afro, corn row, permanents, hot comb straightening, and wigs. After Ms. Sims discusses the anatomy of hair, its normal variations in thickness and oil content, and general hair cleansing and care, there is an extensive discourse on each of the hairstyles mentioned above and related matters, including alternative curling methods.

Whether one is interested in the physical aspects of beauty or in such subjects as alcohol and drug use and abuse, rape prevention, dieting, self-examination of the breasts, mental health, foot care, behavior as it relates to beauty, hypertension (the silent and predominant killer of Blacks), or a host of other subjects which might be of interest or concern to Black women, this book addresses them. It should prove to be a standard reference work for Black women and for those whose occupations involve service to Black women.

From reading the book, it becomes obvious that there are many common sense aspects, as well as many intricacies, to maximizing one's potential for physical beauty. The extent to which one uses a systematic approach and gives attention to detail undoubtedly bears a relationship to the end result. Therefore, any woman can, after reading the book, decide, after taking into consideration her objectives, responsibilities, available time, financial means, personal needs, priorities, and past practices, which of the approaches in this book she may wish to follow. Ms. Sims has stressed, and I concur with this, that in any event, to understand and strive for physical and mental health is a prerequisite for the good life. ALL ABOUT HEALTH AND BEAUTY FOR THE BLACK WOMAN communicates Ms. Sims's view that in addition to "a common past" and "a shared present," Black women, with a high degree of self-knowledge, self-appreciation, and self-care, can have an even greater future.

NORMA J. GOODWIN, M.D.
Senior Vice-President
New York City Health and Hospital Corporation

ACKNOWLEDGMENTS

Before I began to write this book I conducted a series of probing interviews with Black women of all ages and occupations, from all walks of life, living in different parts of this country. I wanted to learn what kind of information would best serve my readers. The extraordinary interest and candor of those interviewed inspired me to extend the boundaries of this book far beyond mere equations of cosmetic beauty. Therefore, first and foremost, I want to thank those women: Elsie Archer, Claudette Branch, Gladys Bryant, Charlene Dash, Julie Dash, Rhudine Dash, Ann Edwards, Diana Falis, Jessie Gibson, Thelma Green, Vy Higginson, Carol Hobbs, Nina Houchen, Alberta Lloyd, Denise McDonald, Milly Moorehead, Willette Nelson, LaMarr Renee, Karen Robinson, Audrey Smaltz, Lois Williams, Enevia Wilson, and Valerie Wilson.

In order to present you with the most accurate and relevant information from the field of contemporary medicine, I sought the assistance of many eminent women and men, dedicated physicians who patiently and unstintingly answered all my questions. Of these, my very special thanks to Dr. Helen O. Dickens, Professor of Obstetrics and Gynaecology and Associate Dean of the School of Medicine, University of Pennsylvania; Dr. Greta F. Clarke, Dermatologist; Dr. Alvin S. Keith, Podiatrist; Dr. Helen B. Barnes, Professor of Obstetrics and Gynaecology, University of Mississippi Medical Center; Dr. Alvin E. Friedman-Kien, Professor of Dermatology, New York University School of Medicine; Dr. George C. Branche, Internist; Dr. Lois Chatham, National Institute on Drug Abuse; Dr. Aaron B. Lerner, Chairman of the Department of Dermatology, Yale University; Dr. Herbert Berger, Director of Medicine, Richmond Memorial Hospital, New York; Dr. Richard A. Williams, Internist, Martin Luther King Hospital, Los Angeles; Dr. John A. Kenney, Jr., Chairman of the Department of Dermatology, Howard University, Washington, D.C.; Dr. R. Chester Redhead, Dentist; Dr. Joseph I. Paris, Gynaecologist; Dr. Arthur L. Garnes, Chief of Plastic Surgery, Harlem Hospital; Dr. Arthur Williams, Director of the Department of Oral Surgery, Harlem Hospital; Dr. Errol A. Thompson, Chief of Otolaryngology Service, Harlem

Hospital, Professor of Clinical Otolaryngology, Columbia University; Dr. Herman C. Jordan, Associate Director in Ophthalmology at Harlem Hospital Center; Dr. David Burns, Medical Officer for the Clearing House for Smoking and Health Division of the Center for Disease Control, Atlanta, Georgia; Dr. Norman Orentreich, Dermatologist; Dr. Phillip Casson, Associate Professor of Plastic Surgery, New York University Medical Center; Dr. Robert Auerbach, Dermatologist; and Dr. Norma J. Goodwin, Senior Vice-President of Community Health and Ambulatory Care, New York City Health and Hospital Corporation.

I want to single out for special praise Dr. Charles Brown, President of Manhattan Central Medical Society, and Dr. Gerald E. Thomson, Director of Medicine at Harlem Hospital, both of whom allowed me to call them countless times on divers matters and who guided me to many important medical specialists.

Other experts and professionals in the fields of health and beauty whom I want to thank heartily for affording me the benefit of their information and opinions are Carmela Daniega, City of New York Nutrition Clinic; Dr. Thomas F. Johnson, Professor of Physiology, Howard University, Washington, D.C.; Joyce Hart, Co-ordinator of the Post-Mastectomy Program, American Cancer Society; Ruth Ann Stewart, Assistant Chief of the Schomburg Center for Research in Black Culture; Nena Rico, nail specialist; Susan Robbins and Patti Gross of the Information Office of the Population Council; Mr. Robert E. Bochat, Assistant to the Director of the Institute of Reconstructive Surgery, New York University Medical Center; Mr. Joel Gerson, Vice-President, Christine Valmy Salons, Inc.; Mr. Allan Luks, Executive Director of the New York City Affiliate of the National Council on Alcoholism; Shiela Rossi, Account Supervisor for the Rowland Company; Mrs. Edna Kallinen, Director of Lydia O'Leary's Covermark Application Assistance Salon, New York City; Dr. Memory Elvin-Lewis, Chairman of the Department of Microbiology, Washington University School of Dental Medicine, St. Louis, Missouri; Kathleen Stanford-Grant, Director of Pilates System of Muscle Contrology at Henri Bendel, New York City; Mr. John Henry Jones, News Editor of the American Cancer Society; George Buckner, President, Hair Fashions East, New York City; Andre Douglas, Style Consultant, Hair Fashions East, New York City; Camello "Frenchie" Casimir, Proprietor, Casdulan Hair Salon, Harlem, New York; Mr. Stephan Janofsky, Librarian, New York Academy of Medicine; Dr. Dorothy V. Harris, Professor of Physical Education, Pennsylvania State University and General Director of the Research Center for Women and Sport; and Detective Theresa Enterlin, Sex Crime Analysis Unit, New York City Police Department.

I want to acknowledge a very special debt of gratitude to Dr. Mamie Phipps Clark, Executive Director of the Northside Center for Child Development, New York City, and her husband, Dr. Kenneth B. Clark, President of the Metropolitan Applied Research Center, New York City. Not only did they furnish me with considerable specific help but their exemplary moral and social leadership has been a major inspiration.

Many thanks must go to my husband, Michael Alistair Findlay, whose constant enthusiasm for this project encouraged me to persevere for the four years it has taken to complete.

I am most grateful to the writer Tony Tuttle for introducing me to Lisa Drew of Doubleday & Company, to her for believing in this book, and to my editor Louise Gault for, above all, her understanding and patience.

Last but not least I want to thank my typist Michael Cooper and my able research assistants Linda Rodin and Patrecia Sawyer West.

PREFACE

———◆———

Concepts of beauty are among our most ingrained prejudices. In the last decade, Black and white America experienced a barrage of Black Power and "Black Is Beautiful" propaganda that has helped not only the white world but us ourselves to redefine beauty in terms of our natural heritage and our God-given physical and spiritual grace. Now, the majority of our people are prepared to renounce all feelings of inferiority or ambivalence concerning our appearance and know, truly, what the wisest of our elders have always known: that our colors and our features are second to none under the sun.

The physical countenance, however, is only a key to inner beauty, not an end in itself. I had originally planned to call this book *The Beautiful Black Woman*, but as my thinking and reading plunged me into all areas of our Black female ethic I soon realized that that approach was too one-dimensional, and to concentrate only upon the outward signs was to ignore many of the attributes we possess or aspire to.

Our most precious gift is life itself. Adorning that gift is our color. Despite the fact that in the past and, sadly, in the present, the very high cost of our color is sometimes our freedom and even our lives, we must also acknowledge that the color itself and the solidarity it creates is, next to life, our most treasured possession.

I believe firmly that beauty transcends color and I also believe, paradoxically, that my color is the best. Perhaps every woman of every race needs that thought.

We have all been provided with the raw elements of beauty. Elegance, grace, refinement, confidence, style, and cordiality are well within the grasp of every Black woman and these are the stuff of which beauty is made, not a well-turned nose. A healthy body and mind are the first prerequisites, and then and only then can we consider the aspects of cosmetic beauty. If you remember only one thing from this book, I want it to be the necessity for regular medical examinations to prevent and control illness, not how to put on eyelashes. Without health, there simply can be no beauty.

I have attempted to find answers to the many questions I have asked over the years, questions that some of you have told me you also ask and that I believe to be of paramount importance to us as Black women. From why our skin is Black to hypoallergenic cosmetics to the quiet killer hypertension, I have written about facts I hope you will not only read but use.

No woman can succeed as a politician, as a housewife, as a businesswoman, as a fashion model, as a secretary, or as anything if she lacks basic information concerning herself. Each woman must face the honest facts about her physical assets and liabilities in both appearance and health and proceed to remove whatever obstacles she finds.

To do this, each individual woman must be selfish, think only of herself for a while, care about her looks and her diet and her blood pressure. In this strife-ridden century we must not lose our self-esteem, and self-esteem can only come from self-knowledge.

No matter what age we are, life begins today. As Black women, we have captured the limelight and we cannot dwell on all the social injustices of the past. We have to nurture our position at center stage and exploit it far beyond the boundaries of mere equality. No Black woman should want to be equal to a non-Black; she must want to be much better! We must strive not only for acceptance and participation but for forceful, creative leadership in this world.

I would like you to follow the process of self-learning that I had to develop for my career. The business of being beautiful is more a workaday process than a miracle of birth. All Black women can be extraordinarily beautiful all the time if our wills are strong. Affluence is not a help; it is no hindrance either, but a moderate income is no liability toward becoming a totally enriched and enriching Black woman.

Within this book you will find the basic tools for a sensibility of physical and mental well-being that goes far beyond "looking good." As I share with you my experience as a model, public speaker, businesswoman, wife and mother, you must recognize that this is supported by four years of research and hundreds of hours of consultation with health-care and beauty specialists. From talking to many of you in your homes, in stores, at work, in colleges, and high schools, I found that our basic needs were quite similar.

This book does not tell you how to look or act like a model or a movie star. What it does is help you choose a system for your looks and life style that increases your ability to get the maximum out of life.

N.S.
New York City

Chapter I

OUR SKIN

We possess a vital organ approximately twenty feet in size that weighs about seven pounds. The skin. Each square centimeter of skin contains a yard of blood vessels. Every blood vessel acts as a thermostat and dilates or contracts to maintain the correct body temperature. Over two million sweat glands in the skin constantly regulate the chemical and fluid balance of the body. Our skin also consists of countless glands and nerve endings; thus it is a prime sensory organ.

The skin divides itself into three layers. The hypodermis is a layer of fatty tissue that lies beneath the dermis, or true skin. The dermis contains nerves, blood vessels, sebaceous glands, smooth muscles, and hair follicles. Covering this is the epidermis, the visible surface of the skin. Even at birth, the epidermis is marked with wrinkles, ridges, and furrows and is covered with openings, called pores, through which moisture passes out of, or into, the body. The skin is flexible although its elasticity changes according to age and location. (Skin at the joints is particularly elastic.) The skin is always growing and replacing itself; the surface skin cornifies and is shed. All our nails and our hair are natural appendages of the skin and have much the same chemical structure.

Skin Color

Anthropologists are investigating a theory that all the races of man descend from one Black "protorace" that originated in Africa. As members of this race dispersed into less sunny climates, a process of natural selection occurred whereby only those with lighter skins survived because they were better able to absorb the sunlight and synthesize the vitamin D needed to avoid diseases such as rickets. We do know that there is no difference in the basic properties of the skin between Black peoples and other races. Texture, thickness, and the quantity of sweat and sebaceous glands are consistent in all human beings. Our skin color is determined by pigment which is in turn derived from melanin (Greek: *melan*=black). There is no consensus among scientists relating to the exact cause of melanin distribution, but it is currently believed that although all individuals have an equal number of melanin-bearing cells, melanocytes, the appearance of white skin is caused by an uneven distribution pattern of these cells. Our melanocytes are evenly distributed, perhaps larger, and certainly more active.

Special Skin Conditions

Because of our hyperactive pigmentation system we are prone to three skin conditions:

DARKER PATCHES

The following areas of our body tend to be darker than others. Individuals may vary from the virtually invisible to the very conspicuous: knees, lower buttocks, elbows, shoulders, ear lobes, back of the neck. This condition is permanent. It is irreversible. It is perfectly normal. If you find it unsightly, that is unfortunate as it is part of our distinction. I must caution you against attempting to lighten these areas by such activities as brush-scrubbing. This will achieve the opposite result. The skin, when aggravated, becomes darker. If you wish to avoid increasing the dark patches, remember that daily friction caused by rubbing elbows, knees, and buttocks on hard surfaces such as desks, chairs, and floors must be shunned.

LIGHTER PATCHES

Trauma to the skin, even slight as caused by pimples and scratching, can heal to a lighter (hypopigmentation) color as well as a darker (hyperpigmentation) one. Hypopigmentation often takes the form of a patchy, freckled appearance, but this type of discoloration usually fades within one year if it has resulted from a minor injury. The only way to avoid such blotchy marks is to leave surface eruptions alone as much as possible.

ASHINESS

This phenomenon is commonly found on the limbs but is by no means confined to them. It is induced by the skin's rapid loss of moisture. This is caused by changes in temperature and humidity. Some of us are in the habit of applying a body oil to counter this condition. That does not restore the moisture to the skin; it only temporarily disguises the ashy appearance and seals the pores. It is essential that you apply a moisturizing product, cream, or lotion. Do not rub it in but let the skin absorb it naturally.

Keloids

When our skin is damaged or broken, a keloid may form during the healing process. A keloid is a thickened dark growth of fibrous tissue usually larger than the original area of damage. Our skin heals faster than most and for this advantage we become subject to keloids. They may occur anywhere on the body but especially on the chest and the back, and they will persist unless treated by a qualified dermatologist. Treatments commonly practiced to flatten keloids involve the use of dry ice, X-rays, and steroid injections. In extreme cases surgery may be performed, but there is a high risk that another, larger keloid will form in the same place. Although keloids can be rendered less obvious, some trace will always remain. Keloids have been known to form spontaneously where there has been no exterior damage to the skin. This usually occurs on the chest where the skin is tightest and is aggravated by the strain of heavy breasts improperly supported. Keloids can also be encouraged by persistent wearing of heavy jewelry on the arms and neck. The skin becomes imperceptibly damaged and keloids form.

Special Skin Problems

Our skin color makes us susceptible to certain common skin problems that identify themselves strongly and often persistently.

Acne

The principal cause of acne is hormonal change that the body endures during adolescence. However, women of all ages can contract acne for a variety of reasons and it is by no means restricted to teen-agers. Any hormonal change can stimulate acne, including that produced by oral contraception and pregnancy itself. Acne is caused by an oversecretion of sebum (oil) in the skin ducts that when clogged become infected. Sometimes this happens as a result of constipation when the sweat glands in the skin that function to eliminate impurities become overloaded. Many of us still believe that there is a connection between acne and the ingestion of candy and fried food. This is a highly overrated theory, but it is known that women prone to acne should avoid iodine, found in seafood. Whatever the cause, you can seriously lessen the risk of acne by keeping the skin absolutely clean at all times. Acne is a medical problem, not a cosmetic one. Because our Black skins are more sensitive to pigment change, the treatment for acne should not be harsh. If the problem develops, first try a brand-name product and follow the directions correctly. In ten days there should be signs of improvement. If not, you must see your doctor immediately.

Allergies

Local skin disorders are frequently caused by an allergic reaction. You can become allergic to absolutely anything—animal, vegetable, or mineral. It is quite wrong to assume that your allergy can only be caused by new or foreign materials. We often become suddenly allergic to a flower, pet, or food that we have been in contact with for years. If you cannot isolate the offending matter, consult your doctor and mention everything you may suspect, no matter how silly it may seem to you.

Chloasma

Perhaps the most common and most serious skin complaint that plagues Black women is chloasma, sometimes called melasma or, more commonly, "mask of pregnancy." This is a darkening of pigmentation across the center of the face. Light skins are even more susceptible to this state than very dark skins but it can affect anyone. It is caused by hormonal change and if it happens while you are pregnant it will probably disappear in the months following birth. It is far more dangerous if it occurs while you are taking birth-control pills. In this case, immediately contact your doctor as soon as it appears. If you do not receive professional advice at this stage, the chloasma can become permanent and irremedial.

Stretch Marks

These are caused by a permanent loss of the elastic tissue in the skin. They may be a result of any rapid weight loss or weight gain—which you can avoid —or pregnancy. To avoid or at least limit the possibility of pregnancy stretch marks, I suggest the following:

1) Exercise is very necessary at this time, but do not indulge in *strenuous* activity.
2) Avoid massaging the stomach area. If the stomach or breasts are subjected to prolonged massaging, the skin can tear and stretch.
3) Always keep the skin moist; do not let it dry out.
4) Ask your doctor if you should wear an approved pregnancy girdle.

The Advantages of Our Skin

As Black women, our skin is blessed with certain unique properties. Although scars take longer to fade, wounds are faster to heal. The greatest advantage is that our skin ages benignly. Many factors contribute to this, including genetics and environment, but the answer probably lies in our great capacity to withstand the damaging effects of the sun. The sun is the principal villain in the battle to save the skin. We can trace many maladies, from premature wrinkles to skin cancer, to the harmful rays of the sun.

The Sun

It is essential that we do not consider ourselves totally immune from the damaging ultraviolet rays of the sun simply because our skin can tolerate three times the exposure that white skin can. Our skin can sustain damage that will not be visible to the eye but that occurs within the epidermis, or lower layers of skin, and that can be very painful. No matter how dark your skin, you will benefit from using a sun-screen product that blocks out the damaging rays of the sun. This will not necessarily prevent you from achieving a deeper tan. If your skin color is light to medium, you should use a protective lotion when sunbathing, one that contains moisturizing ingredients, not just baby oil which in fact magnifies the sun's effect. When pregnant, stay out of the sun. If chloasma develops and is combined with exposure to direct, strong sun, it can become permanent. Also, if your birth-control pill contains a high percentage of estrogen, stay out of the sun and reduce the risk of chloasma.

Water

Before bathing in the sea or chlorinated swimming pools, always apply a generous amount of baby oil to your skin. Although the salt or chlorine do little damage while the body is immersed in the water, the oil will effectively seal your pores. It is damaging to let chemical or natural (saline) residue dry on the skin after bathing. If possible, soap the body lightly after sunbathing if you have been swimming, and always rinse under a shower.

Skin Health

Soft, supple, rich, warm, attractive skin is acquired and sustained only by correct cleansing procedures. The frequency with which we clean our bodies is not necessarily as important as the methods we employ. We wash for three reasons:

1) To rid the skin's surface of visible, accumulated dirt.
2) To disinfect the areas of the skin and reduce the risk of bacterial infection.
3) To replace the skin's natural moisture.

The following discussion of skin types and bathing applies to the body. Cleansing of the face and scalp are dealt with in the chapters "Our Face" and "Our Hair."

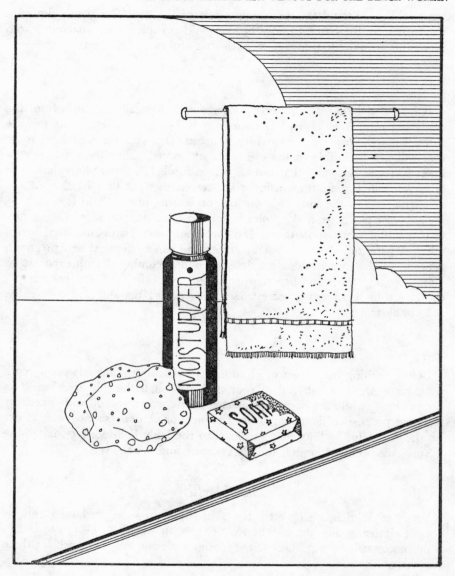

As Black women, our bodies fall into one of two skin-type categories:

A) If you have never, or only rarely, experienced the ashy tinge that indicates skin dryness, assume that you have a *normal-to-oily skin* that is resilient and fairly flexible.

B) Many of us have a skin that is prone to ashiness and that exhibits a characteristically taut appearance. This indicates a *normal-to-dry skin* tendency.

A) CLEANSING PROCEDURES FOR NORMAL-TO-OILY SKIN

Your active sebaceous glands are constantly depositing their secretions of sebum on the surface of the skin, even while you sleep. Unless removed regularly, this oily film combines with bacteria to create a wide range of problems from body odor to acne.

The body must be washed every day. The choice of bath or shower is up to you. To guarantee a clean, healthy skin you should bathe or shower twice a day. If you follow my instructions seven days a week, you will have an exceptional skin:

a) Use hot, but not scalding, water to open your pores.

b) Only wash with a pure soap (Ivory is a good example) that does not contain chemicals or perfume or detergents.

If you have extraoily skin, use a high-alkali or medicated soap such as Cuticura or Clearasil. These contain active oil-removing ingredients and are designed for use especially on areas such as the chest and back where the skin is thickest and contains a large number of sweat glands. So-called deodorant and antibacterial soaps may make you feel fresher but their odor-reducing effectiveness is highly debatable.

c) Absolutely avoid additives. Oils, powders, salts, crystals, and bubble-bath preparations retard the pores' ability to open and release excess oil.

d) If you have a very oily skin you may need a loofah—a rough-textured, fibrous sponge found in any drugstore. A long-handled natural bristle brush will help you reach your back.

e) When washing, soap the entire body lavishly. Use medicated soap only on problem areas. Firmly massage the suds over the skin's surface.

f) Rinse thoroughly in warm water and remove all traces of soapsuds. Dried residue will clog your pores. Rinse again in water as cool as you can bear to clean and close the pores.

g) Towel-dry vigorously to remove all excess moisture.

h) Apply a mild astringent such as witch hazel to extraoily parts of the body. Definitely do not use any form of concentrated alcohol which will dehydrate the skin totally.

If taking a tub bath, remember that the only way to rinse properly is with running water, not the water you have washed in. If you prefer to shower, you must lather the body outside the direct flow of water so that the soap can settle and work.

Your normal-to-oily skin suffers most in conditions that combine heat and humidity. A hot kitchen or a long summer day will produce the same sticky result. The only way to counteract this and sustain a healthy skin is by frequent and thorough washing. Nothing else will remove that surface accumulation of oil.

B) CLEANSING PROCEDURES FOR NORMAL-TO-DRY SKIN

Because your skin loses to the air more moisture than is regularly secreted by the sebaceous glands, it is essential that you habitually replace this water. I have designed this cleansing system to do precisely that.

a) Find at least ten minutes every day for bathing. Preferably this should be in the morning on rising, but the amount of time spent in the bath is more important than the time of day.

b) Hot water carries away the body's oils, so use only warm water.

c) Wash with a mild, pure soap, such as Ivory, free of medicating or deodorizing agents. Your skin may not be able to withstand the potentially abrasive chemicals found in medicinal and deodorant products.

If you suffer from a very dry skin, try a superfatted castile soap (Johnson & Johnson's Baby Soap) or a glycerine soap (Pear's Neutrogena).

Superfatted soaps are rich in oils such as coconut, lanolin, olive oil, and vegetable oils. They are high-lathering and while they cleanse they remove a minimum of the skin's natural oils and replenish that oil supply.

Glycerine soaps are transparent and soft. Unlike almost all other soaps, they are very low in alkali content and alkali is harmful to dry skin. These soaps melt quickly and are quite expensive because glycerine is a valuable substance. Superfatted soaps are longer-lasting and not expensive.

d) While the bath is running, pour in one ounce of a pure, nonperfumed, nondetergent emollient such as baby oil. Exposure to or immersion in water is not alone sufficient to feed the skin. Oil is essential to trap that moisture and seal it into the epidermis. I suggest you avoid luxuries like colored bath crystals and bubble-bath products because, although they may appear to soften the skin, the dyes, perfumes, and chemical contents may irritate. The major value of these preparations is psychological.

e) Soak in the bathtub for at least five minutes immersed up to your chin. Keep doors and windows closed to simulate a sauna-type atmosphere and allow the steam to open your pores.

f) Using a soft washcloth or natural sponge, lather the whole surface of the body. Those who recommend the use of loofahs or bristle brushes to remove dry, flaky skin are imparting dangerous advice. Such implements create more irritation than they remove and are not necessary if you soak and wash correctly.

g) Rinse thoroughly. This is the most important part of your regimen. Do not rinse with the water you have soaked in, but shower the suds off with a light force of warm (not hot) water. Remove all traces of soap. If any is left to dry and clog the pores, you will experience ashiness and itching and you might as well have not bathed at all.

h) Pat yourself dry with a soft towel. Never rub.

i) While the skin is still slightly damp, apply a moisturizer such as Vaseline Intensive Care Lotion. This will add water to the skin and add oil to prevent quick evaporation. To take full advantage of the lotion, you must let your naked body absorb it at room temperature without rubbing. This will take five to seven minutes. If you use an emollient like baby oil or Vaseline petroleum jelly, this will not be absorbed but simply grease the skin surface.

If you simply cannot bathe every day and must rely partially or entirely on showering to clean your skin:

1) Avoid harsh water pressure.
2) Soap the body profusely while standing away from direct spray.
3) Rinse and rinse again.
4) Apply body lotion.

Although the steam generated by the shower will open your pores, it is no real substitute for soaking in the bathtub because it is important that water not only contact the skin but enter it, and for this, immersion is most efficacious.

As Black women with normal-to-dry skin, we must cope with harmful atmospheric circumstances such as air-conditioning, steam heat, and low humidity in winter. All these evaporate the natural oils and moisture in the skin. After repeated exposure to dry heat or dry cold inside or outside the home, your skin must replenish its food supply. The best way to do this is to pat on a body lotion before sleeping. A room humidifier can be of great benefit to your skin and will prevent it from drying out overnight. A large pot of water placed on top of the radiator will often do just as well. Make sure that the window is slightly open, even if it is only a hairline.

All types of Black skin, dry and oily, may suffer from excessively dry, scaly areas at the elbows, knees, ankles, and feet. I recommend the use of a cream such as Pretty Feet to be massaged into these areas for three to five minutes before bathing. It will gently remove rough skin although it is free of alcohol, nongreasy, and nongritty.

Our Skin and the Aging Process

Three major factors are responsible for the deterioration of the skin's appearance as our age increases:

1) ULTRAVIOLET LIGHT

Because of our color we are better able than other races to withstand the damaging effects of the ultraviolet rays emanating from the sun. The substance melanin is responsible for our dark pigmentation. Melanin is exceptionally dense and virtually insoluble. Highly durable, it is one of the few materials still present in mummified corpses 2,000 years old. Melanin absorbs part of the sun's radiation. The remaining ultraviolet rays penetrate the epidermis and stimulate chemical and physical changes in the glands below the dermis. The skin gradually becomes drier and the result is wrinkling. Our skin has a reputation for sustaining a youthful appearance because our melanin screens out much of the harmful radiation.

2) INTERNAL AGING

As we become older, important changes occur in the bone structure of the body and the muscles themselves. As the frame for the skin shrinks, the skin itself suffers. This process is natural and irreversible.

3) PROTEIN AND HORMONE DEFICIENCY

Two important substances, collagen and estrogen, are produced by the body in decreasing amounts with age. Collagen is a protein product that controls the elasticity of the skin. As the body secretes diminishing amounts of collagen, the skin gradually becomes less supple. Estrogen is the sex hormone that controls the functioning of the sebaceous glands. When we pass our mid-twenties, our estrogen output slows down and eventually the activity of the sebaceous glands declines to the point that there is a marked inability of the skin to oil itself.

To Deal with Aging Skin

The stores are glutted with products that attempt to seduce the consumer with wily rejuvenation devices. These products usually lay claim to a miracle ingredient that is either bizarre or scientific-sounding. You will only be disappointed if you let the advertising claims relieve you of your money. Some substances that might temporarily lend the look of freshness to the skin can do nothing substantive about the varied aging factors that affect the skin. If you try to help time take its course gracefully and naturally rather than attempting to turn back the clock, you will be far better pleased with the results. Since it is dryness of the skin that in age contributes heavily to a wrinkled appearance, concentrate on continually feeding oil and moisture to the skin. Any basic water-bearing lubricant will do (moisturizing creams are 60–70 per cent water) if used judiciously and constantly. Always let the pores absorb—do not rub in—and apply after every bath and each night before bed. This will prohibit the skin's tendency to crease and will keep it pliant for as long as possible.

In addition to this, your over-all health is a major factor in dealing with aging skin. Sound and sufficient sleep, regular elimination, a balanced diet, and correct exercise will establish and retain a personal metabolism for you that will be reflected positively by your skin.

Skin Specialists

Only a physician should be consulted in the event of serious skin disorders, never a beauty specialist or anyone without a medical degree. Physicians who specialize in problems of the skin and hair are known as dermatologists.

Care of Damaged Skin

BURNS

Immediately irrigate the burn area with lukewarm to cool water. If possible, submerge the skin in water or shower the burn area. If the burn is major, do not apply any ointments, oils, or antiseptics. Simply pack the burn with clean sheets or towels and call the doctor immediately. If the burn is minor, the application of a cold, damp compress will relieve the sting. Spread the skin with lard or butter to quickly replace fluid loss.

CUTS

Wash hands thoroughly before treating the wound. Wash the wounded area with a mild soap, rinsing with running water away from the wound. Cover with the cleanest soft cloth available and tighten according to the amount of bleeding. If the bleeding is copious or persistent, call a doctor. If the cut is minor but the area becomes hot or inflamed (this may take several days), infection is present and you must seek professional medical help.

Our ability to heal quickly and the consequent tendency toward the formation of keloids and other pigment aberrations mean that even the most apparently superficial wounds require close attention and any discoloration should be brought to the attention of a doctor.

The following simple mixtures for dressings will provide speedy relief from skin irritations. They should not be considered alternatives or substitutes for prescribed or packaged medication but as emergency measures.

Mild inflammation	Milk and water
Harsh inflammation	Cornstarch and water
Insect bites	Vinegar and water
Itching and irritation	Milk of Magnesia and olive oil (half and half)
Swelling	1 tablespoon Epsom salts to one quart warm water

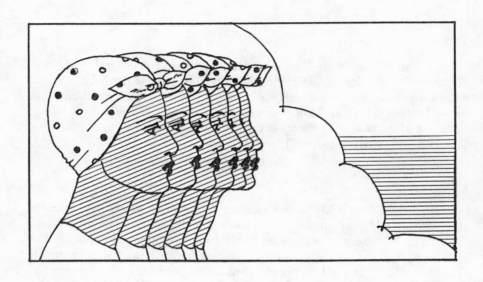

Chapter II

OUR FACE

———— ◆ ————

Racial characteristics are highly marked in the features of the face but the texture, structure, and density of facial skin is common to all races. Our quintessential feature is, of course, our color. It has been estimated that there are at least thirty-five color divisions for the Black race as opposed to only three (brunette, blond, redhead) for Caucasians. For this reason I cannot give advice about appropriate shades of eye shadow, for example, and hope that it will apply to all of us. What I will do is examine in detail every part of the face and consider how best it can be cared for and beautified.

A. FACIAL SKIN

The skin on our face and scalp is not entirely the same as that found elsewhere on our body. It heals more quickly and has a higher concentration per square inch of sebaceous glands.

Before we are able to care for the face properly we must know what kind of skin we possess. Since the large number of sebaceous glands in the face are very active in lubricating the skin, it is normal for our face to be slightly oily. Skin types are based upon the degree and distribution of this oiliness.

Dry skin. The skin is insufficiently lubricated resulting in a tight, flaky, or fissured surface. If your face chaps regularly with the onset of cold weather, you have dry skin.

Oily skin. When the skin is sufficiently lubricated, one is not necessarily aware of it. If the secretions are too great, a greasy film constantly accumulates.

Combination skin. This is most frequently exemplified by dry forehead and cheek areas with increased oiliness around the nose, mouth, and chin. Because of its color, our skin easily reflects the light. Do not confuse a tendency to shininess with oily skin.

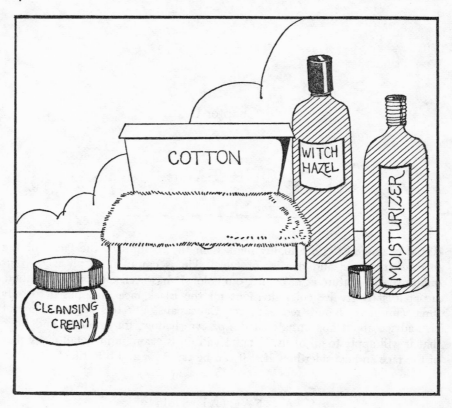

Facial Skin Care

The foundation of facial care is cleanliness and the foundation of cleanliness is soap and water. In order to build on these foundations and create and maintain a clear, beautiful complexion you must have, and know how to use, certain products.

MOISTURIZERS

These are made in both cream and lotion form. They consist of a high percentage of water mixed with mineral oil in an emollient base. The emollient binds the water and oil, and on the skin the water is absorbed as a food for the skin while the oil lubricates the skin surface and prevents evaporation. Soap alone dries out the skin and moisturizers are needed to build up the skin's fluid content. They are also a much-needed premake-up base that provides a smooth complexion prior to the application of cosmetics. As moisturizers I recommend Pond's Moisturizing Cream, Jergen's Extra Dry Skin

Formula, and Vaseline Intensive Care Lotion. These are relatively free from those additives that usually serve only to perfume the product and can cause skin irritation. The main purpose of "extra ingredients" in moisturizers is to boost the price.

CLEANSING CREAMS AND LOTIONS

These cleansing products are not luxuries. Many dermatologists do not consider them necessary because it is true that you can completely clean the skin with soap and water. But in order to remove all the dirt and soiled make-up that accumulates on the skin nowadays, we should complete four or five soap-and-water washings of the face. Not only is that tedious and time-consuming, but I believe injurious to the skin. A correctly formulated cleansing cream is designed to melt on application, spread easily, and flush dirt and make-up from the pores. It consists of emollient base, mineral oil, and solvent ingredients that break up and dislodge grime from the orifices of the sebaceous glands. Our cosmetics such as face powder, rouge, foundation base, lipstick, and cake make-up contain chemicals specifically designed to bind them easily onto the skin. Therefore we need a strong solvent to remove them completely. A good cleansing cream will readily dissolve the greasy binding materials found in cosmetic products and the polluted air itself. It will have an irritation factor far lower than multiple soap-and-water washings and it should leave on the skin a protective emollient film that reseals the skin against irritants. Because water in such a cream only dilutes its cleansing properties, I prefer to use Albolene unscented cleansing cream, which contains no water.

ASTRINGENTS

Products known as skin toners, skin fresheners, and astringents are basically alcohol in an oil solution designed to seal the pores and act as a pleasant antiseptic. Beyond this they simply provide us with a tight, tingling sensation that we are conditioned to equate with cleanliness and freshness. While recommending their limited use to those with normal-to-oily skins, I must caution you that any product with an alcohol content greater than 20 per cent will overdehydrate the skin. Witch hazel, which is about 15 per cent alcohol, is the best astringent to use for both dry and oily skin.

STERILE ABSORBENT COTTON

Although this sounds very medicinal and is, in fact, manufactured for medical use, it is inexpensive and available in every drugstore. Although it may be easier, when applying creams or removing make-up, to grab facial tissues or bathroom tissue, they are in the long run abrasive to the skin and in the short run not absorbent enough to do the job properly. Cotton balls are too small and unmanageable for most of our purposes. The most practical way of using sterile absorbent cotton is to buy the largest size and when needed tear off from the roll enough to make a double six-inch pad. This can be folded, refolded, and disposed of as you use it. Above all, never use a color-dyed product, paper or cotton, to wipe the skin. The dyes and perfumes may prove to be dangerous.

TOWELS

Because your face contains many orifices through which bacteria can enter your body, you must always use a separate washcloth and towel for your face —never the one you use for your body. These should be of a softer, less coarse consistency.

WASHBASIN

Your face can become no cleaner than your sink, so make sure that the whole basin area is frequently scoured and disinfected with an abrasive cleanser. Rinse thoroughly with hot running water. This will kill germs that breed in and around plumbing areas and are anathema to a clear skin.

APPLICATION TECHNIQUE

Always apply a soap, cream, lotion, or cosmetic to the face with your fingertips only. Move in an upward direction from the base of the neck out from the center of the face and toward the hairline. Our facial nerves and muscles benefit from this stimulation sympathetic to their axis.

CLEANSING PROCEDURE FOR DRY SKIN

If you have a quite dry skin, use a superfatted soap such as Basis or Johnson's Baby Soap. Usually, any mild, nondeodorant soap (Ivory) will suffice.

1) Wash with soap and water, applying the lather in a circular rubbing motion to the neck, face, ears, up to the hairline.
2) Rinse thoroughly in clean water.
3) Pat dry with hand towel.
4) Massage cleansing cream into the skin until almost invisible. You may prefer a lotion which is easy to apply and perhaps more economical. Both cream and lotion form have the same cleansing properties.
5) Remove cream, grime, and make-up with sterile cotton pad. Soak the pad in warm water, then squeeze. Repeat, wiping face until no soil residue remains on a clean pad.
6) Gently pat a tiny amount of moisturizer on the face, neck, and ears.

This will help to sustain the fluid content of your skin while you sleep. No matter how dry your skin, use of heavy, so-called "night" and "throat" creams is to no avail because they clog the pores and prevent the skin from breathing naturally.

IN THE MORNING:

Wash thoroughly with soap and water, rinse in clean water, and pat dry.

Apply a moderate amount of moisturizer to the face and wait five minutes before applying any make-up. This time allows the cream to be fully absorbed by the skin. (If it mixes with the cosmetics, the value is lost.)

Cleansing Procedure for Oily (Normal) Skin

1) Massage a cleanser (cream or lotion) into the skin, covering all exposed areas of the face and neck.

2) Wipe face thoroughly with cotton pad. The dirt and make-up will come off easily if the pad is dampened in warm water and squeezed dry. Keep wiping face until no residual grime appears on the pad.

3) Wash the face, neck, and ears to the hairline in warm water. Use a pure soap such as Ivory and lather well.

4) Rinse in clean, cool water to close the pores.

5) Blot dry with a hand towel.

6) Shake a few drops of astringent (preferably witch hazel) onto a cotton pad dampened with cold water and apply to the face, avoiding eyes and neck. The neck has few sebaceous glands and will suffer from astringent application—become dry and tight.

IN THE MORNING:

Apply and remove cleansing lotion or cream. Wash in soap and water; rinse in clean, cold water.

Pat on witch hazel, wait two minutes, then apply light amount of moisturizing lotion. Let it be absorbed and wait five minutes before applying any make-up.

Cleansing Procedure for Combination Skin

BEFORE BED:

Follow steps 1 through 5 for oily skin, then:

6) Rub a moderate amount of moisturizing lotion on entire surface of face, neck, and ears.

7) Shake a few drops of witch hazel onto a cold, damp pad and remove the moisturizer only from the oily areas of the face, e.g., chin, nose, and forehead.

IN THE MORNING:

Apply and remove cleansing lotion and wash in water with a mild soap. Rinse thoroughly in clean, warm water. Repeat 6 and 7 (above), then wait a few minutes before applying make-up.

AGING OF THE FACE

The face and the hands share the dubious distinction of showing age more profoundly than other parts of the body. This is due to the deteriorating consequences of sunlight upon the muscular and glandular system of the face. Those parts of the flesh most exposed to light will appear to wither soonest. As we know, those parts of the body that rarely see the light of day often retain a firm appearance even into old age. As Black women, we suffer less the damaging effects of the sun but we are by no means immune. We can do nothing about the skin's loss of elasticity and the gradual reduction in the amount of natural oils secreted by the sebaceous glands. These glands tend to predominate in parts of the face with an underlying bone (chin, nose, and forehead) and are less abundant in the skin of the neck, eyes, and cheek hollows. The latter areas are consequently the first to dry out and furrow.

THE TREATMENT OF AGING FACIAL SKIN

Without surgery it is not possible to smooth or tighten the skin for anything but a very brief period of time. You can, however, postpone wrinkles and enjoy a fresher appearance if you never, ever allow the facial skin to dry out.

The natural cycle of the skin is from very dry at birth, rapidly increasing to extreme oiliness in adolescence and early twenties, then reverting to very dry as one passes sixty. No matter what skin type you had when young, it will change and gradually become drier. Check every few years to be sure that a once-oily normal skin may not now need a nightly moisturizer since a few prominent lines have become conspicuous. Nothing can rejuvenate the facial skin, but an ample diet of moisture and oil will greatly benefit a skin growing drier with age.

SPECIAL FACIAL TREATMENTS

If you dedicate yourself to the basic cleansing procedures that I have outlined, you will develop a clear, healthy, normal skin. Because most of us subject our faces daily to the ravaging ills of urban pollution, we feel that we need extra help. There are, of course, a host of beauty products that claim to transform a good skin into a wonderful, glowing complexion. In my opinion there are quite definitely procedures that are very beneficial to the countenance of the skin. Many others are either worthless or downright harmful. The official attitude of most dermatologists is that for nonproblem skin, anything more elaborate than soap and water has at best only a psychological effect. Without wishing to dispute them, I can only suggest that the procedures I recommend certainly aid the appearance of my skin and if followed judiciously, I believe will make the difference between simply a clean skin and a smooth, voluptuous complexion. The scurf, or outermost dead layer of skin, is replaced every three weeks, so for any beauty treatment to be effective it must be followed regularly, not haphazardly.

BODY CONDITION

I cannot emphasize too often or too strongly the need for sufficient sleep, proper exercise, and correct diet. Your face will literally show the results.

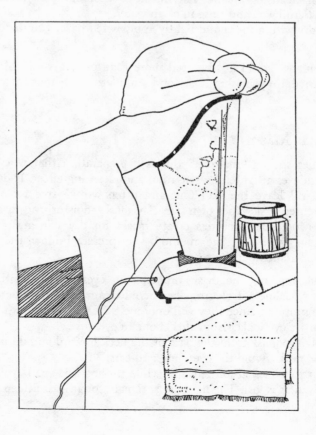

The Facial Sauna

The purpose of a facial sauna is to utilize the properties of steam so as to deep clean the skin by flushing out the pores. This may be done with a commercial sauna kit or a simple pot of boiling water. Because the instructions that accompany many kits are incomplete and there are dangers involved, you must follow my directions.

1) Generously apply cleansing cream to the face and neck. Massage into the skin. Remove excess cream.
2) Bend over sauna and cover entire head and sauna with a large towel.
3) Keep your face at least eighteen inches away from the surface of the water. Closer than this may scald the skin.
4) Keep eyes shut at all times.
5) Cease when the face perspires profusely or feels uncomfortably hot. Never stay longer than ten minutes.
6) The surface of your skin will now be covered with a film of impurities mixed with cleansing cream. This must be thoroughly removed with soap and water. Scrub well and rinse in clean water.
7) Pat dry with a towel and lightly apply witch hazel (diluted, if your skin is dry).

Facial saunas should not be used more than once a week. More frequent use will dehydrate your skin if dry and stimulate the glands to overactivity if oily.

The Facial Mask

Sometimes spelled "masque," this is a preparation that when applied to the skin achieves a tightening sensation and cleansing effect. It does not deep clean but will leave the skin taut and often wrinkle-free for a few hours. There are three basic types of mask: clay mask, moisturizing mask, and peel-off mask. Most manufacturers create masks for dry skin and for oily skin. Choose your type and the method you prefer. Follow the instructions carefully and remember these tips:

1) Before applying the mask, protect your eyes and lips with a generous amount of Vaseline petroleum jelly. A cold cream or cleansing cream will not do the job properly, since they will only melt. Be sure to smooth the Vaseline into the entire eye socket from cheekbone to eyebrow.
2) Apply the mask from the base of the neck upward and do not forget the back of the neck. Avoid the eyes, lips, and ears.
3) Keep your face absolutely still while the mask is on. If you eat or talk, the effectiveness is lost. The mask must remain for at least fifteen minutes.

4) Never use soap to remove a mask but simply warm water and a clean washcloth.

A mask is most beneficial immediately following a facial sauna. If you do this, omit the application of astringent after the sauna. As with the sauna, you should not use a mask more than once a week.

MOISTURIZERS

Many people imagine that if they have oily skin they do not need a moisturizer. That is simply not true. Because the moisturizer is mostly water, you cannot overload the skin's pores and all skins need water. You must use a moisturizer after a facial sauna or mask. Unrestricted use of moisturizing cream or lotion will keep the skin supple and well fed, especially when it is necessary to counteract the dehydrating effects of air-conditioning and steam heat. Always dab a small amount of moisturizer on the face and allow it to be absorbed before sleeping. If you have a very oily skin, look for the special moisturizers developed for this condition.

UNSAFE OR INADEQUATE FACIAL TREATMENTS

Hormone creams. I will not argue with those authorities that claim hormones such as estrogen can be absorbed through the skin. If absorbed in large enough doses, estrogen will apparently cause the skin to swell and hold water, which may lead to a slightly more youthful appearance. Estrogen is not a simple substance but the female sex hormone that plays such an important part in the cycle of life and birth, so that an imbalance of this hormone can lead to most unpleasant bodily changes. For this reason, the Food and Drug Administration (FDA) considers it unsafe to absorb more than 20,000 hormone units per month. This is the equivalent of only two ounces of cream because each ounce is supposed to contain no more than 10,000 units. Manufacturers are required to label these hormone creams with safety instructions, but many use ambiguous language and of course it is very easy to use more than the maximum dosage. Many professionals are agreed that the safe dosage is not sufficient to cause any substantive change in the appearance of the skin, so as a consumer you are faced with the choice of either adhering to the instructions and realizing no difference in your skin or exceeding the proper amount and risking serious disorders. That is no choice, and you may lose more than your money, so steer clear of these products.

Protein- and vitamin-enriched creams. In order for our bodies to manufacture healthy skin it is important that we not be deficient in protein-based substances such as collagen and vitamins A and E. A normal diet will provide you with all you need and it will be duly absorbed by the digestive system and put to work where needed. The FDA reports that vitamin A can be absorbed via the skin only if actively massaged for several hours. You are unlikely to find that information on the jar. In most cases these products make extravagant claims for substances with unfamiliar names. Usually these substances are present in the body in sufficient quantities for a good skin. As a rule of thumb you may be sure that it is always better to ingest proteins and vitamins as we do in our food every day rather than attempt the expensive and often fruitless procedure of forcing them into the skin from the wrong direction.

Exfoliation (peeling). There are a variety of methods for removing the outermost layer of skin, the scurf. These include lotions, gels, creams, abrasive particles, and surgical procedures. All should be avoided by Black women. If you care for your skin correctly, the scurf sheds naturally and regularly. Because of our melanin structure, any trauma to the surface of the skin, no matter how minor, can cause pigment change (dark areas, light patches) or permanent pigment loss. Never contemplate any form of skin abrasion or peeling or even the use of widely available commercial products for exfoliation without the advice of a dermatologist. For the same reasons, avoid the use of facial brushes and coarse washcloths. Only bring the face into contact with the softest-textured fabrics. Never poke the skin with such implements as metal pimple extractors.

Alcohol. As we have already seen, the alcohol content of witch hazel is high enough for the oiliest skin and low enough for a dry skin. Never use raw alcohol, rubbing alcohol, or wood alcohol on the facial skin. Your pores and glands will rapidly dehydrate, and your concern for eventual damage must outweigh the temporary stimulation it may provide. If you do not have witch hazel available and must use a toner or astringent with a higher alcohol content (in excess of 20 per cent), always dilute by applying a few drops of the liquid into a well-dampened cotton pad.

The pH factor. Many advertising claims for facial products now use the letters "pH" followed by a number. This always looks and sounds very impressive. In fact it is a simple scale from 1 to 10 by which scientists indicate the degree of alkalinity or acidity of a material: pH4 indicates high acidity and pH9 high alkalinity while pH7 is about neutral with equal balance between acid and alkali. Since alkali is necessary in cleansing products but excess alkalinity will dry out the skin, it is indicated by advertisers that a low pH number is most desirable. This is true if you have a very dry skin. Otherwise, most soaps have a pH of about 7 and will not harm your skin. I pay little attention to the pH factor and simply avoid products that have deodorizing or perfuming additives that may irritate.

New Products

If you encounter a new commodity or treatment for the face and are tempted to try it, you must follow the instructions and use it consistently.

Only then will you be able to ascertain its effectiveness, if any, and quickly pinpoint adverse side effects, should they occur.

PERSISTENT FACIAL CARE

No regimen will work if tried halfheartedly. If your skin is a source of concern, turn that concern into the energy and discipline you need to sustain a regimented care schedule. Nobody can afford to skip a morning wash or an evening cleansing; bacteria will form, pores close, and your dirty skin becomes a problem skin. No amount of miracle creams or facial treatments can compensate for improperly cleansed facial skin.

Common Facial Skin Problems

Even complexions that receive scrupulous care can develop unsightly blemishes from time to time. Avoid excessive self-treatment since this can lead to discoloration. In minor cases, home care is possible.

BLACKHEADS

These accumulate in the pores of the skin and consist of dirt mixed with the skin's oil. When the oil oxidizes at the surface of the skin, these waxy plugs turn dark. If caught in their early stages, some may be very carefully coaxed out. Open the pores with steam from a facial sauna, then wrap your fingertips in sterile gauze or cotton and very gently squeeze. Immediately apply an antiseptic astringent. Never use your bare hands or fingernails, metal extractors, or pins. If the blackhead does not emerge easily, you will bruise the tissue by applying too much pressure. Deeply imbedded blackheads should be removed by a dermatologist.

WHITEHEADS

These tiny cysts occur when the oil glands are clogged and hard, fatty material in tiny sacs is built up in each pore. If they do not disappear with very gentle scrubbing, do not remove by any other method, especially squeezing. See a dermatologist.

PIMPLES

There are sundry causes for pimples including infection from improper cleaning of the face, allergic reactions to food, fatigue, and glandular changes. Dry out the blemish with a drying cream or lotion such as Clearasil and keep the surrounding area thoroughly clean. Wash with a mild, medicated soap and warm water. Rinse with cold water and apply an astringent. Keep hands, fingers, fingernails, and articles of clothing away from the face. If pimples become very inflamed, consult a physician.

FLESH MOLES

Many of us develop harmless small dark growths on the face and these increase with age. Commonly called flesh moles, they are clinically defined as *dermatosis papulosa nigra*. They do not require medical attention unless they cause irritation or change in appearance. If they present cosmetic concern, a dermatologist may be able to remove them.

DERMATITIS

Abuse to the skin and various forms of internal and external irritation can lead to dermatitis, which refers to any serious inflammation of the skin, and in Black women can cause discoloration. The affected area may be imperceptible but for a few tiny dark spots, or it may be marked by scales, scabs, watery discharge, and eczema. This can be prevented by practicing good hygiene and keeping strong soaps away from the face. An allergic reaction to a particular cosmetic product or piece of jewelry sometimes produces dermatitis. Always consult a physician.

Rare Facial Skin Problems

VITILIGO

This is the complete loss of pigment from the skin and of course in our case the result is profoundly noticeable. Although the cause is unknown, certain cases have responded well to treatment.

DISCOID LUPUS

Similar to vitiligo, this is a progressive loss of color on the face and scalp caused by a chronic, ulcerating skin disease. This is more often found in women than men and, although the precise cause is unknown, treatment is possible.

Facial Skin Specialists

Only a dermatologist (a physician with special skills concerning the skin and hair) should be allowed to diagnose and treat normal to major skin disorders of the face. Very minor problems may be treated by a qualified cosmetologist if he or she does no more than professionally carry out the care and cleansing treatments I have described in this chapter. A cosmetologist has no medical training but has received skin care training at a state-licensed beauty school. Be wary of anyone posing as a cosmetologist who has no credentials from a State Board of Cosmetology or who seeks to use electrical machinery or surgical instruments on your skin. If in doubt, refer to the American Medical Association, local chapter. Long a field dominated by white women, I am pleased to see a growing number of skilled Black women practicing this profession.

Cosmetics for Skin Disorders

Serious, unsightly skin problems, whether temporary or permanent, can be effectively disguised by the judicious use of make-up. Most physicians recommend Lydia O'Leary's Covermark products which are tinted opaque creams, waterproof and sunproof. The range of colors is not yet as varied as it could be to suit all our complexions, but there are specialists where the product is sold who help to match your natural color. These products do not rub off and resist cracking. If applied correctly, they avoid a masklike appearance. Birthmarks, postoperative scars, and stretch marks all can be disguised.

Make-up for the Face

I frequently encounter instructions for the application of cosmetics that presuppose the reader has a face that conveniently corresponds to one of a

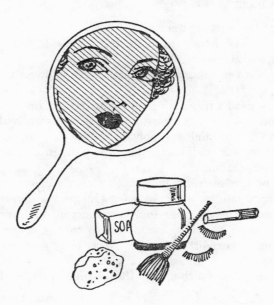

number of fictional categories. Our faces are not really round, square, oblong, or heart-shaped at all. Our skulls vary little in formation and it is the relative position and size of our facial features that create the illusion of a particular "shape" of face. Usually such make-up information stresses the importance of clever drawing or shading so that we may emphasize good features and reduce bad ones. Although convincing to read, this kind of advice is very difficult to put into practice without professional assistance. Still, no matter how skillfully applied, such make-up is quite useless unless you are on the stage, in front of a camera, or only seen from a distance of fifteen feet. For normal, close-up day and evening wear, it looks exactly like camouflage and may deceive no one but yourself. In addition to that, such information is inevitably written with Caucasian features in mind and unless you wish to try to alter your looks in that direction, they have no relevance for the Black woman. Even some Black cosmetic companies have created products that they claim should be used to try to slim the face and nose and make the cheekbones bonier. For us, that simply is neither dignified nor necessary. If you possess a broad, flat nose, it is not a mistake of nature that must be rectified but a strong identifying racial feature of which to be proud. Above all, make-up procedures for the Black woman must recognize our color and create a complexion with both continuity and flexibility. In the following pages I am going to discuss in detail the color and properties of available products, how to choose them and how, as a Black woman, you must apply them. My aim is to impart enough sound specifications that you will be capable of creating your own personal style.

The Make-up Base

This consists of two separate items:

Foundation. Can be liquid, cream, or clear gel and is packaged in bottles, jars, tubes, cakes, and aerosol cans.

Face powder. Can be compacted in cake form or loose in a fairly deep box.

In addition, you need a magnifying mirror at least six inches in diameter; a clean, very soft make-up brush for dusting; plenty of cotton swabs (Q-Tips or Johnson's Cotton Buds); and a supply of white, flat, round, foam-rubber sponges. The last item is readily available in any drugstore and is invaluable for many make-up operations.

The purpose of the cosmetic base is to create an even skin tone and provide a working surface for other make-up. Our complexion changes during the day from a dull state on rising to a brightness in the afternoon back to dull during the evening. A good base minimizes these changes and also protects the skin from surface dirt and germs. Never leave your base on for more than eight hours; it is very unhealthy to keep the same make-up on all day and night with simply a touch-up for the evening. Remove it completely, clean your face and reapply the base.

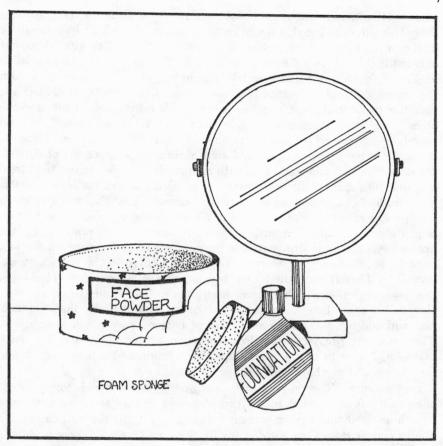

TYPES OF BASE

The clear gel foundations are the most difficult to work with because they dry fast and it is not easy to achieve a color consistency. Many also have a red tint that is not sympathetic to our skin colors. Foundations that are medicated or hypoallergenic will be too light for most of our skins. Foundations containing moisturizers are good for women with dry skins, but you still must apply a moisturizer separately before the foundation. My preference in face powders is for the loose powder because I find the compacted powder must be rubbed onto the skin and this often disturbs and streaks the underlying foundation.

CHOOSING YOUR BASE COLOR

Foundation. This should match your facial skin color as closely as possible. Never use a foundation that is lighter than your skin. In fact, in order to make a close match you must choose a tint very slightly darker than your own. This will even the skin tones. In the store, try the color where it will be used—on the face. It is ridiculous to try it on your hand or arm where not only is the color slightly different but the skin itself may be less porous. In all likelihood you will not find a match straight out of a jar because even with the advent of Black cosmetics the color range is inadequate. If that is the case, buy two foundations, one the nearest shade on the lighter side and the other the nearest shade on the darker side. Dot a tiny amount of dark on your forehead and add the same amount of light. Rub gently and blend. If the result is too light, clean off and start again with a larger dot of dark. If too dark, clean off and start again with a larger dot of light. If you have tried this and still cannot come near to your own color, examine the hues available in cream lipsticks, cream eye shadows, and cream rouge. This will give you a much wider range to choose from and all can safely be mixed with foundation. Federal regulations regarding the ingredients used in products for the lips and eyes are more stringent than for products used elsewhere on the face or body, so you need not worry about using lip color on the cheeks, for instance. In Detroit recently I met a woman with a very dark black—not brown—complexion who had never been able to find a foundation remotely close to her color. I suggested that she take the darkest brown liquid foundation and add, on the face, a small dab of charcoal-gray cream eye shadow. The result was a perfectly blended foundation for her skin color. To match my color, I have to take a brown liquid foundation and a light beige liquid foundation and mix both with a copper-red cream rouge.

Face powder. The purpose of face powder is not so much to contribute color to the foundation as to set it in place and prevent streaking and excessive shine. It should also impart an adhesive quality to the foundation and absorb perspiration. Face powders for Black women are even more limited in color than foundations. I can suggest Revlon "Moon Drops" Translucent #1, #2, and #3 (light, medium, and deep), all of which are just slightly tinted tan to brown. Other so-called "translucent" or "transparent" powders are supposed to be neutral in color but on some of our complexions impart a whitish tinge. Always remember that you need less face powder than you think—just a touch.

TO APPLY A SMOOTH BASE

1) Your skin must be very, very clean.

2) Pat moisturizer on your neck, ears, eyelids, and lips. Gently smooth over the face.

3) Leave moisturizer on for five minutes, then blot off excess with paper tissue.

4) With a clean cotton swab, dot a small amount of foundation on

forehead, center of nose, center of cheeks, eyelids, under the eyes, under the chin, on the ears, and behind the ears, if this area is to be exposed.

5) Using only the very tips of your fingers, blend the foundation onto the skin with many small, light, quick strokes. Do not rub, press, or drag the fingers. Your touch must be featherlike and rapid. The first time you try, it may not look right, but it is worth practicing a few times because it is your "touch" that is all-important with make-up for looks, speed, and efficiency.

6) For the neck, just graze with a few light long strokes to the collarbone.

7) Take a large open facial tissue and cover your entire face. Press lightly onto the face and remove. Do not rub or jerk.

8) Apply the face powder with a large pad of absorbent cotton. The powder puffs that come with the product are inadequate. Dip your cotton pad lightly into the container and press very softly onto the skin surface.

9) With a soft make-up brush, dust the face lightly to remove surplus powder.

Oily Skin

1) Do not neglect the moisturizer. Without it the foundation will sink into the pores and appear too dark.

2) Between steps 3 and 4, lightly apply face powder or apply the foundation with a slightly damp, flat rubber sponge.

3) Instead of blotting your foundation with a facial tissue (step 7), use a damp cotton pad and repeat after step 9.

Dry Skin

Instead of blotting excess moisturizer (step 3), let it remain and blend with the foundation.

Minimum Base

After step 3, take a cotton swab and lightly dab liquid foundation only on lighter areas of the face. Using a flat rubber sponge, blend with quick strokes upward and outward. Omit steps 6 through 9. An alternative to this is to use no foundation at all but, after step 3, apply compact (pressed) powder very lightly with flat rubber sponge. This is especially good for women with excessively oily skins.

Natural Look

Proceed with steps 1 through 7. Take a soft, clean disposable towel (preferably not paper) and firmly wipe your whole face. Use a circular motion of the hand and reach into eyes, nose, and chin areas. You will be left with an invisible foundation.

Additional Suggestions for the Base

Always shake the bottle well if you use a liquid foundation. The elements sometimes settle and this creates a very irregular consistency and color. If you use cream foundation from a jar, stir it well before using.

One of our most frequent mistakes is to apply cosmetics by low-intensity artificial light. When seen in daylight or high-intensity light, this make-up will suffer. If you cannot apply your base near a window and use natural light, then at least use a 150-watt light bulb. Every aspect of your make-up color—contrast, depth, and finish—is altered by different intensities of light.

If you experience the emergence of shiny areas on your face a couple of hours after applying the base, do not add powder to reduce the shine, and avoid repeated touch-ups with foundation. Carry a packet of dry facial linen blotters. These are treated, 3"×4" tissues that, when gently pressed to the face, will remove perspiration and surface oils without disturbing the make-up. If the skin is very oily, use a damp cotton pad with a few drops of witch hazel to blot the shiny area and dab a very tiny amount of foundation on the area. Blend, and lightly press powder over. To cover a temporary blemish such as a pimple, take a spot of foundation from the rim of the bottle or jar or inside the cap (wherever it is slightly congealed) and using an orange stick or the blunt end of an eyebrow pencil, place over the blemish. Wait three to five minutes, then tap lightly to blend.

Base Products to Avoid

Bronzing tints that come as gels or in aerosol cans stain the skin an unnatural color and are unpredictable in terms of pigment stability. They frequently produce a most unnatural color that cannot be removed even with cleansing cream and multiple washings. Aerosol sprays designed to set or finish your base are dangerous to use near the eyes and are either inadequate or much too sticky.

Any product that prevents the face from perspiring should not be used. Your face must breathe when wearing make-up and most make-up is designed to interact with your perspiration.

Bleaching creams can cause permanent pigment loss. I have encountered too many women with heartbreaking marks from bleaching creams to recommend them under any circumstances. If you are tempted to try such a product, you must have your doctor's advice and supervision.

Theatrical make-up is not designed for normal use and contains many ingredients necessary for stage and camera lights which are not good for your skin.

Undertoners are generally not effective for our skin colors. Careful use of moisturizers will prepare the skin for the foundation just as well, if not better.

B. THE EYES

There are substantial differences between our brown eyes and those that are any other color. The choroid section of the eye, located behind the sclera or "white" of the eye, is so pigmented that clear sclera is tinted and may appear muddied or slightly yellowish in some individuals. This yellow tinge may increase with age as fatty deposits build in the sclera. Glaucoma is a disease of the eye that attacks us at an earlier age and much more frequently than other races. Glaucoma is caused by an increase of pressure within the eye and this is linked to pigment quantity of the eye. Also, our high incidence of sickle-cell anemia accounts for many serious eye problems. Yet despite these apparently discouraging facts, certain leading ophthalmologists believe our brown eye to be anatomically superior to that of a Caucasian. Although this still awaits positive proof, researchers point to the very low incidence among our people of malignant melanoma, a form of eye tumor very common to other races.

Care of the Eyes

DIET

In parts of Africa, vitamin A deficiency is such a serious problem that blindness results. No American diet, no matter how unbalanced or meager, is so bereft of vitamin A that the eyes are affected.

EYEWASH

Only use plain water, ever. Home and commercial preparations are not sufficiently sterilized and you risk introducing a malignant growing organism into the eye.

EYE DROPS

The less put in the eye, the better. Although eye drops will not damage the eye, they are designed to have a cosmetic effect and cannot permanently soothe or heal. Most contain a vasoconstrictor that by causing the blood vessels in the eye to contract, the sclera appears briefly as white, clear, and sparkling. However, this is paid for later when the blood vessels have to dilate and the eye becomes red, dull, and tired.

SUNLIGHT

Never gaze directly at the sun. Even if your eyes do not register strain, you should wear sunglasses if facing the sun directly for more than a few minutes. Always keep your eyes closed when sunbathing. The result of extended exposure by the eyes to harsh glare is that your night vision will become impaired. When buying sunglasses, avoid pale cosmetic tints. These are not strong enough to occlude light. Use dark blues, browns, grays, or greens.

EYE SPECIALISTS

The only professional trained to take care of all aspects of eye health is an ophthalmologist, a doctor of medicine. This person should be visited once a year. Your first visit should include:

1) Microscopic examination of both eyes;
2) Pressure test for both eyes;
3) Check of left and right eye correlation;
4) Sight test for reading and distance.

Costs vary with location, but $30 is average for this first visit. A small price to pay for sight.

An optometrist is not a doctor of medicine and is only qualified to test your sight and prescribe corrective lenses. The examination that you receive at an optometrist or vision center will only determine how well you see and will not lead to a diagnosis of why your sight may be bad or reveal any dormant eye ailments.

An optician is simply an expert in the field of lenses, telescopes, prisms, and mirrors. Opticians are not necessarily able to examine, diagnose, or cure eye problems.

Definitely do not buy your first pair of glasses without consulting an ophthalmologist and definitely do not contemplate contact lenses—soft or hard—without a thorough eye examination by an ophthalmologist.

WARNING SIGNS

Floating black spots before the eyes are usually a benign common trait that we become accustomed to, but if you regularly experience any of the following, see your doctor:

Frequent sties	Dimness
Fuzziness	Halo around lights
Distortion of space	Color difficulties

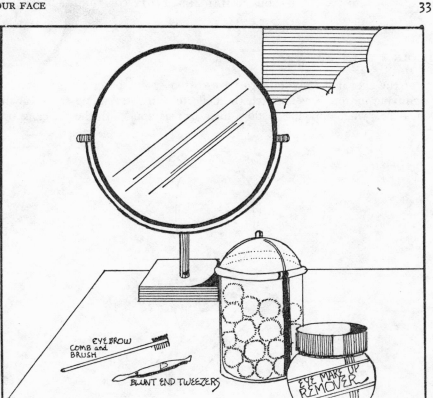

EYEBROW COMB and BRUSH

BLUNT END TWEEZERS

EYE MAKE UP REMOVER

Make-up for the Eyes

The eyes are extremely vulnerable and for this reason are protected by bony sockets. Our brows and lashes screen foreign matter and prevent perspiration from entering the eyes. Never let your make-up be a cause of denying the eye any of this protection. Be very careful when using brushes, tweezers, and pencils near the eyes. Never, ever attempt to apply or remove eye make-up in a moving vehicle. A sudden stop or start may cost you an eye. The skin of the eyelid and surrounding area is the thinnest anywhere on your body. It can quickly dry out and succumb to irritation. Always put on moisturizer before applying and after removing make-up. Use only the softest brushes on the eye.

Tools

For the eyes it is important to have cotton swabs, blunt tweezers, and a magnifying mirror. Never stretch the delicate skin surrounding the eye with your fingers when applying shadow, liner, or mascara. With the judicious use

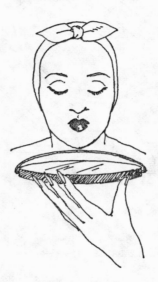

of the mirror you do not have to contort face or body in order to see what you are doing and still be able to do it. Hold or lay the mirror absolutely flat and horizontal underneath your chin and slightly forward of it. Hold your head erect with your eyes open and staring directly ahead. Look down and very slowly tilt your head forward until you can just begin to see into the mirror. This way your eyelids will be fully extended and your eyes will still be open.

Color

Most cosmetic eye products are developed to complement eyes that are hazel, blue, green, or gray. Not dark brown. Consequently the majority of these products are in shades such as pale blue, light green, lavender, rose, etc. Against a dark skin these tones are not at all flattering and make our eyes appear to protrude unless the wearer has light skin and nonbrown eyes. Look for colors that augment your own eye color. I use black, dark browns, charcoal grays as well as navy blues, bottle green, and deep purple.

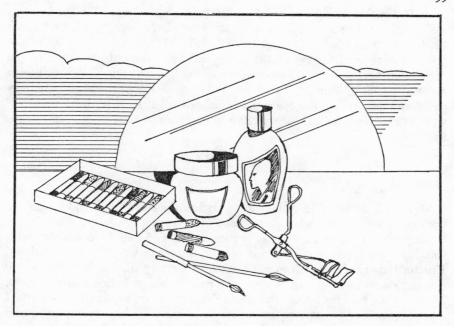

Eye Make-up Products and Their Application

EYE SHADOW

This may be a cream, crayon, or powder. The creams are hard to use, but the crayons are easy to control and gentle on the skin. I prefer a powder because it is long lasting and does not crease on the eyelid. The powder is also good for oily skins. If an applicator such as a brush is required, it usually comes with the product.

The secret of applying eye shadow is the same as that for foundation— never draw or spread, but feather it on and blend with many tiny light strokes of the brush or finger. First dab a small amount of shadow on the center of the eyelid close to the lashes. Blend from the inner corner of the lid and sweep across and up. Keep the eyebrows raised while doing this and apply shadow only to the part of the eyelid that covers the eyeball. Do not cover the receding shelf between eyebrow and eyeball and avoid applying too close to the nose.

EYE LINER

Eye liner is designed to stress the size and shape of the eye and make the lashes appear thicker. Avoid all blues and greens and favor the browns, blacks, and charcoal grays. Eye liner is either in liquid form or as a cake that is applied with a damp brush. I find the cake easy to control if the brush is well cared for, cleaned, and has no stray hairs. Draw a very fine line across the base of the eyelashes (not on the lid itself), starting a hair's-breadth from the inner corner of the eye and stopping exactly at the outside corner of the eye, no farther. Some Black women are in the habit of using black or brown eyebrow pencil to "line" the bottom inside rim of the eye. This is extremely dated and only makes the eye appear smaller than it is. It is also a very dangerous habit since no make-up or sharp object should be that close to the eye itself.

MASCARA

Mascara is designed to make your eyelashes thicker, darker, and longer. As with eye liner, it can be bought in cake form with a brush applicator but is also manufactured as a cream in bottles, tubes, and penlike containers with spiral-grooved applicators. The more liquid forms are less easy to control and I prefer the cake-and-brush method since by wetting the brush appropriately one can determine just the amount and consistency of mascara one requires. Most women find the spiral-grooved applicators to be the easiest to use and I would recommend that type to anyone in a hurry. With head forward and eyes directed down into your magnifying mirror, hold the brush directly beneath the base of the upper lashes. Draw the brush swiftly upward and outward through the lashes, following the direction of the curl. If you apply a second coat, wait at least five minutes after the first. To cover the lower lashes, hold the brush or applicator vertically and stroke down on each lash. Be very sparing with mascara on lower lashes.

FALSE EYELASHES

I have never had sufficient reason to use human hair lashes since synthetic lashes are just as good-looking, less expensive, and easier to work with. Lashes are usually sold in sets with top and bottom strips of lashes for each eye. Because they can be readily regulated, I use individual lashes, but, if you do this, be prepared to spend quite a long time putting them on.

When sold in sets the bottom-set lashes are much closer to our own upper lashes because they are better spaced, attached to a thinner strip, are less bushy, and tend to be nearer the length of our own top lashes. Darken the white strip with a dark brown eyebrow pencil. They can be rolled to become curly like our own lashes by placing when damp on a small clean sheet of paper and then rolling the paper around a slim object such as an orange stick. Secure with a rubber band and leave overnight. If you use top-set lashes, brown is the best color. Black top-set lashes are generally too strong for normal wear. Avoid light browns which simply disappear against our skins. Also, never wear top-set false lashes beneath the eyes.

All false eyelashes are sold with glue, but since it may not be sterilized and is white in color I use Duo (brown) Surgical Adhesive.

Applying false eyelashes cannot be done in a hurry. Learn to manipulate your tweezers and never use your fingers, which are too large to be efficient for this delicate operation.

Upper lashes. Place a tiny amount of glue on a toothpick and spread it across the inside of the eyelash band. With head and mirror in the same position as for applying mascara, grip the outer edge of the lashes with the tweezers and carry toward the eye. Position the free end of the lashes ⅛ inch from the inside of the eye and gently lay the lashes across the base line of your own lashes. The band should be barely touching your eyelid. Do not attempt to push or position with the fingers. If you miss, start over again. Always wait three minutes for the glue to dry before applying other lashes. False lashes are very effective and look more natural if you trim at either end so that at the outer and inner corners of your eyes your own lashes predominate. Blend together with mascara.

Lower lashes. Hold your mirror directly in front of your face and with head erect, drop the jaw and open your mouth. Grip lower lash with tweezers in the center and place just *under* your own.

Individual lashes. Squeeze a spot of glue onto a paper. Grip the end of a top lash with the tweezers, the nylon base facing toward you. (Remember that upper lashes curl up, lower lashes curl down.) Dip the base in glue and apply to the base of your own lash. Never glue the whole false lash to the whole real lash. Place the thicker lashes toward the outside of the eye, just as your own grow.

To remove false eyelashes. If you experience pain when starting this procedure, moisten the base of the lashes with baby oil on a cotton swab. This helps to loosen the glue, but the oil must be cleaned off the lashes later. One of the reasons that I use surgical adhesive for my false lashes is that it peels off very easily. Grip the outer corner of the lash strip at the base with the balls of your fingers (not the nails) and firmly pull across. For removing bottom lashes, repeat this procedure after loosening with baby oil applied underneath the lashes.

To clean false eyelashes. Place in shallow cup or saucer and barely cover with rubbing alcohol. Let sit for five minutes. Remove and place on a tissue. Stroke with cotton swab to remove glue remnants from the base. Dry for at least one hour before reapplying. If the lashes are excessively soiled with glue and mascara, soak overnight in two tablespoons of Ivory liquid dishwashing detergent. Remove with tweezers and soak for five minutes in clean water, then scrub gently with a soft toothbrush.

TO CURL EYELASHES

The only safe method is to use a clamplike instrument designed for this purpose. Make sure you buy one that has a rubber protective pad on the jaws. Always follow the instructions but use before, not after, applying mascara. Hold on the lashes for at least thirty seconds and immediately set with mascara. Do each eye at a time and avoid blinking.

EYEBROWS

Black women have naturally well-shaped and correctly defined eyebrows. The hair is soft and easy to control. We should not be at all anxious to try to radically alter the brows we were born with. Because the eyebrow hair is shorter and more fibrous than elsewhere on the body, it has a much slower growth cycle—about three months. This is one good reason to consider carefully before adopting an extreme eyebrow style. If it involves removing part or all of the eyebrow, it will take a long time to regrow. Also, since you will not (or at least should not) be wearing make-up at all times, you must imagine what your altered brows will look like without make-up. You may look quite ridiculous with half-shaven eyebrows. We must definitely avoid the high-arch, half-moon styles that are very old-fashioned and perfectly unbecoming; they are guaranteed to make the youngest face age ten years. This is also true of half-brows, pencil-thin brows, and no brows at all. We have strong, shapely, distinctive eyebrows. Let's keep them. If you indulge in extreme alterations of your eyebrow shape, they may never return to their original, appropriate shape.

EYEBROW SHAPING

The eyebrow should not extend past the inner corner of the eye nor more than ¼ inch beyond the outer corners. It should rest atop the bony promontory protecting the eye. The texture should be soft and fluffy with no exaggerated growth or loss. All you need for this is petroleum jelly and a pair of clean-slant or blunt-ended tweezers. These are the easiest to use since they allow a firm grasp on each hair. You do not need a razor or scissors. The only safe and sure method of shaping brows is by plucking. Scissors never cut close enough and should not be wielded that close to the eye. A razor alters the shape of the growth pattern, creates stubble, and removes too much at a time. By plucking you remove only what you want, very slowly, and regrowth is natural. Do not try to bleach the brows. Brow bleaches lighten our skin and turn the brow hair yellow.

Shape one brow at a time, using your magnifying mirror:

1) Massage a thick coat of petroleum jelly into the brow. This opens the pores to minimize pain while plucking. This is even more effective if you apply while in a hot bath; the steam also opens the pores.

2) Petroleum jelly must remain for thirty minutes.

3) Wipe off excess.

4) Moisten a cotton swab and roll the end in a small quantity of soap. Using swab as a pencil, draw on your brow the shape and size of the brow you require, careful to draw in the direction of hair growth. The soap will dry white and indicate area NOT to be plucked.

5) With another cotton swab, apply petroleum jelly again to hairs you wish to remove.

6) Commencing with the lower hairs, pluck out singly, pulling in direction of growth. Move toward the bridge of the nose and leave to the last the hairs on top of the brow. Pluck both brows before removing soap so that an easy comparison can be made. If you feel a mistake has been made, do not increase the problem by plucking haphazardly but wash the brows and start these instructions over again.

7) Dab brows with witch hazel to close the pores. Your brows will remain sore and bumpy for thirty minutes. Do not apply color until swelling has declined.

8) Our brows do not match, so it is futile and quite unnecessary to attempt a perfect pair.

EYEBROW CONTROL

If you are satisfied with the shape and length of your eyebrows but the hairs are too curly or grow in the wrong direction, you will need an eyebrow brush-comb. This is a small instrument with a comb and brush on either side of one end and is available in any five-and-ten-cent store. In addition to this, it is useful to have a medium-hard bristle toothbrush with a flat face.

1) Apply a moderate amount of petroleum jelly to the brows. Substitute moisturizer if about to put on make-up.

2) Comb for at least one minute in desired direction.

3) Brush with toothbrush for at least five minutes.

EYEBROW MAKE-UP

The color of your eyebrows must relate to the color of your eyes, not the color of your hair. If your hair is dyed, do not dye your brows or paint them a light color. This produces an undesirable clownish effect.

Products for the eyebrows are pencil, powder, or liquid. Avoid the liquid, which simply paints the hairs and the skin and looks very false.

Eyebrow pencil. You never need a black pencil. If your brows are rich and full you probably need not color them at all, and if they are sparse the black pencil will be too obvious. Use charcoal gray, dark brown, or sable. Keep pencil very sharp and draw tiny hairs with slim, quick strokes. Press firmly, then lift off quickly and lightly. Never draw in continuous lines.

Eyebrow powder. Again, never use black, just charcoal gray, dark brown, and sable. Place a small amount on the brush and gently blow to remove excess. Apply with firm, small, quick strokes fading to the outer edge of the eyebrow. After putting on powder or pencil, remove some cotton from the end of a cotton swab and with remainder gently stroke brow to remove surplus color.

If you have unruly eyebrows, keep them in shape by dabbing on a very small amount of glycerine soap or Duo's brown surgical adhesive. Stroke lightly and swiftly in the desired direction.

EYEBROW GROWTH

If your brows are sparse, or you wish to hurry the regrowth process, massage them with petroleum jelly every night and leave on while you sleep. This is especially effective when bathing since the pores open and can be stimulated. Always clean off petroleum jelly thoroughly.

PROFESSIONAL TREATMENTS

Many beauty salon personnel are eager to give you their versions of the latest eyebrow fashions with little or no regard for the true quality, quantity, or shape of your own eyebrows. Watch what they do and insist on one eyebrow at a time. Check frequently in the mirror to make sure the shape is to your liking and not just theirs.

Eyes and Eyebrows

These are the most difficult features to make up successfully. We vary so much that I cannot set rigid guidelines, but I will suggest some devices that are useful for certain types of eye shapes and eye conditions.

WIDE-SET EYES

Concentrate your eye shadow, mascara, and liner on the inner half of the eye. Blend well but very lightly to the outer edge. Your eyelashes should be even in length. Do not pluck the inner brows.

CLOSE-SET EYES

Start color at the center of the lid and leave inner lashes free of mascara, but apply two or three coats to the outer edge. Your liner should not extend beyond the outer corner of the eye. This looks very awkward and obvious. Wear the shortest, curliest lashes available with the very shortest on the inside. Thin the brows slightly out from the bridge of the nose.

Protruding Eyes

Never use light eye shadow. Keep it dark and powdered, avoiding glossy sheens. Use a strong eye liner but keep it close to the lash base. Your lashes should have a prominent curl.

Puffy Eyelids

Use a matte-finish eye shadow and avoid pearlized color and "highlight" eye cosmetics.

Bags or Circles under Eyes

Most women make the mistake of attempting to disguise these conditions by darkening or lightening the area. Both methods simply attract attention. Uniformity of color is what you should strive for. Match these areas with your foundation and give a matte finish with powder. Dot a small amount of foundation on with a cotton swab, starting under the bottom lashes, and blend from the inner to the outer eye and down to the cheekbone. If you blend up, the "tired eyes" will only show more.

Eye Make-up and Corrective Lenses

Glasses. The shape and color of your frames will be more obvious than your make-up, so take that into consideration when choosing colors. Part of your make-up is obscured, so keep it to a minimum and shun color effects that will contrast with your frames. Put your glasses on from time to time while applying make-up.

Contact lenses. Always put them in before applying make-up. This way you can see what you are doing and also avoid carrying particles of cosmetics to your eye via the lens. This often happens when a woman puts her contact lenses in impatiently after finishing her make-up.

Do not use lash-lengthening mascara or dust lashes with powder. Both increase the risk of foreign particles entering the eye and creating irritation. This may happen not only when applied but throughout the wearing time.

To Remove Eye Make-up

Most modern eye cosmetic products include nonwater-soluble binding agents. They cannot be removed with soap and water or normal cleansing cream. There are two types of cleansers that have been developed just for this job. Eye make-up removers are either bottled liquids or saturated pads sold in jars. The liquids are not economical to use because of the amount needed to clean, and they may sting the eyes. I use the pads, which are concentrated and less messy. If they feel slightly dry or if I have heavy make-up to remove, I add a few drops of baby oil to the pad. In fact, a four-inch lump of cotton saturated in baby oil works as well as the presaturated pads. When removing the make-up, never wipe into the eye. Always move the pad away from the eye: up and out from the top lid, down and away from the lower eye. Start at the inside corner of the lid and wipe across to the temple. If it does not come off at first, never rub vigorously. This will only irritate the skin and grind the make-up into the pores. Continue to stroke quite gently with new pads. If after removal there is too much oil left around the eye, dab with a wet cotton pad, never paper tissue, which is too abrasive.

EMERGENCY TREATMENT FOR THE EYES

Specks of grime, unless they immediately create a burning sensation, are best removed by rapidly blinking the eye. This moves the speck to the eye corner where it can be lifted with the point of a folded handkerchief.

If the eyes are exposed to a burning liquid chemical such as lye, immediately flush them thoroughly with a nontoxic liquid such as water or milk. This must be done at once.

If you suspect that the cornea may be damaged, do not touch or probe. Close the eye and cover lightly until professional help can be sought.

If the eye feels damaged but nothing can be determined, compare the shape of the eyes with the eyelids closed. If one is flatter, the eyeball may be perforated and a doctor should be called.

C. THE CHEEKS

Make-up

COLOR

As the names imply, "rouge" and "blush" products were developed to add color and complement strictly Caucasian skins. We would probably not bother to use them at all if the advertising pressure were not so insidious. When we do use these products most of us are guilty of employing red much too indiscriminately for our dark skins. Unless of very light complexion we should ignore the vivid principal colors such as red, pink, and orange, and learn to experiment with natural shades of plum, bronze, and umber.

TYPE

Powdered rouge is my favorite and definitely must be the choice of anyone with an oily skin. Instead of using the brush supplied with the powder, just touch it to the face with a cotton pad.

Liquids look tempting but are hard to control and have a marked tendency to streak no matter how skillfully applied.

Creams and gels are the most practical. Only use a tiny amount.

APPLICATION

First you must locate your true cheekbones. With eyes closed, place the tips of your index fingers at the outer corners of your eyes. Move them down very slowly until you feel the bony protuberance. Apply the color here and blend toward the temples. Never draw or smear the color, but just dab lightly and sparingly.

Most manufacturers of these products try to encourage the use of their colors on other parts of the face such as the chin or the forehead. This is rarely an improvement and inevitably looks very artificial.

D. THE LIPS

Unlike the rest of the face, our lips contain no lubricating oil glands. Consequently our lips are often in danger of dehydration, especially if the air lacks humidity. Under these circumstances even wetting of the lips with the tongue only increases the rate of dehydration. We must find alternate ways of moistening the lips.

As Black women, we are conscious of the fact that our lips are proportionately larger than those of other races and in many cases are darker than the general complexion. Sometimes our lower lip is significantly lighter than the top lip. This is very common and not at all unnatural.

Lip Care

Brushing the teeth also cleans the lips but it is very necessary to keep them free from sores and chapping with appropriate moisturizing agents. The moisturizer you use for your face is not sufficient to protect the lips. I suggest frequent use of medicated creams such as Blistex. Chapsticks may be too harsh; creams are absorbed more readily and soothe gently.

Make-up for the Lips

SHAPE

You absolutely cannot alter the size or shape of your lips with cosmetics. Any measures that you feel might accomplish this are tedious and utterly contrived. It is all too obvious when a Black woman attempts to "draw" lips smaller or better-shaped than her own. If you cannot be proud of your lips but wish not to draw attention to them, steer clear of all lip make-up completely. This includes foundation and lip gloss. Simply keep well lubricated with moisture.

COLOR

Darker-skinned women should avoid pinks and oranges. Almost any other color can be used effectively on the lips if it matches the tone of your own skin. Whatever the color of your lipstick, it should not contrast greatly in tone, be darker or lighter, than the rest of the face. If you cannot find a manufactured color that does this, experiment on the back of your hand by mixing a little of your foundation with your favorite lip color. I often use a dark burgundy or brown translucent lip gloss to tone down a red lipstick and achieve a natural but very attractive lip color.

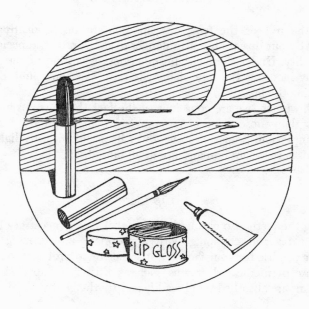

PRODUCTS FOR THE LIPS

Lipstick now comes in creams, liquids, and pencils as well as the traditional stick. The pencils and liquids are not made with color sufficiently suited to our skin color and the creams lack body. None of them provides the even coverage that a stick was designed for. Lip glosses come in cream form and are either clear for just a shine and protection or are translucent and tinted to add extra color.

HOW TO APPLY LIP MAKE-UP

Even if you wear nothing on the face but lipstick you must first apply a moistener, a medicated cream, and then foundation. This will reduce the amount of time you have to spend freshening up your lip color and help you retain a firm, smooth look all day.

1) Take a flat, sable-tipped lip brush. Check that the hairs are straight and even.

2) Stroke the lipstick gently with the brush to gather color.

3) Hold your magnifying mirror six inches from your face and part the lips.

4) Outline the lips in four measures: from left corner to center bottom; from center bottom to right corner; from right corner to center top; from center top to left corner.

5) Fill in with bold, sweeping strokes of the brush.

Follow the same rules to apply lip gloss and cover only that area which has already received lipstick.

With modern cosmetics there is no need to blot the lips. In fact, this will only dull the make-up and remove color. Face powder should never be applied to the lips. It causes lipstick to cake and crack.

Care of Make-up Equipment

All face towels and washcloths should be white. Color dyes can run and some contain harsh ingredients. The best way to prevent infection is to wash your towels and washcloths separately from your regular laundry.

Clean implements are essential for the creation of fresh, smooth make-up. At least once a month take all your face sponges, powder pads, and powder puffs and wash in hot, soapy water. Squeeze and let dry.

All tools that are used near the eyes and mouth, including tweezers, lip brushes and applicators for mascara, eye liner and eye shadow, should be regularly disinfected and cleaned. Add rubbing alcohol to a hot solution of soap and water and let all these tools soak for thirty minutes. Wash and rinse, then dry on paper towels.

Areas where make-up tools are kept, such as bathroom shelves, drawers, and plastic bags, must be regularly cleaned with soap and water. Not only does this hinder the spread of germs to the face, but it keeps your implements new and fresh and able to help you do the very best make-up job. You cannot expect to apply make-up evenly with brushes that are caked with crusty old cosmetics.

E. THE EARS

Like the eyes, our ears may prove to be superior to the Caucasian. It is certainly an acknowledged fact now that otosclerosis, a disease of the middle ear that is very common in whites, occurs much less frequently among our people.

Ear Cleaning

The only object that your ear should ever feel is a washcloth. Cotton swabs, fingernails, and all pointed objects such as hairpins must be kept out of, and far from, the ear canal. If pimples and blackheads in the ear are a problem, saturate a small piece of sterilized cotton with astringent and press into the ear canal. If you have long, sharp fingernails, cleaning your ears can be a problem and I suggest using white cotton gloves moistened with soap and water. Syringing of the ear to clear wax deposits should be done by a doctor.

Ear Care

At the first inkling of regular nasal obstruction or hearing impairment, see your doctor. There is a correct way to blow your nose, incidentally, that prevents forcing infected material from the nose into the ear canal, which happens when you blow both nostrils hard at the same time. Instead, close one nostril at a time and gently blow the other.

Because of our tendency to contract keloids, the most common ear complaint from Black women is that of hypertrophic scars on the ear lobes resulting from injudicious piercing of the ears. Because we do not know until it happens how keloid-prone we are, my advice is avoid piercing your ears. If you must wear earrings for pierced ears, at least go to a doctor. It will not cost more than elsewhere and you can be sure that any complications will be dealt with. Amateur ear-piercing leaves scars and infection that can linger a lifetime.

Earrings

Because even minor trauma to our skin can cause hyperpigmentation, avoid earrings that are tight enough to leave the ears sore. Even if keloids do not form, any bruising of the ear lobes can result in a permanent blackening of the lobe area. Remove your earrings whenever possible and never wear them all day and all evening. Remember to include the ears and especially the ear lobes when you moisturize the rest of the face.

F. THE TEETH

Our teeth are vital living organs that consist of three layers: the enamel, a relatively thin but very hard covering for the crown; the dentin, a softer, ivorylike substance that forms the body of the tooth; the dental pulp that occupies the center of the tooth.

Other than the color of the gums, which has no significance, there are absolutely no differences between the structure of our teeth and that of any other race.

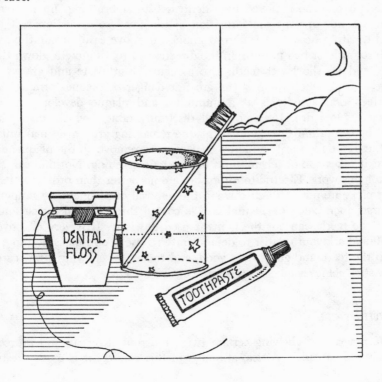

Tooth Care

EATING

There is no doubt that the acidic substances found in carbonated beverages and high-carbohydrate foods attack the tooth enamel. Avoid sugar and starch in abnormal quantities.

CLEANING

In the past we were encouraged to believe that tooth decay resulted simply from food particles remaining in the crevices of the teeth. If this were true, frequent brushing of the teeth or rinsing of the mouth would prohibit dental disease. The facts are more complex. Food particles combine with saliva and mouth bacteria to create a gummy mass known as dental plaque. This plaque destroys the cement between the fissures of the teeth, loosens teeth from gums, and produces the toxins that cause abscesses. If not regularly removed, plaque moves out of reach of the toothbrush, calcifies, and turns into tartar, which can only be removed by a dentist. Casual brushing, no matter how often, will not prevent the formation of plaque. Use a medium-soft brush, straight, with a head that is narrow enough to move easily inside the mouth. Brush for at least two minutes in the direction of tooth growth, down the top teeth, and up the lower teeth. Use a regular toothpaste and always brush before retiring when there is the greatest danger of plaque forming. While you sleep oral activity is at a minimum and plaque development is encouraged. Most drugstores now sell disclosing tablets which when chewed reveal by coloration the extent of plaque remaining after a normal brushing. Use these initially until you know that you can remove all the plaque, even if at first it takes five or ten minutes of constant brushing. Nothing can substitute for this work. Electric toothbrushes are no better than ordinary ones and water picks are not at all effective in the removal of plaque; they simply flush the larger food particles. Dental floss, a coated thread useful for cleaning between the teeth, can cut the gums if used unwisely. It is very effective and you should ask your dentist to demonstrate its use. Toothpicks do more damage to the teeth and gums than good, and the act of chewing a raw carrot or celery stick achieves much better results.

TOOTH STICKS

The practice of chewing certain twigs and roots to clean and protect the teeth is widespread in Africa, although in this country it is mostly restricted to the inhabitants of Appalachia and the Ozarks. It is a habit that cannot be assumed but must be practiced from birth since the jaw muscles required for the practice are formidable and must be trained. Extensive research is presently under way to investigate what remedial properties the chewing sticks may contain. Already in India and in England there are toothpastes on the market derived from chewing sticks. Of course many different types of wood are used, depending on region and local fancy, but some doctors have tentatively suggested that there may possibly be some antisickle-cell-anemia properties in some chewing sticks as well as obvious dental benefits. The practice of chewing the stick itself is beyond doubt damaging to the gums, but it is possible that one day the stick substances will be widely used medicinally.

Teeth Whitening

Tooth enamel is exceptionally resilient and any agent strong enough to bleach the enamel would also cause deterioration. Correct cleaning of the teeth will make them as white as they can possibly be. No toothpaste product, whether paste or liquid, can actually whiten the teeth.

Fluoride

Fluoride is an active strengthener of teeth but is most effective if introduced early in life during infancy. Fluoride in toothpaste is helpful, but its effectiveness can be overestimated since it is a more potent strengthener of the teeth if ingested anatomically as part of our drinking water.

Gums

Sore gums are neglected gums. To prevent plaque from forcing teeth and gums apart it is necessary to brush the gums also. Use a rotary motion. Massage the gums frequently with the fingers or the rubber tip attached to some toothbrushes. If your gums bleed, tell your dentist; it may indicate a serious problem.

Halitosis

Bad breath is not simply the result of improperly cleaned teeth, smoking, or drinking. It may be a symptom or a warning sign of a more complicated condition such as tooth decay, stomach trouble, postnasal drip, tonsilitis, or sinusitis. If you have persistent bad mouth odor, do not just try to disguise it with mouthwash or drops but mention it to your doctor or dentist.

Dental Diseases

Tooth complaints can be generally divided into two categories. The first, dental caries or decay of the tooth resulting from plaque, and the second, gingivitis, which affects the gums, can both be aggravated by poor nutritional habits, lackadaisical brushing, and contempt for professional care.

Teeth and Pregnancy

During the first three months it is not unusual for the active endocrine system to induce bleeding of the gums. This is not serious. But it is a sheer myth that pregnancy induces cavities or that the unborn child is building its own teeth at the expense of the mother's. Women often discover after pregnancy that their teeth are in bad shape and blame the pregnancy. More often than not the woman has neglected her teeth for a year because of morning sickness and other preoccupations. She does not visit the dentist and brushes carelessly, if at all. You must continue good teeth-hygiene habits in pregnancy, and because your child is forming its teeth, nutritional considerations are very important for both mother and child.

The Dentist

You cannot hope to retain healthy teeth into old age unless you visit the dentist once a year at the very least. Fear prevents most of us from making the appointments we should. We forget, of course, that modern methods of anaesthesia render the visits virtually painless and we torture ourselves with the anticipated pain which is always much worse. A first visit to the dentist should include the following:

1) Questions about your general health;
2) X-rays of your teeth;
3) Thorough examination;
4) Explanation of any existing conditions such as cavities, caries, gingivitis;
5) Methods of treating such conditions;
6) Cost of treatment and method of payment;
7) Removal of tartar (cleaning).

Tooth Extraction

Many of us avoid the dentist for financial reasons, little realizing that we are compiling a giant bill for the future. Preventive medicine in the form of regular visits to the doctor and dentist is always cheaper than the cost of treatment resulting from a condition that has developed because of neglect.

Often we resign ourselves to the fact that if a tooth becomes bad we can simply have it removed. This is dangerous, unnecessary, and more costly in the long run. You use all your teeth. The number is the result of a balance that Nature evolved, and as soon as you upset that balance an inexorable chain of events begins. You inhibit the ability to chew your food correctly and your digestion suffers. Eventually the facial skin near the cavity collapses and can wrinkle quite prematurely. Unless the gap is obvious, some women never get around to having a plate fitted. If you do have an extraction, be fitted at once and at least save the shape of your mouth and jaw area. When we compare the relatively low cost of an extraction to the large amount needed to save the tooth, we often forget to include the long-term costs incurred by buying, fitting, replacing, and maintaining artificial dentures. It might just be less expensive to save the tooth. If your dentist indicates that a tooth or teeth must be removed and you hesitate to let it occur, at least see another dentist and get a second opinion. That is your right and it is well worth it to save your teeth—the only ones you will ever have.

Dental Surgery

An orthodontist is a dentist who specializes in the direction of tooth growth and the reshaping of malformed teeth. An oral surgeon specializes in correcting misaligned jaws in order to correct the patient's bite. Neither of these procedures is just a beautification matter. Distorted teeth and jaws adversely affect one's ability to speak and chew and can cause a wide variety of disorders from tooth decay to lisps to ulcers. If you require this kind of work, your dentist will be able to locate the best local clinic or hospital.

Yellowing Teeth

This can be caused by smoking or age or a combination of the two. Nicotine from cigarettes stains the teeth but not as badly as from pipes and cigars. As we grow older, the tough enamel on our teeth is worn away and cannot be replaced. The ivory color of the underlying dentin then shows through and imparts a yellowish tinge to the teeth.

The Future of Tooth Care

Research is progressing on laser-beam-applied porcelain sealants that fully protect the teeth from all exterior damage, but until that becomes common we just have to brush hard and correctly and, no matter how loathsome it is in your imagination, make that dentist's appointment. And keep it.

Chapter III

OUR HAIR

—◆═◆═◆—

All hair is composed of nitrogen, sulfur, water, iron traces, and amino acids. This keratin structure, like that of the nails, is very similar to the structure of skin. Because our skin, through its unique pigmentation, is a very strong identifying factor racially, it is not surprising that the hair also should exhibit certain distinct qualities not found in other races. Disparagingly referred to as "kinky" or "woolly," our tightly curled hair strands may have evolved in our

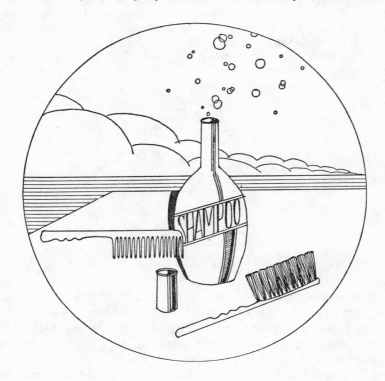

African ancestors as a natural protection against the equatorial heat waves of the sun. The closely knit growth pattern and special texture of our hair allow optimum ventilation of the scalp while at the same time inhibiting the more harmful effects of the sun's radiation. This theory has special significance if we bear in mind that the principal function of hair is not decorative but the regulation of body temperature and the protection of the body as a whole. Our tightly curled hair contrasts strongly with the Orientals' tendency toward very straight hair and the Caucasian occupies a middle ground where curly hair predominates. Of course, many Black women in this country and around the world have hair that cannot be so neatly categorized. As early as 1853 the English anthropologist Rowland Alexander observed:

> . . . if the African nations be examined, every possible gradation in the hair will be perceived, from the short close curls of the Kafir to the crisp but bushy locks of the Berberine, and again to the flowing hair of the Tuaryk or Tibbo. . . . The Ashantees and others have hair which is rather curled than wooly, and is occasionally so long as to reach to the shoulders. . . . The Foulahs or Fellatahs, natives of Sudan, have crepid and crisp, sometimes wooly hair. . . . The Mandingoes in Senegambia have the genuine black, or frizzled, or wooly hair of the Negro. . . . The flaxen locks of the Somali females (stained like those of the Lujean girls) render them conspicious. . . . The Calla tribes shave the head, preserving a lock of hair on it for every man they have killed. . . . The Nubians have long, strongly frizzled or slightly crisp (but never wooly) hair. It is sometimes of a shining jet black, but in other cases of a color intermediate between the ebony black of Sennar Negroes and the brown of the Egyptians.

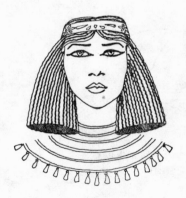

When examined under a microscope, the hair shaft of a Black woman or man appears to be relatively flat and sickle-shaped whereas the hair shaft of a Caucasian is round and that of an Oriental is oblong and kidney-shaped. Some hair specialists believe that the flatter the hair shaft, the curlier the hair. Generally, our hair is very porous, quite coarse in structure with much natural body and a very strong wave pattern. All types of hair grow from a curved root and then rise perpendicular to the skin. Ours then twists upon itself to form whorls and loops and an intertwining that gives the shaft a curve resembling that of a fine watch spring. The relatively dull sheen of our untreated hair may be due to the large concentration of microscopic air bubbles (present to some degree in all types of hair) that diffuse and refract light in such a way as to impart a matte rather than a glossy appearance to the hair; hence our predilection for lubricant oils and creams for the hair. Despite the fact that our type of hair is so frequently compared unfavorably with Oriental and Caucasian types of hair, little research is being done at an advanced level to analyze all the factors responsible for our hair shape and texture. However, despite the fact that our hair may ostensibly be less manageable than that of other races, we cannot submit to the general (white) viewpoint that it is qualitatively inferior. Even a totally objective observer would have to admit that our hair:

1) From a functional standpoint does a better job than any other of protecting the scalp;

2) Grows stronger longer (i.e., older Black women) than all other types of hair;

3) Despite the required effort can be worn in the widest possible range of styles (from corn row to chignon), unlike any other type of hair.

These are just a few things in favor of our hair; we will encounter others later in this chapter. Naturally, I believe there to be nothing inferior about our beautiful hair—quite the opposite!

A. THE ANATOMY OF HAIR

Within the dermis or lower skin are found the *papillae*, thickened cones of nerves and blood vessels that nourish the roots of the hair. Cylindrical-shaped cells form in the papilla and grow into a *follicle*, the hair root. This in turn develops as hair through the dermis and emerges from the epidermis when it becomes visible. As the hair comes into contact with air it oxidizes and hardens. Hair is hydrophilic, sensitive to humidity and all atmospheric changes. In dry weather hair extends and in damp weather it contracts.

Our very first hair makes its appearance during the fifth month of life of the fetus. This is a very fine downy hair called *lanugo*. This semideveloped hair is lost either before or shortly after birth to be replaced by our secondary scalp hair that then gradually becomes coarser. From birth on, our hair grows at the approximate rate of one inch per month.

The hair in cross section reveals two different strengths of keratin, the fiber protein of which hair and nails are made. The core of the hair is the *medulla*, a narrow column of cells of soft keratin. The function of the medulla is not known and it may be frequently broken along the length of the hair or even absent altogether. Hair does not seem to suffer when it is absent, although pigment of the hair is often found in this layer. The medulla is surrounded by the bulk of the hair shaft, the *cortex*, which is protected by a thin outer layer of *cuticle* and *cuticle scales*. Both the cortex and the cuticle are made of hard keratin. The cuticle has no pigment but the cortex is the main bearer of pigment. It was formerly believed that the hair shaft had a central "canal" by way of which the hair could "breathe" and "vital juices" flow. This is not the case. The hair consists of dead cells and an arrangement of minuscule air bubbles. Because these cells are mostly keratin, a protein rich in sulfur and resistant to strong acids, the hair is susceptible to alkaline agents.

The relative shortness of our hair is traceable to the manner in which the cuticle scales are arranged along the shaft of all hair in an overlapping manner not unlike that of the bark on a palm tree. Thus the shaft is not of uniform thickness in any type of hair, but in ours especially there are points of extreme narrowing which present structural weaknesses allowing for easy fragmentation. Contrary to its appearance, our hair is most fragile and requires very gentle treatment; it will not tolerate abuse. It is not true, however, that our hair is any drier than that of other races. All hair is lubricated by the sebum (oil) secreted by the sebaceous glands found in profusion near all hair follicles. This sebum not only protects the hair from dryness but prevents the spread of bacteria and helps to maintain the correct body temperature as well as functioning (as in perspiration) to rid the body of waste substances. These manifold functions are just as active in the sebaceous glands found in the scalps of Black women and men as those of other races. Thus it is a physiological fact that the scalps of Black people are just as oily as the rest. It is the texture of our hair and its lack of luster that make us interested in scalp lubricants, not the actual moistness of the scalp.

Of course, illness and hormonal change (as during menstruation or menopause) will affect the circulation of the blood that in turn acts upon the blood vessels serving the hair papillae. In this manner the growth, texture, and appearance of the hair can be changed by any alteration to the bloodstream and aided by good over-all health, nutrition, and exercise. In addition to the sebum from the sebaceous glands themselves, the hair is also moistened by amino acids that regulate the moisture within the cortex and retain sufficient moisture for optimum development. These amino acids are fed by the blood directly into the capillaries of each papilla.

The growth of the hair is a constant process and it is normal for us to lose between fifty and one hundred hairs every twenty-four hours. An individual hair grows from two to five years (this is called the *anagen* period and is fastest in summer), then stops growing and enters a resting (*telogen*) period that lasts a maximum of six months. During this time the hair gradually weakens its hold in the follicle and is either brushed out or forced out by a new, emerging hair shaft. If the hair shaft is destroyed, a new hair will inevitably appear. If the hair does not reappear, the follicle itself has been damaged. So long as the follicle is not destroyed (in which case the hair loss is permanent), medical attention can usually remedy interruptions in the growth pattern.

The nature of your hair is determined by your race (heredity), and its health is strongly related to the health of your body as a whole (heredity and environment). However, this has been a general discussion and it is an acknowledged axiom that no two persons have identical hair characteristics any more than they could have identical fingerprints. The shape of the root and the chemical composition can vary enormously even in two heads of hair that appear to be perfectly similar. It is our job to get to know the special characteristics of our own hair and learn to care for it accordingly.

B. BASIC HAIR HYGIENE

The American Black woman may have hair which is fine-textured and blond or virtually black and coarse. All possible degrees between these two extremes are also represented, including all shades of browns and reds. Nevertheless, every one of us must be indebted to the genius of a pioneer inventor-manufacturer in the field of hair-care products for the Black woman. Singlehandedly, Madame C. J. Walker created ways and means for us to care

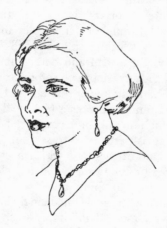

for our hair that are now very standard procedures. The daughter of former slaves, Madame Walker began her research into hair care for Black women in 1901 and set new standards for the maintenance of healthy hair and scalps. Among other things she invented the hot iron (straightening) comb and founded a beauty culture business that still employs hundreds of thousands of Black women around the globe. She died, the first female Black millionaire, in 1919.

Hair Washing

If you comb and brush your hair correctly every day, you probably need only wash your hair every eight or ten days. Of course, if you have excessively oily hair or gray or white hair, sooner than that is advisable. The main reason that frequent (daily) washings of the hair are damaging is that hair is weak when wet and unless meticulous care is taken, breakage very easily occurs when the hair is hurriedly rinsed, untangled, styled, and pinned or curled. Although our hair when dry is very elastic and can resist the normal stretching entailed by daily brushing and combing, it becomes very fragile when wet. Dermatologists recommend daily washings only if the hair is worn in its natural state (not straightened or styled) and if great care is taken in grooming the hair when damp.

Choosing a Shampoo

These days we are bombarded with hair-cleansing products that claim not only to improve one's love life but also to cure the most obscure scalp diseases. All we should require our shampoo to do is remove surface grease, dirt, and skin debris from the hair without adversely affecting the health of the hair or scalp. After washing, the hair should be fragrant, lustrous, soft and manageable and, more important than any of those qualities, clean. The fatty oils (lipids) diffused throughout the scales in the hair keep the hair moist and soft. Any strong alkaline solution will destroy these lipids and leave hair brittle and dry. Cake soap and detergents are quite high in alkali and should be avoided. Many shampoo products are now vying on the market with each other, claiming low or neutral "pH factors." As I mentioned in "Our Face," a low pH number means a high acid content; a pH7 is about neutral and a pH9 is high in alkaline content. Most regular nonadditive shampoos are pH7, which is perfectly safe for our hair. I prefer and recommend the most popular kind of shampoo which is an unadulterated clear liquid without built-in rinses or conditioners. Such a clear shampoo may be oil- or soap-based, but all are easy to apply, quick to lather, and simple to rinse. Unless suggested by your doctor, avoid medicinal shampoos and, in fact, any shampoo that claims to do more than simply wash your hair since in most cases the additives necessary for "stimulating," "conditioning," or "medicating" impair the basic property of the product—to cleanse. Shampoos that contain food sources such as protein are relatively poor cleaning agents and usually leave the hair with an unnecessary coating. Many leading hairdressers have reported to me that such combination shampoos have created a lot of problems with their Black customers' hair. Shampoos come in many forms other than liquid and can be a lotion, paste, or gel without losing effectiveness, but I must warn that anyone expecting good results from a dry or aerosol shampoo will be disappointed. Always read the label before buying, and choose the plainest, most straightforward product. (All you must expect from it is cleansing properties.) I prefer and recommend Johnson's Baby Shampoo for all kinds of hair—normal, dry, and oily. If you have extremely dry hair, try a vegetable-oil-based castile shampoo.

How to Shampoo

1) Thoroughly rinse the hair in lukewarm water.

2) Apply a generous amount of shampoo and massage into the hair with the fingertips only, making sure you follow the hairline and include the entire head and nape of the neck. Avoid abrading your scalp with fingernails and if they are very long, use soft cotton gloves or a sponge for this step. When wet, our hair contracts to almost half its length and thus easily becomes matted. For this reason it is imperative that the shampoo be vigorously massaged into the scalp to penetrate all the hairs. Do not use the palms to massage in shampoo; this will only mat and break the hairs.

3) Rinse thoroughly in clean warm water (not hot). Even if you lather twice it is most important that each rinsing be absolutely thorough.

4) Repeat step 2.

5) Your final rinse should be threefold. First, running warm water to remove every vestige of the shampoo. Second, a rinse in cool running water while running your fingers gently through your hair. Third, a final rinse in warm water until the hair is squeaky. If you are shampooing while in the bathtub, do not submerge your head to rinse; this will only increase the dirt on your hair. Keep a large plastic container by the tub and rinse from that, always using fresh, clean water.

If you wear your hair naturally and wish to shampoo every day, lightly oil the hair first, rinse in warm running water, and lather only once with a diluted solution of very mild shampoo.

Use of Hair Rinses

Hair rinses were developed as acidic solutions prepared to restore the acid balance of the hair after the use of high-alkaline shampoos. When lime soap was used as a shampoo, Black women often rinsed afterward with vinegar or lemon juice and this practice is not uncommon today. If you use a noncombination mild shampoo and rinse with clean running water, as I have suggested, you should have no need of a special rinse. If you insist on using a rinse, do read the label very thoroughly; it may contain artificial pigment for especially oily or dry hair. A rinse should only be left on for limited duration. The only rinse I feel safe recommending to you is the old-fashioned one: one cup of fresh lemon juice (or vinegar) mixed with one cup of cool water.

To Apply Rinse

1) Pour the solution onto the hair from the nape of the neck forward.
2) Gently massage with the fingertips throughout the hair.
3) Let stand for three minutes.
4) Rinse out completely in cool running water.

Hair Conditioners

Because of the styling and processes that our hair endures, most hair specialists and doctors agree that about 80 per cent of all Black women require the regular use of hair conditioners. A conditioner is generally defined as being a substance that can be absorbed by the cortex of the hair shaft through the cuticle, not something that simply coats the cuticle scales. The aim of a conditioner is to give body and lubrication to the individual hair shafts. Most conditioners contain proteins or oils or waxes or combinations of all three. Other than conditioning shampoos (which I do not recommend), conditioners may be based in creams, gels, liquids, or powders. Conditioning agents that Black women should definitely avoid are henna (principally a coloring factor) and balsam. Both of these simply coat the hair shaft, then strip it of oils, leaving the hair very dry. If you are in a quandary about what type of conditioner to use for your hair, seek the advice of a knowledgeable hairdresser or dermatologist. My preferred conditioner is Wella Kolestral Concentrate.

To Apply Conditioner

1) Follow the instructions and only leave on for the required time. Longer may not hurt but it certainly will not help.
2) Speed and assist the penetration of the conditioner by applying moderate heat with a heating cap or dryer, but remember:
   a) Set dial to warm, not hot.
   b) Cover head with Saran Wrap and a shower cap.
3) If you use a quick conditioner, a hot towel wrapped around the head will do the trick. Probably the best method for increasing the effectiveness of a conditioner is to use steam heat and several appliances are made for this purpose.
4) It is imperative that you know whether the conditioner is to be rinsed out or left on. Some women have damaged or lost their hair because they have left conditioners on indefinitely.
5) If the conditioner is to be rinsed out, follow my steps under "How to Shampoo," and do not begin to dry the hair until it literally squeaks.

To Dry the Hair

A hot drier can be very damaging to our hair and should only be used by a professional. At home never set a drier higher than "warm." Never brush the hair when wet—only comb. Brushing gathers, pulls, and snaps hairs. Wet hair is easy to handle without a drier as follows:

1) Blot and squeeze water from the hair with a soft towel. Do not rub the hair; this will lead to breakage.

2) Insert comb vertically into hair but stop short of the scalp. Gently move the comb out (not "up") and allow the hairs to slide off the teeth of the comb. Stop when you feel the hair tugging. For this, you must use only a large, gap-toothed plastic comb with rounded teeth.

3) If the hair is badly tangled, use a "finger comb." Using only the cushions of your fingertips (not the nails), gently pull out and free the tangles.

4) Part the hair and divide into small sections. Squeeze and blot dry each section with a towel and pat gently.

5) For very messy tangles, use a large comb. Move in small sections at a time and work from the end toward the root, not vice versa, concentrating on only a few hairs at a time. No matter how short the hair, a finger or two should always anchor the root to prevent breakage and loss when undoing tangles.

Patience when drying and untangling the hair is always rewarded. If you try either operation in a hurry, the result will be a botched job that will not only look terrible but may lead to hair damage.

C. HAIR GROOMING

The comb originated in Africa; both wooden and ivory combs, some fantastically ornate, have been found in Egyptian tombs. The state of our hair is directly related to the type and condition of our combs and brushes and how we use them. The material from which a comb is made is not so important as its shape. Your comb should have a definite handle to prevent slippage. The teeth must be smooth and rounded, not sharp. This is the single most important thing to look for. Avoid wire or metal-tooth combs. The hair shaft curls around these teeth and is very easily broken. Wooden picks are not safe; as they splinter, causing hairs to break. Ideally you should have one wide-toothed comb for wet hair and a finer-toothed comb for styling. There is no point in washing your hair if you are going to untangle or style it with a dirty comb. Combs must be washed as often as your hair.

Your hairbrush can either be a hero or a villain, depending upon your choice and usage. If the brush ends are flat, diagonal, or pointed, it is of no use to you: it will irritate the scalp and tear the hair shaft. The best brush for our hair has bristles which are firm, well spaced, and, most important, rounded. Only two types fit this category: a natural bristle and a plastic (rounded) bristle. Since the former is not sufficiently flexible, I do not recommend it for wet hair; only use a plastic brush which has sufficient "give" to avoid pulling and tugging out hairs. I use a hairdresser's plastic brush when my hair is natural or wet and a bristle brush if my hair is dry or straightened. Try both to see which suits your style and grade of hair, but remember to examine the bristle ends very carefully and make sure they are rounded. They should also vary in length and be graded in each tuft with the longest in the center. In the store, try the brush on your arm. If it hurts or scratches there, it will certainly do the same to your scalp. Your brush must be kept clean, especially if you carry it in a bag with other cosmetic tools and preparations. Both comb and brush collect debris from the hair and elsewhere and must be clean at all times.

Our hair can split easily and break often. For this reason, only brush or comb for grooming and styling, not as a fetish or to stimulate the hair or scalp. The more that is done to our hair, the greater is the risk of damage. If it is kept clean and well groomed, it will thrive if left alone.

Lubricants

As I mentioned earlier in this chapter, our scalps are no drier than those of other races and neither is our hair. An oily film along the hair shaft keeps moisture in, keeps the hair flexible, and should give a lustrous appearance to the hair as well as protecting the scalp from bacteria. Our desire for scalp lubricants is unfounded on physiological fact unless the individual has a naturally dry skin, in which case she probably also has a genuinely dry scalp, but it is not a racial trait. The structure of our hair absorbs light and the result is a dull rather than shiny surface. Greasing the hair will only serve to give luster to the hair surface, but it will not stimulate hair growth; it will not prevent hair loss; it will have no beneficial effect on the health of hair or scalp unless you suffer from excessively dry hair. The stimulating effect of the massage that occurs when the scalp is oiled may possibly improve the circulation in the scalp but that has not yet been conclusively proven. Neither petroleum nor lanolin nor vitamin oils or creams have been proven effective. Despite these facts, we will still continue to oil our hair and scalp and there is a better way to do it. I prefer to use a very light cream but many preparations are popular, including heavy greases (oil and water). Only use a very tiny drop on the tip of your index finger. Part the hair and rub gently on the scalp, bringing it slowly up to the ends of the hairs. Do just a small part at a time. Never oil the hair more than once a week or your pores will clog and the accumulation of oil on the hair and scalp will attract rather than repel dirt and bacteria. Women who grease their hair frequently find it very hard to shampoo and rinse to squeaky cleanliness and consequently their hair is never really clean; this state of affairs is really disastrous for the preservation of a full, healthy head of hair, and in addition it looks quite dreadful when grease is plainly visible on the scalp, ears, forehead, and neck. If you suffer from dandruff, do not use any special conditioner or lubricant without professional advice; you can easily aggravate the problem until it becomes virtually insurmountable.

D. BASIC HAIR CARE

Dry Hair

Black women are subject to a number of conditions other than heredity that can cause dull, brittle, lifeless hair. Occupational hazards such as steam, dust, and chemicals are frequently cited by experts as well as excessive heat and chemical treatments of the hair for cosmetic reasons. Even if the hair is inadequately groomed, the distribution of sebum from the sebaceous glands will be erratic and the shaft of each hair will not receive an equal portion. Hair luster depends upon, firstly, the adequate secretion of oil by the glands and, secondly, the adequate distribution of that oil over the entire hair surface. The latter can only be accomplished by judicious brushing and combing. Internal disorders, especially those that affect the blood, may produce changes in the hair texture from strong to weak and from vibrant to lifeless.

CARE OF DRY HAIR

1) Shampoo once per week at the most, preferably once every ten days. Use a mild, oil-based shampoo and follow my instructions for washing and rinsing.

2) Follow shampoo with the application of a true conditioner that will penetrate the hair cuticle. Avoid "body" conditioners that will simply coat, then strip the hair shaft.

3) With the conditioner, use just moderate to warm heat to activate, never any hotter, and stay with the heat the minimum required time.

4) Blot dry with a towel while in a cool airstream. A warm to hot dryer will strip the natural oils from the hair and make it very susceptible to breakage while it is drying.

5) If you straighten your hair, try to avoid any chemical straightening procedures. If using a hot comb, make sure each strand is well oiled before pressing and use only a light press.

6) Absolutely avoid hot curlers, hot rollers, heating caps, and hot dryers.

7) If you use any kind of rollers, you must use end papers and never use sponge rollers; these absorb oil and moisture from the hair.

8) Once every week, lightly oil scalp and hair shafts with a *light* oil or

cream. Resist the temptation to use a heavy grease; this will only attract dirt and require frequent washings which are bad for dry hair.

9) Avoid the regular use of lacquers and hair sprays. When you must, choose only those products that are oil-based.

Dry hair is weak and breaks easily. Brushing and combing must be done only as needed and with great care. Think twice before subjecting the hair to permanents, bleaches, or dyes; these procedures just weaken the hair shafts even more. You must bear the nature of your hair in mind when selecting style. A corn row must not be too tight or left in too long if you have dry hair, and if you have an Afro, only brush or comb it as needed for grooming; excessive tampering will only weaken the hair.

Oily Hair

Excessively oily hair is caused by an overabundance of secretions by the sebaceous glands in the scalp. It is usually a hereditary problem, although it can be caused by changes in the body condition (pregnancy, menstruation) or in the environment (very hot weather). Women who have oily hair notice an increase in oiliness a few days after washing the hair and find it hard to manage. Sometimes this condition is accompanied by dandruff.

CARE OF OILY HAIR

1) Use great caution when choosing a shampoo. Many that are labeled "for oily hair" contain much alcohol and salicylic acid that simply overdry the hair and create another equally undesirable condition.

2) Wash the hair in hot water, following my directions for rinsing. Wash your hair whenever it begins to look or feel greasy or at least once every week.

3) After washing the hair, apply my lemon-juice or vinegar rinse. This will gently strip the hair of excess oils.

4) You do not need a conditioner; your hair has enough natural oil.

5) Blot your hair dry and use only a cool airstream for drying. Hot air will stimulate the oil glands.

6) You may use a chemical straightener but be sure to choose the mildest possible. Harsh chemicals at this stage can be retained by the hair and mix with your natural oils to produce unmanageable results. If you straighten with a comb, use a warm press, but grease the hair sparingly with a mild, light cream.

7) Do not oil or grease the hair and scalp.

8) Do not massage the scalp.

9) Too much combing and brushing will stimulate the sebaceous glands, so do so only for grooming.

10) Try not to use hair sprays and lacquers on a regular basis, but for occasional use, choose a nonoil-based product.

11) Try to match your hairstyle to your type of hair. The easiest for your oily hair is to brush it back close to the head and wear in a bun or braided. An Afro, for instance, will demand a lot of attention to keep it looking good.

12) Bleaches, dyes, and permanents are more successful on, and least damaging to, oily hair than any other kind.

Fine (Thin) Hair

This is my kind of hair. The medulla may be missing or may be very fractured and the hair shafts are small and lie close to the scalp. This kind of hair is often difficult to style and is usually inherited, although it can be caused by certain illnesses as well as by excessive use of chemical straighteners. A woman who recovers from some form of hair loss usually grows back this type of hair. Whatever the claims of an expert or product, thin hair cannot be made to grow thicker.

CARE OF FINE HAIR

1) Wash in a mild shampoo every ten days and rinse very well.

2) Use a rich, penetrating conditioner such as Wella Kolestral Concentrate and avoid the type that appears to add body but simply coats the hair with adhesives that seem to make the hair look thicker temporarily but, in fact, leave a dangerous legacy of dehydration that just further thins the shaft.

3) Use a warm-temperature heating device to make the conditioner penetrate.

4) Blot your hair dry with a towel and set your dryer on moderate to warm.

5) Use only the mildest chemical relaxers to straighten the hair. Never use a hard press with a straightening comb. If you attempt to make your hair utterly straight it will only look thinner than it is if plastered to your scalp. Our hair needs some natural curl to give it body.

6) When using curlers, leave them on for as long as possible but do not try to help the curl with heated curlers; they may not "take" because of the fineness of your hair. Small rollers will make your hair appear thicker and a setting lotion will help them to hold.

7) Most hair sprays will only coat and separate fine hair.

8) Your hair will suffer if you choose a style that requires teasing or back combing. A corn row may make your hair appear thinner than it is. If you do wear this style, make sure the braids are fairly loose. When styling an Afro with fine hair, only braid the lower half of the hair strands. When combed or blown out, the unbraided top half will have more body. Straight long hair-

styles often exaggerate fine hair unless worn close to the scalp and in a chignon. The shorter the hair is, the thicker it looks. Instead of a layer cut, a blunt cut (hair of even length) increases the appearance of thickness.

9) Thin hair tends to be weak, so avoid or use with great caution, permanents, bleaches, and dyes.

10) Only if your hair and scalp are also very dry should you use any lubricant. In any case, just use a light cream; a thick grease will glue the hair strands together and the over-all effect will be of even thinner hair.

11) Hairpieces and wiglets are excellent for filling out fine hair.

Thick Hair

No woman with thick hair should complain! Those who do receive no sympathy from me, or most other Black women around the world. Thick hair is what most of us desire and envy, since it connotes strong, healthy follicles and hair shafts. I am well aware, however, that this type of hair does present specific problems when it comes to washing, grooming, and straightening. It is often difficult to style, and hairdressers try to leave women to the last who have this grade of hair, then rush the job.

CARE OF THICK HAIR

See my instructions for general washing and rinsing and drying, conditioning, and grooming. It is imperative that you rinse very well—three or four times.

1) If you want straightened hair, your hair can take all processes. Still, avoid very harsh chemicals and very hot combs; both wreak havoc even on the strongest hair.

2) When rolling, use large rollers and strive for a loose curl; a small curl will make your hair look even thicker. Thick hair will hold a curl well, so there is no need to fiddle daily with touch-ups from a hot comb; this inevitably leads to damage.

3) Combing and brushing may be difficult but cannot be hurried. Have patience and do not try to force out tangles, but separate them with your fingers.

4) Of course, the corn row and the Afro styles are well suited to your hair, which can be worn in almost any possible way. If you wish to play down the thickness or bushiness of your hair, choose a cut that will give the appearance of finer hair. It may also be more manageable.

5) Perspiration, especially with straightened hair, may be a big problem for you. Wash frequently and avoid chemical straighteners. Your hair can probably take more washings than any other kind, so take advantage of that and keep it always clean and groomed.

Gray Hair

Gradually graying of the hair, at any age, is a normal physiological change. It is progressive and permanent, usually starting at the temples, then across the head until the entire scalp is affected. The exact cause of this loss of pigment is not known, although many theories are still advanced, the most popular speculating that the nervous system is responsible and that anxiety plays a major role in this change, while others equally accepted state that hormonal or vitamin deficiency is the major cause. Premature grayness is often hereditary and it cannot be proved to be linked with any form of weakness or deficiency. Personally, I find natural gray hair one of the most elegant marks of distinction for a Black woman, one that well matches our rich complexions. It is a trait to be proud of and should be emphasized, not disguised.

CARE OF GRAY HAIR

1) Use only a mild shampoo and rinse well.
2) Only use conditioners if your hair is also fine or dry.
3) Treat your hair gently and remember that too much heat, especially from straightening combs, can turn your hair a yellow color. The hot comb should only be barely warm enough to accomplish the press—no hotter. Chemical straighteners should be avoided since your hair may not be growing as fast or abundantly as before and the harsh chemicals can further retard strength of the hair. Use a very mild relaxer.
4) Do not dye your hair. It will grow out far sooner than you expect and the contrast is very obvious when the roots are lighter than the rest. As an alternative, use nonperoxide brighteners that are safe for gray, silver, and white hair.
5) If you decide to try to change the color of your hair, bear in mind that black, dark brown, and chestnut hues will probably age your face and make it appear too hard. Lighter colors tend to give a more youthful appearance, so do not try to dye your hair from its naturally light tone to a much darker one, but choose a light shade that is becoming to your age. Be very careful not to choose a color more than one or two shades lighter than your own, however, because this is very apparently artificial.
6) Corn rows look very bad in gray hair but Afros look splendid. I prefer to see a gray-haired woman wear medium-length hair off the face. Short hair is best tight to the head or worn with a bun.

Thinning Hair

Our hair tends to be shorter and thinner at the temples and all around the hairline to the nape of the neck. All women experience this thinning at a certain age, regardless of race, but we are also prone to it for a variety of factors that are largely our own fault and can be remedied:

a) Do not pull children's hair tight into braids and ponytails. This strain at an age when the hair is still soft and quite weak starts the cycle of abuse that results in thinning hair.

b) When wearing our hair straight, we do not wash sufficiently thoroughly at the hairline for fear of making it bushy. Dirty hair collects bacteria and the follicle can become diseased and die.

c) Constant grooming with unclean combs and brushes can also spread bacteria.

d) Because the edges of our hair are troublesome when straightening, we are guilty of "touching up" the temples or sides with a hot comb or hot grease or leaving harsh chemicals on for far too long—all of these things lead to hair loss.

e) Scarves secured very tightly at the temples and nape of the neck can also contribute to the problem.

f) Various hairstyles involve constant traction with the follicles at the edges of the hairline, leading to temporary or permanent loss at these points.

As we grow older and hormonal changes occur, we cannot expect our hair to grow as fast or as strong or to be able to replace itself as it did when we were teen-agers. Always treat your hair gently at any age, but do so especially if you are twenty-five and definitely if you are over thirty-five. Damage to the hairline at this age usually cannot be rectified.

Care of Thinning Hair

1) Follow very closely my general instructions for hair care.

2) Use no chemical straighteners at all.

3) For straightening use only a light warm press with a minimum of oil. The combination of hot oil and a hot press is fatal; the oil melts and can cause permanent damage to the hair root.

4) No massage. This only encourages hair to fall out.

5) Do not wear rollers or curlers too tightly or for long periods of time.

6) Avoid buns or ponytails that pull the hair constantly back from the forehead.

7) Do not tease the hair, and when combing and brushing, be very gentle; do not tug or pull.

8) A short hairstyle that does not strain at the hairline will prevent pulling at the hairline (the weight of long hair does this) and will give the appearance of fullness to thinning hair.

9) If you notice at any time an appreciable increase in the rate of thinning, you must consult a doctor.

E. HAIRSTYLING

In tribal Africa, from antiquity to the present day, it is often the custom to utilize hairstyling as a method of communication concerning the identity of the wearer. Traditional ways of wearing the hair have been established to announce availability for marriage, engagement, marital status, the birth of a son or daughter, religious favor, prowess in hunting or war, and position in the tribal hierarchy. In America today, such indices are not widely practiced, although often we tend to presuppose an individual's political and behavioral tendencies (from radical to conservative) based upon the way she wears her hair.

Black women's hairstyles have undergone much change in the last ten years as "processed" hair went out of style and the natural Afro became popular, along with the exotic corn row. Now we are experiencing a nonnostalgic but very common-sense return to straightened hair. Inasmuch as our hues of color vary widely, so do our hairstyles. The choice of a particular way to wear one's hair is a very personal, particular choice and should be dictated as much by one's emotional, political, or occupational status as by rules found in fashion magazines for particular "shapes of face." I have very little faith in such gross generalizations. In fact, with my broad brow and high forehead, had I followed the "rules" I should have worn my hair in bangs or with a center part. Had I done that, I probably would not have had a modeling career at all! I wanted to show my face and enjoyed a very severe hairstyle, and it worked. You must experiment, but not daily or you will ruin your hair changing styles all the time. Pay little attention to friends or relatives unless they themselves have achieved success in this area. Even if it is supposedly "right" for fashion and your "shape of face," a hairstyle that makes you feel uncomfortable or self-conscious should be abandoned. The most important thing is that you should feel attractive and comfortable and be able to manage proper care of your hairstyle.

Hairstyle Care

AFRO

This requires constant combing and must be conditioned every time you shampoo (which should be once per week). When you lubricate the scalp, massage and bring the oil to the ends of each strand. Keep your hair trimmed for uniformity and shape. Never use metal combs or picks. Any implement you use must have well-rounded teeth and have no sharp or jagged edges. If your hair is fine, only braid the lower half and when it is all combed out, this will give an added illusion of fullness. In the mornings, if your Afro is matted, never rake a comb or brush through it. Moisten slightly with equal parts of oil and water and gently pull out with the tips of your fingers. Do not use your fingers or nails to comb but simply pull very gently.

Corn Row

Many of us are guilty of leaving this style alone for weeks on end. It must be taken down and shampooed at least every ten days or else bacteria will accumulate and gradually destroy the hair roots. When you take down to wash, also lubricate and massage the scalp. If you attach beads or other ornaments to your corn row, you must remove them before sleeping.

Straightened Hair (Chemical)

Never attempt this yourself at home. The risk of permanent damage is simply too great and your hair is too precious. You should seek a reputable beauty parlor, speak to a customer who has had this treatment successfully, and stay with the same establishment so that the operator knows your unique hair characteristics. This process should not be undertaken more than four times per year and, while in effect, never attempt to color your hair or use a hot comb to "touch up." The hair is made weaker by this chemical straightening and requires conditioning every time you shampoo.

Straightened Hair (Hot Comb)

Never hard press the hair; a gentle press is sufficient. Be careful not to overlubricate the hair with heavy grease that will only attract germs and dirt —one oiling when the hair is pressed is enough. The hot comb tends to split the hair ends and your hair should be regularly trimmed (by a professional) if you use this straightening process.

No matter what style we choose, it has to be created and sustained by certain treatments or processes. If left to grow naturally with only a minimum of grooming, our hair would become damaged and fragile. Our hair needs frequent washing and conditioning and individual styles require additional attention. There is no "best" way to wear our curly hair. Improperly cared for, the "natural" Afro can damage the hair as much as careless use of straightening techniques and it is a fallacy to believe that hair "breathes" and that therefore a "natural" style is healthier than straightening. In fact, I find when my hair is not pressed I experience more trouble and hair loss than otherwise. Either way, hard work and patience and diligent care are required by the wearer. Damage to the hair does not usually occur because of a particular style or even because of the products or procedures used on the hair, but because of human error in the use of such products and carelessness in handling particular styles. Over all, we should consider ourselves fortunate in that our naturally soft and delicate hair can be satisfactorily transformed into a multitude of different styles and lengths.

F. HAIR TECHNIQUES

For countless centuries, Black women have straightened their hair, not necessarily in emulation of Caucasian styles but as a practical, manageable, attractive alternative. During and immediately after slavery, Black women in this country would straighten their hair by first heating a piece of flannel before the fire, then oiling the hair with lard and pulling the strands through the hot flannel. In this century, thanks to Madame C. J. Walker, there are two reliable methods of hair straightening in use throughout the country: the chemical method and the hot comb method. In general, the doctors with whom I have spoken prefer the hot comb method for safety and recommend that chemical straightening not be undertaken more than four times per year.

Hot Comb Straightening

Sometimes known as the *pressing method*, this involves a generous application of hair oil to freshly washed hair (to minimize burning), which is then subjected to pressure from root to end by a heated metal comb. This comb should pass freely along all the strands of hair. After this treatment the hair is usually set in curls. This pressing will last until the scalp's own moisture or a thorough washing makes the hair revert to its naturally curly state. This is my preferred method of straightening my hair because it is relatively clean, simple, and quick. There are, of course, many dangers, the chief of which is that of burning the hair with a comb that is too hot and is pressed too hard on the hair. The scalp also can suffer injury in this manner. The oil may melt and, with a hot comb, damage the cuticle of the hair as well as the hair follicle. In order to avoid this, always have the comb warm—not hot. Make sure there are no excess greases or perfumes or pomades on the hair, that the hair has been thoroughly shampooed, and do not lightly or quickly attempt to touch up parts of the hair with a hot comb. The pressing method should be used by all women with fine or thinning hair, gray or artificially colored hair, and women at the time of pregnancy and menopause. Even if your hair is very lush, thick, and resilient, never have a hard press with a very hot comb.

Hot Comb Don't's

1) Don't attempt this method at home unless you have been trained by an experienced professional. Many operators may be willing to teach you pri-

vately or you can sign up for a short course at a hairdressing school. It may look simple to you and you may think you will save money by doing it at home, but most women who do invariably use TOO MUCH HEAT. The hair looks great for a few hours but the damage may be incalculable and only come to light much later. Special skills are required and if you do not have them, leave it alone.

2) Don't hot comb the hair when it is wet. Even if you are only doing a section of your hair, it must be well washed and well rinsed and very dry before applying the comb. Breakage will occur if there are traces of soap or shampoo in the hair, and you may be baking in these chemicals as well as bacteria and grime.

3) Never put a hot comb to your hair without first testing it. You should have a clean towel at hand to wrap the comb in when it has heated up. If the towel is scorched, the comb is too hot. Hold the comb up to a light and if there is any trace of smoke, replace it in the towel to cool.

4) Don't apply heavy grease to the scalp before pressing. This will disguise the heat of the comb and you may badly singe both hair and scalp. Apply a cream lightly to the hair only—just enough to keep it supple. Totally dry hair will burn even with a fairly cool comb.

5) Never apply a hot comb to touch up chemically straightened hair, even if it is reverting at the root. The combination of the two processes is too much for your hair to handle.

6) Don't use a plug-in electric comb at home. They are deceptively difficult to regulate and will either be too cool or far too hot. Always use a comb heated on a stove or special burner.

You must, when using this process at home, choose a well-lighted area that gives you plenty of room to sit and stand and with a table at a convenient height for your equipment. You also need a large mirror at an adequate height. It is very bad to heat the comb on the kitchen stove and then rush to another part of the house to find a mirror. Accidents often happen that way, and not only to your hair. Invest in a small heating device from a hairdressing supply house and keep all your equipment in one place. If you are comfortable, you will not be so tempted to rush and botch the job. It is also quite unsanitary to straighten your hair in the place where you normally cook food.

Chemical Straightening

This method has become increasingly popular in recent years and some beauty salons no longer will use the hot-comb method, favoring chemical straightening because it is supposed to be quick and easy to handle. (It is also quite expensive, so there may well be a profit motive in its appeal to beauty-salon owners and operators.) Basically, two separate chemical procedures are performed. First, a *relaxer* is applied to the hair which softens and changes the vitality of the hair shaft. Secondly, a *neutralizer* is applied that stops the action of the relaxer and, by oxidization, rehardens the hair into a new, straight position. The chemicals used are mostly alkaline in nature and allow the hair to be altered by diminishing the hair's natural elasticity.

The procedure should commence with a thorough cleansing of the scalp, although I have too often noted operators who apply the chemicals directly to soiled hair; this can be ruinous. Some hairdressers avoid shampooing the hair with the claim that the hair is weaker when wet and the scalp more tender. This is certainly true, but if the shampoo is mild and the cleansing action without massage or abrasion and the drying thorough, then the hair will certainly benefit from being clean before the straightening process is commenced. The scalp and the forehead must be protected with a coating of grease, then the alkaline (relaxer) cream is combed through the hair until it is visibly straightened. A rinse is then used as a neutralizer and, rolled in curlers, the hair is dried under a dryer. It is important to be aware of the fact that if the neutralizer is not applied or applied too late, the relaxer will eventually cause hair disintegration and loss. A very strong chemical is used to relax the hair and it should only be handled by an operator thoroughly conversant with your hair type and history. A mild solution should be used on a woman with fine hair whereas stronger hair can take a stronger solution. Good judgment on the part of the operator is essential to avoid temporary or permanent damage. No solution is totally harmless if abused or misused by carelessness or accident. The margin of error between the point of complete straightening and the onset of damage to the cuticle and cortex is very small indeed, which is why I strongly suggest that this treatment be done in two stages—the first a simple test with a very mild solution to partially straighten the hair and determine just how well it holds up to the chemicals. I have spoken to too many Black women around this country who have suffered serious hair loss from this method not to be very skeptical about it. It should definitely NOT be attempted in the home by anyone other than a fully trained and qualified practitioner. Great skill and judgment are needed for this method to be used safely with success. Never should it be tried on dyed or damaged hair. Unless the hair is badly burned by the hot-comb method, that method is fairly safe, temporary, and reversible, whereas chemical straightening attacks the core and fiber of the hair itself and can cause very serious ruin if attempted by the amateur. Go to a good beauty salon and always have a patch test done first on a small area of the head. Usually some of the chemical is placed behind the ear a day or so before your appointment. If there is any irritation, you may be allergic to the chemical and cannot and should not use chemical straightening methods. Never let a hairdresser talk you into this method simply because it is easier and more profitable for her or him. Make sure the operator thoroughly understands your type of hair and is willing to let you talk frankly with other clients whose hair he has been straightening chemically for some time. Also, in fairness to the operator, you must tell her or him what other procedures you use on your hair, how often it is washed, combed, and brushed, and if you have any present bodily condition such as illness or pregnancy that might preclude the use of chemicals. The operator must give you full instructions regarding aftercare of your chemically straightened hair as well as what particular side effects to be watchful for. It is wise to stay with one operator who can spot any minor changes in your hair that might herald serious problems. If you hop from one shop to another, these signs will not be detected. Never dye your hair if it has been chemically straightened, and avoid the hot comb completely. A competent chemical straightening should have no bad side effects and last from six weeks to two months, depending upon the rate of growth of your hair.

Chemical Treatments to Avoid

Hot permanent waving using electric apparatus and hot alkaline solutions often requires up to four hours of heating the scalp while it is tightly bound. Physicians warn against this procedure not only as it may damage the hair and scalp but because it is risky for women who may be suffering from high blood pressure, lung problems, and anemia.

Cold permanent waving entails the use of strong, harsh alkalis, sulphides, and thioglycolates that are tricky to neutralize and can do permanent damage to the hair root and shaft.

Curling

Our African ancestors had many ingenious methods of curling their hair including the use of fabric, mud, and twigs. Although we can form a curl in our hair with our fingers, the tension in the cortex will always seek to return it to its former position, so it is not possible to form curls permanently without a special treatment of which today there are three:

Water waving simply involves wetting the hair and rolling individual groups of strands around rods or rollers, then drying the hair either artificially or at room temperature. After the hair is dry and the rollers removed, the hair will retain a wave or curl. This process has to be repeated frequently and will not work well with individuals who have oily hair since the sebum acts as a barrier to the water.

The Marcel wave technique is named after a nineteenth-century Frenchman who invented a curling iron and a maneuver that revolutionized hairwaving. Nowadays in this country it is still very popular in our communities. The marcel irons are scissors-shaped with loose handles that allow the iron to revolve. The iron is heated, clamped on the hair, revolved, and released.

Electric rollers are now widely available in kits that combine sophisticated uses of steam or dry heat and that can also apply conditioner to the hair while it is being waved. Follow the instructions to the letter with these kits but never leave hot rollers in for more than five minutes.

Hair is easier to shape when presoftened by water or oils. The final size of your curl or wave will be determined by the size of the rod, roller, or curler you use. The larger the roller, the looser the curl.

Curling Hints

1) You can break and split your hair by pulling out curlers quickly and carelessly.

2) If your hair is fine, dry, or damaged, never wind it very tightly.

3) The only rollers that you can sleep in are large ones placed at the top of the head and these only if the hair is loosely wound.

4) Always use end papers to reduce friction between your hair and the rollers. Winding is easier and curls are more even.

5) We should never use sponge rollers. They create a great amount of friction with our type of hair and absorb much of the much-needed natural oils in the hair. When removed they have a very strong pull and can break our fine hair.

6) Be very careful not to dig into or scrape the scalp while using pins and rollers and other implements to hold the hair.

7) Electric rollers and curling irons should be used sparingly, not every day. A heat-regulated curling iron is best, one that is specially coated to prevent the hair from sticking.

8) When removing curlers, do so very gently and unwind in one correct direction only. If you are impatient, you may pull out hairs from the root. The greater the care and neatness you acquire while setting the curl, the easier it will be to remove the rollers.

9) I cannot overestimate the importance of keeping all hair-care tools such as rollers, pins, and nets clean at all times. You should wash them in hot soapy water at least twice a month, rinse thoroughly, and let dry on a towel.

Coloring

As Black women, we possess natural hair colors that range from a pale sandy blond to jet black. Most of us, however, have a bitter dark brown or off-black hair color with brown highlights. Hair is pigmented in much the same way as is the skin and tends to conform to the pigmentation patterns in the skin and of the eyes. Aside from the physical damage that certain kinds of permanent hair coloring can create, as Black women we must be well aware of what hair colors are really apt for our skin tones and I do not believe that "anything goes." To slightly enrich or darken one's hair (which is easy) or further highlight and lighten the shade (which is more difficult) are both quite within the realm of elegance and practicality. It is folly, however, to suppose that we can change the color of our hair from black to white with impunity and not look quite ridiculous. We may imagine that the effect is dramatic but sadly it is frequently clownish. Just as a blond Caucasian will look very peculiar with dyed jet-black hair, so do we commit a travesty to our unique racial coloring by trying to reverse nature.

Our African-Egyptian forebears discovered the use of hair dyes and would rub the vegetable dye "henna" into their hair and nails to give a red tint to brownish pigment. Henna is still a popular natural dye, although it did not reach western Europe until 1890. I would caution against the use of this dye because, apart from its chemical properties which are not entirely sympathetic to our hair types, it builds up an acidic paste on the hair cuticle and over periods of time this results in a quite unnaturally hard texture and a brittle, artificial auburn color.

Because of the delicate texture of our hair and its absorbency, many professionals in the field do not recommend permanent dyes for Black women. When it is done, it must only be performed by a very skilled technician who is fully aware of your hair's particular properties. In order for any dye to be permanent, the hair must first be stripped of its pigment and this involves applying chemicals that react with the keratin of the hair shaft itself. This is a delicate and potentially formidable procedure that can only leave the hair weaker even if the dye job is successful. The perfect dye, if one can be found, would not injure the hair or irritate the scalp and would create a color that was very natural in both daylight and artificial light. No home dye can guarantee any of the above and very few professionals are willing to accept any such responsibilities, especially with our hair. All the natural oils and surface of the cuticle scales have to be removed by solvents such as ammonia, sodium, and potassium. Great care has to be employed when applying these chemicals to the hair since they are potentially damaging, as are the ingredients of the dyes themselves: hydrogen peroxide, ammonium hydroxide, ammonium persulfate, sodium peroxide. Unless you have utter confidence in your operator, have seen his or her work on other women, are sure that the new color or tint will blend with your skin tones, and you have fairly strong, thick hair, I do not suggest a permanent dye. Remember, the color in the bottle or on the chart or in the photograph will not be nearly the same as the color on your *head*, next to *your* skin. Always have a skin patch test before the actual dyeing. Certainly never attempt to dye hair that has been chemically straightened.

TEMPORARY HAIR COLORING

All of the above holds true for this category except that some such dyes act only to coat the hair and do not penetrate the cortex and thus have less potential for damaging the inside of the hair shaft and the life of the hair.

Color rinses are acidic rather than alkaline and therefore work with, not against, the normal nature of the hair. They harden the cuticle and do not penetrate to the cortex. The natural color is left in the hair. Still, use these with caution and never carelessly. Only use the kind that can be easily removed by washing.

Color sprays combined with regular hair spray are very messy, rub off on almost everything and even so can contain harmful chemicals. Frequent applications are necessary and they are uneconomical as well as potentially unsafe.

Color crayon for the hair can be massaged or brushed onto the hair strands and if applied expertly can be effective for retouching roots that are growing in.

Semipermanent hair colorings claim to be more effective than rinses but often last little longer than three or four washings. These do change the structure of the keratin balance in the hair and can be as dangerous as permanent dyes.

Metallic dyes are poisonous and should be avoided at all costs.

Oxidation dyes are now called "hair tints" by the industry since it is felt that "dye" has negative connotations (with good reason!). In fact, these tints are just as permanent and change the molecular structure of the cortex.

Bleaching, or "stripping," is a process required when a dye has been unsuccessful or has damaged the hair or in order to dye from a very dark color to a very light one. The most effective and least harmful agent employed in this process is hydrogen peroxide, but bleaching is a delicate operation that requires a fully trained operator. The chemical is a strong one and if misapplied can wreak havoc.

After Coloring

During the dyeing process the hair is inevitably softened and weakened. First of all, the rinsing must be very, very complete to rid the scalp of all traces of dye or tint or rinse. Before styling the hair it must be reconditioned. Do not depend upon dyes that have built-in conditioners; the value is nil. After dyeing, the cuticle is very dry and brittle and must be fed more oils. If you wish to straighten your hair, do it only with a light warm-comb press, never a chemical.

Gray Hair

Because it is weaker, gray hair must be handled very delicately if dyed and a bluish tint should always be used before proceeding further.

Cutting

There is a perpetual myth repeated daily by Black women that our hair is stunted and needs trimming (or cutting) to encourage growth. I must put my foot down very strongly indeed and declare that the visible hair is *dead*. It cannot be stimulated or encouraged; it has no living cells. Of course, its chemical components can be changed by the action of other chemicals as in dyes, straighteners, water, and lubricants, but hair is not a living thing. The follicle at the base of the scalp is alive and the papilla below the follicle consists of living cells, but once the hair emerges it is dead. Cutting the hair will make it more manageable, perhaps more attractive, and will remove unsightly split ends, but *it will not stimulate growth*.

SHAPING

We cut our hair to suit certain styles that we prefer and nowadays many women choose a shorter style that is easier to groom and wash and maintain than long hair.

TRIMMING

When the ends of the hair shaft have lost their porous quality and split often and become damaged, occasional trimming resolves this problem.

THINNING

This may be necessary for those of us fortunate enough to have thick, bushy hair that requires a reduction in bulk. This does have some pitfalls, however, since the flat strokes of the thinning razor slice open the cortex, cut through the cuticle and expose the center of the hair shaft not only to the environment but also to damage from combing and brushing and from chemicals present in shampoos.

SINGEING

This method should be outlawed. It is based on the false premise that the medulla is hollow and canal-like, carrying "natural juices" from the papilla throughout the hair's length. It was thought that singeing the hair "sealed the ends" and thus prevented the "juices" from escaping. This neat fairy tale is pure fiction. In fact, what happens when the hair is singed is that gases are formed and trapped in the hair shaft, pressure builds up, and the ends split.

Not every hair grows at the same rate and the cycle of hair growth and replacement is continual; therefore, continual cutting is required to keep the hairs of even length and prevent the hair from becoming ragged and untidy. As we grow older, the hair grows at a slower rate than its normal one inch per month and if, as Black women, we prize our hair, we should think twice before drastically changing our hair by cutting it very, very short because it may take a long time to grow back.

It is really self-defeating to try to cut one's own hair. You cannot see your head from every angle and cannot manipulate scissors correctly all over your head. Most women who try it once spend a lot of money and time having a professional correct their mistakes. Stick to the salons.

G. TOOLS FOR THE HAIR

In order to maintain our hairstyles and keep our hair well groomed, certain implements are needed and a word about the choice and care and use of these is in order since so much unfortunate wear and tear can result from ignorance about our tools.

Hairpins

Small and large hairpins and bobby pins must always be rubber-tipped. If the tips are half off or missing, the hair shaft will be torn and the scalp scratched. Hair oil tends to loosen the tips, so examine them often and throw them away as soon as they are damaged. If you use pins a lot, ask your hairdresser to order a large professional box; in bulk they are inexpensive.

Rubber Bands

These are sly destroyers. They can slice and cut and break and pull out hairs. Only use coated ponytail holders that are available in many colors and can be found in five-and-ten-cent stores and drugstores. They are not as elastic as regular rubber bands but hold the hair neatly and tightly. Do not pull the hair or twist it into a very tight clump before using the band because this pulling action will continue all day. Never leave the band on longer than twenty-four hours and if you have difficulty removing, cut carefully with nail scissors.

Hair Sprays

Sprays and lacquers, if used with great regularity, can dry out the hair and make it brittle and broken. If you have dry hair, look for an oil-based spray. There are a number on the market specifically for Black women that cater to normal and dry hair. If your hair is oily, a regular spray will suffice, but still use in moderation.

Hairnets

If not worn too tightly, hairnets are most beneficial at night for keeping the hair in place. If you do tie up your hair at night, avoid a rough abrasive fabric such as wool; use silk or cotton. Perhaps the best method, especially if the hair is oily, is to put two large Kleenex tissues on the scalp and then a hairnet to hold them in place.

Electric Appliances

We develop many expensive devices for the hair which are supposed to be labor-saving but are not well tested on human subjects over long periods of time and are especially unproven for Black women. I advise using only such appliances (irons, curlers, rollers, dryers, heating caps) in emergencies and not as a daily diet. Often the effect is quick indeed but lasts only a short while.

H. HAIR HEALTH

Hormones

Undoubtedly the hormonal balance of the body will affect hair growth, but that balance is very delicate and is related to the whole body's metabolism and must not be carelessly tampered with. The application of hormone preparations to the hair itself will have no effect since the hair has no capacity to live. Ingesting hormones for the sake of the hair should only be done with a doctor's approval.

Diet

Other than a regular, well-balanced diet, I do not believe any one food in special quantities can affect the quality of the hair. Carbohydrates, proteins, minerals, and vitamins are all necessary in varying degrees for the maintenance of healthy hair, but only a trained professional can spot a hair defect stemming from a particular dietary deficiency and it is quite wrong to attempt self-diagnosis in this manner. If you notice a sudden change in your hair quality and believe it linked to your diet, see a doctor.

Massage

The scalp has a greater accumulation of blood vessels than many other parts of the body; thus it has been widely believed that stimulation of this area will bring about increased hair growth or quality. There is no proof that sebaceous glands or the papillae are affected by massage. Manual or mechanical massage of the scalp can be very relaxing, but it is a moot point whether or not it helps the hair. If you have thinning hair, massaging is a sure way to loosen it; so in those instances, avoid massage. When you do massage your own, or someone else's scalp, be sure to use only the cushions of the fingers—not the nails, knuckles, or palms.

Environment

Hair grows faster in warm weather and the sebum is more plentiful and the blood circulation better. If you have naturally oily hair, wash it more frequently in the summer months. In the winter, the cold is very hard on our hair; it becomes dry and lacks vitality. When we wear head coverings in winter they tend to be tight, squashing the hair and preventing it from being aerated. Excessive wind and sun can dry out the hair as well as the skin, as can the chores we perform around the house. Tie up and protect the hair with a soft, smooth scarf while washing, ironing, and cleaning. This will prevent humidity and dirt from adversely affecting your hair and requiring more washing and processing of the hair than is healthy. Wool should never be worn directly against the hair for long periods of time because it is an abrasive fabric. Cotton or silk should be worn in the summer, and in the winter also under the wool head covering. Salt water is very harmful to our hair, so after swimming in the sea, be sure to shampoo and rinse well; all the salt should be rinsed from the scalp. Before swimming in a chlorine-treated swimming pool, lubricate your hair with baby oil, tie up in a light smooth scarf, put on a bathing cap. Your hair will still get wet but will have been well protected. Shampoo with a mild solution and rinse well. Water alone will not remove chlorine or salt.

I. HAIR PROBLEMS AND THEIR TREATMENT

Our earliest recorded history is replete with concern about hair growth, health, and loss. The Egyptian Papyri—medical prescriptions written over 5,000 years ago—mention remedies for graying hair and male and female baldness. The mother of one Egyptian Queen was prescribed

> The toes of a dog
> Refuse of dates
> Hoof of an ass

to be ground and mixed and applied as a paste to cure her rapid hair loss.

Dandruff

Like many other adverse hair conditions that have their causes in scalp ailments, dandruff is linked not to the state of the hair but the state of the scalp. The signs of this condition are well known to all of us: telltale tiny flakes that accumulate on the back and shoulders of our clothing. This excessive scaling is often accompanied by uncomfortable itching. The clinical term for dandruff is *seborrhea,* an excessive production of oil (sebum) by the scalp that leads to a disorderly sloughing off of cells from the skin of the scalp. Dandruff conditions can be either dry or oily, depending upon the nature of the skin. In both cases, cells are prematurely shed in a haphazard manner. Dandruff can be caused by a wide variety of conditions from lack of proper nutrition and hormonal imbalance to complex allergies. Because the shedding of dead cells by the scalp is a perfectly natural process, it is often difficult to determine how and when a serious dandruff problem arises. The most important factor to bear in mind about dandruff is that it is not a cosmetic condition but a medical condition and can be cured only by medical means. A seborrheic scalp is often rife with bacteria that enters when the skin is opened by energetic scratching with the nails or combs or brushes in an attempt to allay the discomfort of dandruff. Many hair preparations containing grease and perfumes further compound the condition by introducing destructive organisms into these small wounds. Serious cases of dandruff must always be reported to a physician for treatment. Mild dandruff, which may be simply a normal scaling in larger than usual quantities, can be treated with four different types of antidandruff products:

Detergents.—These solutions are usually applied to the scalp five to twenty minutes before shampooing.

Medicated shampoos.—The most effective of these contain either sulfur, salicylic acid, or resorcinol. Many such products can be too harsh, so use with caution.

After-shampoo rinses.—These usually contain ammonium compounds and are aimed at reducing scaling.

Antiseptic lotions.—These often come in the form of medicated hairdressings and contain such stimulants as tincture of capsicum and chloral hydrate.

The object of a good antidandruff product should be to prevent itching, scaling, and excessive oiliness, as well as kill a wide range of bacteria and fungi on the scalp. Our hair and scalps are delicate and it is not likely that a nonprescription preparation will clear up a serious case of dandruff without producing unwanted side effects. If you suspect that you have dandruff, first check to see if the telltale deposits are not simply accumulated powder particles from overgenerous use of hair spray. If you are convinced that they are scalp particles and the condition is not accompanied by swelling or scabs, then by all means try a medicated antidandruff product (only one at a time; do not mix). If your problem has not cleared up within a week or ten days, discontinue use and consult a doctor. Repeated use of most commercial products will prove too harsh for both hair and scalp. When you do use them, always follow the directions exactly. If you have just a very mild case of dandruff, it should be sufficient simply to shampoo more thoroughly and more frequently. If your outbreak is severe and is accompanied by any abnormal discomfort or scalp condition, do not apply any preparation before seeing a doctor. Loss of the hair follicle cannot be rectified and this can occur if a seborrheic scalp is treated with a variety of different drugstore remedies. For mild conditions, use a medicated shampoo, once a week for dry hair and twice a week for oily hair. Do not massage the scalp, and brush and comb the hair only as much as necessary for grooming; too much scraping and scratching and pulling will aggravate the dandruff. Lay off all hair cosmetics such as sprays and conditioners for a while. Leave the hair alone; keep it clean.

Hair Loss or Breakage

Most of us notice very quickly if there is an abrupt change in the quality of our hair. The shaft may become limp, the ends more split than usual, or there may even be thin patches appearing at the perimeter of the scalp or in the middle of the head. Finding hairs on your brush and comb is not a sign for alarm if there are still the usual amount on your head: The process of shedding hair is keeping pace with the growth of new hair. Excessive hairfall is not a sign for great alarm or panic but usually indicates a condition that the individual cannot and should not attempt to diagnose and treat without the advice of either a dermatologist or a professional hairdresser with some medical qualifications. With all due respect to the eminent trade of hairdressing, a woman who starts to experience hair damage or loss should really seek the counsel of a medical specialist. The clinical term for hair loss is *alopecia* and *alopecia areata* refers to partial loss in patches, gradually spreading across the scalp. This may be caused by a wide variety of factors from the incorrect use of a hair product, to a hormonal condition or internal infection. If brought swiftly to the attention of a physician, it is reversible in most cases. Traction alopecia is hair loss resulting from external pressure such as a hairstyle that constantly pulls the hair from the roots, a very tight wig, or a hairpiece that is firmly worked into the hair and tugs constantly at the hair, or hair-straightening procedures that are too harsh. These are all related to habit, not disease, and the condition will clear up if the habit is stopped, although once the follicle is removed, the hair will not regrow. Contrary to popular belief, the state of one's "nerves" or emotional stability has little to do with hair health unless the disturbance manifests itself as trichotillomania, which literally means the pulling out of one's hair with the hands. Local scalp infections, either bacterial, viral, or fungal in origin, can cause hair loss. They must be treated by a doctor and are easily cleared up with the use of antibiotics and other drugs and preparations.

General bodily infection stemming from diseases such as diabetes, syphilis, and some forms of cancer can stimulate hair loss, and of course the major condition must be rectified before the condition of the hair can be expected to improve. Hair loss may be localized in the scalp area, or it may be a symptom of more widespread malaise. Assuredly, one's trained and qualified hairdresser can determine the condition of the hair itself and perhaps the cause of hair damage or loss, if it is localized in the hair shaft; but he or she is hardly qualified to diagnose the condition of your body as a whole or even examine a sample hair shaft and follicle microscopically. Do not take chances with a precious commodity. I know how terribly high doctors' bills are, and you may well consider it a frivolous expense to run to a physician because you have a sore scalp, dandruff, or falling hair; but consider not only how expensive it is but how time-consuming it is constantly to cope with female baldness. And do not forget that a change in the state of your hair may be signaling an unwanted and unwelcome change in the state of your whole health.

Hair-loss Remedies

As I have stated, once the hair follicle is destroyed or otherwise removed, hair cannot grow again in that particular spot. A new follicle can be surgically implanted from which new hairs can grow, but without this procedure no new growth should be anticipated. "Cures" for baldness appeal to the vanity and desperation of women who have had the misfortune to sustain hair loss, but there are no patent remedies that can be used with both safety and assurance. If you need help in this area, absolutely avoid the appeals of the home medicines and drugstore medications and "miracle" drugs. Save time, money, and what hair you still have by seeing a qualified physician, preferably a dermatologist. Determine first of all what is causing your condition and receive candid advice about what can be done. I am going to discuss the only two possible remedies for follicle loss that I feel are both safe and have a high rate of success.

HAIR WEAVING

Advanced methods of weaving human hair onto our own existing hairs with tiny nylon threads produce a cosmetic effect of a full head of hair that is very difficult to detect as artificial. This process may involve the attaching of individual hairs onto one's own or the attachment of groups of hairs (similar in fashion to wiglets and hairpieces). When done by a fully trained professional, no tension is created, so the wearer need not fear her own hair will be unduly strained. The anchorage of the woven hair is permanent but must be tightened from time to time as one's hair grows, since this obviously loosens the attached hair which is moved gradually farther and farther away from the scalp. The best styles for a hair-weave patient are those in which the hair is kept relatively short and curled. This is simple to care for and little adaptation has to be made in the care of the new hair, which you simply treat as you would your own hair.

The major drawback in the hair-weave process for Black women is that the human hair used is Caucasian or Oriental in origin and has to be treated first to match the texture of our hair. There are facilities in some major cities for this kind of treatment and before making the decision to undergo this process with a particular specialist, ask to examine (firsthand, not just by photographs) hair weaves that have been performed on other Black women. Make sure the nature of the new hair is to your liking and matches your own or can be made to match your own. If after a hair weave you experience any discomfort or pain, have it removed and consult a doctor. A good hair weave can produce very satisfying results but it is a delicate process that requires highly skilled, fully licensed and experienced technicians. Make sure whoever performs this on your hair has these qualifications.

Hair Transplantation

It has been over twenty years since the first successful hair transplant was performed and nowadays it is a common and safe method of hair replacement that is advised for most forms of female and male baldness. The clinical term for this procedure is punch autografting. Plugs of skin containing intact healthy hair follicles are removed from areas of the scalp where the hair is abundant and implanted into the bald areas. After about three months, new hair should grow from these follicles. Local anaesthesia is administered during this process. Only a few plugs are implanted at a time and many visits to the doctor are required over a period of months or years before hair transplantation can be completed. Leading specialists recommend that no more than twenty-five grafts per session be implanted in Black women. There are a number of reasons why we have to be less casual than others about receiving hair transplants and we should make sure that the doctor who performs this treatment is aware that:

a) Before any implanting is undertaken, a sample graft should be performed in an inconspicuous area and observed over a three-month period to determine the likelihood of keloids, hypertrophic scars, hyperpigmentation, and hypopigmentation.

b) Preoperative procedure must include a complete blood-cell count and thyroid-function tests. A woman contemplating this treatment must not be misled with the dream of a complete transformation from partial baldness to a rich, luxurious growth of hair. There are limitations to what can be accomplished and you must urge your doctor to be candid about your particular case as well as tell you exactly how long he or she expects the course to take and what side effects to expect.

As Black women, we do have some advantages when tackling this treatment. Those of us with coiled black hairs that have repeated overlappings are likely to need relatively fewer implants for scalp coverage than a woman with fine, straight hair. Also, because our scalp color corresponds closely to that of our hair, any new hair coverage will be more cosmetically acceptable than, for instance, a dark-haired Caucasian woman whose pink scalp contrasts strongly with her hair. Inexperienced and unqualified operators abound in this field, as in that of cosmetic surgery, and the Black community is particularly vulnerable to their unscrupulous methods of advertising and practice. Your doctor must have up-to-date qualifications and be willing to let you see and speak to former patients.

J. WIGS

Far from considering wigs a cosmetic option, the ancient Egyptians intentionally kept their hair closely cropped to facilitate the wearing of wigs, which they believed to be an essential item of attire. The poor wore wigs of wool and the rich wore wigs of human hair. They refined the task of hairdressing to a fine art, but it was practiced almost exclusively upon wigs, not growing hair. Few contemporary wigmakers can match the skill of the Egyptians. Most Western women today do not consider a wig to be a vital necessity, but for many of us Black women it is a most important part of our wardrobe because, if we wish to vary our hairstyles, constant processing is not only very costly but potentially damaging to the hair shaft and follicle. The woman who owns a selection of well-made wigs not only can save the expense of frequent visits to the beauty salon, but she can also suit her hair to her mood or activity quickly and simply. There are two distinctly different types of wigs available to the Black woman:

a) *Human-hair wigs* made from Caucasian or Oriental hair are not only expensive but have to be treated before they can come near to matching our own hair in texture, weight, and color. A few manufacturers do create human-hair wigs for the Black woman, but most that are on the market are oriented toward a strictly Caucasian buyer.

b) *Synthetic wigs* made from modified acrylic fiber can be suited and styled to match our hair, as I have demonstrated with the Naomi Sims Collection. Synthetic fiber wigs, if correctly constructed, should not lose their shape, are washable, and are relatively unaffected by extremes of weather.

The Naomi Sims Collection

For a number of years, as a model I found it impossible to buy a wig product of human hair or synthetic fiber that came near to matching the texture of my hair, which is fairly typical of most Black women's hair. It has a strong wave pattern and is coarser in texture but more porous in structure than Caucasian hair. A number of wig products were vying for the Black consumer simply by offering thin, glossy fibers (quite unlike our hair) in a variety of dark colors. Even they did not nearly cover the full range of our hair colors and certainly did not include the many nuances of color (brown and red highlights, for instance) that are naturally found in the hair of many of us. Unsatisfied, therefore, with the state of the industry, I went to work with a research chemist and, with the help of a wig manufacturer, created a new fiber which I named Kanekalon Presselle®. This fiber does match our hair and it can be washed and styled as easily as any other wig product. The fiber is so manageable and versatile that I can design a complete collection of wigs and hairpieces twice a year. I feel that it is very important that not only should the Black woman be able to buy the very latest styles in her own wig fiber, but also that the classic styles be constantly refined and polished. This is what I try to do with the Naomi Sims Collection. I found a way to construct my wigs so that they are very light in weight and I solved the "artificial hairline" problem by designing a revolutionary new wig cap (I call it the High-Brow Cap) only for Black women. This radical new structure creates a vastly improved and artfully natural hairline for the brow and temples and sides of the head. My wigs are precision-crafted with just enough body to create an elegant, smooth silhouette. Most wigmakers make the mistake of weaving hair in quantity rather than quality and the effect is a totally unnatural bushiness. Of course, I am extremely partisan about my product, but if you are shopping for a wig, you must bear in mind the qualities that I claim for mine. If you find those qualities in another manufacturer's product, by all means buy it if you prefer. The important thing in this area, as in many others, is that the female Black consumer demand a product furnished and crafted especially for her by a company or individual related to the Black experience and not simply be satisfied with a beauty product hastily adapted from a Caucasian prototype.

How to Choose a Wig

Texture

Both the sheen as it appears to your eyes and the feel as it relates to your touch should closely match that of your own hair.

Color

Before departing from a color close to that of your own hair, consider the color of your eyes, your eyebrows, and your eyelashes. Sharp contrasts, especially with our complexions, simply look incongruous.

Style

Do not imagine that you have to settle for exactly the style that is set into the wig. Remember that most wigs should be cut professionally to suit your face. Do not do this yourself, but take it to your hairdresser and have it shaped. Once this is done it is permanent and uniquely suited to you. In some stores there is a stylist in residence who will do this for you as you buy the wig. Many require thinning and shaping.

FIT

Last but by no means least, consider how your choice fits your scalp. It must be comfortable or it will give you more grief than joy. Most wig caps are adjustable to small, medium, or large heads, and I would urge you to look for those caps in which the hairs are mounted on elasticized strips or ribbons rather than solid panels. The strips not only provide a closer fit and allow the air to circulate better through the scalp, but they also let you pull your own hair through to achieve a natural mix. These new caps let you scratch your head, for instance, and you do not feel as if you are wearing a skin-tight, hot, and heavy hat.

How to Flatten Your Hair

It is essential, before you place the wig on your head, that your own hair interfere with it as little as possible.

Short and curly hair can be settled by simply putting it up in a series of flat, bobby-pin curls.

Medium to long hair should be parted down the back. The two sides should be wrapped one over the other and the sides then secured with pins.

Very long hair must be secured with a tight French twist. A bun or a pony-tail will only produce a lump in the wig line.

Ideally, it is best to have one's hair straightened, but in any event, it is essential to wear a nylon wig cap (scalp stocking). This must not be too tight, just firm enough to keep your hair in place. This cap not only helps keep the hair flat but prevents friction and splitting and breakage of individual hairs.

How to Wear a Wig

1) First shake out and brush well.
2) Secure your own hair with a nylon cap.
3) The wig should be put on from front to back, like a bathing cap.
4) Align the front with your own browline or slightly behind. Never let the front of the wig overlap your natural hairline; this looks absurdly artificial.
5) Pull the wig down on both sides and wiggle it to assume a straight position. The ear tabs should fit snugly over your ears and should be adjustable.
6) Secure the wig with hairpins: one in front, one top center, and one in

back. The sides can also be secured with fine pins, or you may wish to make a "gripper" (a crossbar of two rubber-tipped bobby pins) to hold the ear tabs at the side to your own hair and the nylon cap.

The one most difficult attribute to obtain with any style is a natural hairline. You have only two alternatives—to use your hairline or the wig's.

Own Hairline

Only try this if your hair is the same texture and general style as the wig. Pull the stocking cap back so as to leave a small margin of your own front hairline protruding (no more than ¼ inch). Now align the wig with the stocking cap and blend your own hair back into the wig.

Wig Hairline

If you place the wig directly over your hairline (but never in front of it), you will notice that the wig hair at your brow is thick and flat. This is what looks so very artificial. Tease the front with your fingers and give it some body or, with the wig firmly anchored, brush all the hair back, then, with the flat palms of the hands, push gently forward from the crown of the wig to make a wave or dip toward the hairline. Repeat at the sides. Only use rubber or plastic brushes; natural bristle or metal or wire will split the fiber. If after playing with it like this, the hairline still looks false, try another wig! One alternative is to choose a style with the brow cut in bangs. If you style your wig with a part and the gap is of a color at odds with that of your scalp, then blend your make-up foundation and with a cotton swab apply it smoothly to the visible portion of your wig cap.

How to Care for Your Wigs

Human-Hair Wigs

These are quite fragile and cannot take any severe punishment. Always keep on wig stands when not in use and they must be kept wrapped tightly to retain any curl. Only attempt to clean and restyle by taking to a professional hairdresser. Human-hair products do not react favorably in adverse weather, and bleached, dyed, or streaked wigs must be kept covered if exposed to the sun for long periods. If not, oxidization and color-change may occur.

SYNTHETIC WIGS

Most brand-name synthetic-wig products can be washed quickly and easily and as often as needed. Follow the manufacturer's instructions, or:

1) Brush out your wig thoroughly.
2) Soak it for two minutes in a solution of mild shampoo and warm water.
3) Squeeze gently. (Do not wring or twist.)
4) Rinse well in cold water.
5) Turn the wig inside out and place on a towel until dry. If wig is not turned inside out, the weight of the moisture tends to pull out the curl.
6) Place dry wig on a stand and brush into the desired style.

If you experience frizzing or loosening curls with your synthetic wig, try the following:
Lightly apply an oil-based hair spray to the entire wig and brush thoroughly. Follow steps 2 through 5 above. After one hour on the towel, set your wig in rollers while applying hair spray to each section. In twenty-four hours the wig will be restyled and ready to wear.

SYNTHETIC WIG DO'S AND DON'T'S

DON'T   Brush wig while wet
            Style or dry with extremely hot equipment
            Wash in washing machine
            Try to dye or bleach
            Comb with Afro picks; this may tear the wig cap
            Store on wig stand wet *or* dry; this stretches the wig
            Wash in hot water
            Wash in harsh detergents; use only a mild shampoo
               or special wig shampoo
            Dry without first squeezing; the weight of the water will pull out
               the shape.
DO   Aways roll with end papers
            Use oil-based hair spray
            Store in a cool, dry place with tissue both inside and around
               the wig.

How to Care for Your Own Hair While Wearing a Wig

Your hair, especially if it has been mistreated or is otherwise damaged, can benefit enormously from wearing a wig if it is regularly washed and cared for. Since hair does not breathe, as long as your wig is well fitted and is not worn day and night, the hair does not suffer from being enclosed. In fact, this is an excellent opportunity for the hair to rest from the elements and recuperate in a protected environment. Do not believe, please, that prolonged wig-wearing causes baldness. Whatever way your hair is worn or processed, it must be shampooed weekly while you wear a wig and braids must be undone nightly.

Because today's synthetic wigs are simple to wear and easy to care for should not suggest that they can be worn with impunity twenty-four hours a day every day of the year. In addition to a weekly washing, your own hair must be conditioned and groomed frequently. Always wear a nylon cap to prevent the inside of the wig cap from abrading your hair, and avoid the use of dirty or broken hairpins or fastening measures that are too tight. A well-made, appropriately styled, properly fitted synthetic wig can enhance the appearance, cut down on hairdressing bills, and protect the hair and scalp.

Hairpieces

A hairpiece is any synthetic or human-hair addition to one's own hair that does not entirely cover the scalp or constitute a full wig. This category includes wiglets, cascades, falls, ponytails, braids, and curls. They can be used to give the hair the appearance of greater length or fullness or adapt it to a style more elaborate than the existing hair. In addition to wigs, which I wear extensively (exclusively the Naomi Sims Collection, of course!), I also make wide and varied use of hairpieces. Because a hairpiece is seen in conjunction with one's real hair, it is of vital importance that the texture and the color be compatible. There are few sights more distressing than that of a fine Black woman, whose own strong hair is of a specific wave pattern and texture, wearing a hairpiece of Caucasian design that looks like a strap of patent leather. When matching a hairpiece to your own hair, try to do so in daylight. The artificial store light tends to flatten out colors and textures and minimize differences that on the street are uncomfortably obvious. Always examine your hairpiece with a front mirror and a hand mirror to see all around the rear of your head to make sure that it sits quite naturally on your head and blends well to the back as well as the front. Always keep your hairpieces fresh and clean. (Refer to my instructions for wig care.) The danger in attempting to anchor them too tightly with pins and small combs is that one's real hair is drawn out.

To Attach Hairpieces

Most are made with comb attachments for easy insertion. If the comb is made of metal, or is too short, I suggest that you replace it with a soft plastic comb with teeth long enough to anchor the hairpiece into your hair. Your own hair should not be too straight or greasy, especially at the root, for easy anchorage. The kinkier our hair is near the root, the easier it will be to attach a hairpiece.

1) Part your hair where you intend to place the hairpiece with enough "spare" to overlap the base.

2) Make a pincurl at this point and secure it with crossed bobby pins (rubber-tipped). This is your anchor.

3) Slip the teeth of the hairpiece comb under the pincurl and attach curl, "gripper," and comb with a large bobby pin.

4) Comb and style your real hair over and around the hairpiece.

Types of Hairpieces

Wiglets are usually machine-made, have a flat base about four inches in diameter and a fiber length of ten to twelve inches. They can add height to the crown and depth to the hairstyle, and the advantages of wiglets are that they can be lightly teased with hair spray into any number of shapes. They are light and easy to handle.

Demiwigs have a fiber length of six to eight inches and a fairly large base contoured to fit the head.

Long falls usually have a dome or contour cap and a fiber length of up to twenty-six inches.

Wig falls have a five-inch contour cap and a fiber length of about sixteen inches.

Mini falls have a small comb or cap base and a fiber length of about ten inches. All falls can be worn close to the hairline or back on the crown of the head or even near the nape of the neck.

Cascades or *clusters* are permanently curled and can be worn on any part of the head. Normally they have comb attachments.

Braids are very versatile and can be unbraided to make a loose ponytail, bun, or chignon. They can also be made into several small braids and are easily secured with comb attachments.

All falls can be worn close to the hairline or back on the crown of the head or even near the nape of the neck. For a very natural-looking fall, turn the base upside down and attach it to the hair from the side opposite the comb; the hair lies normally and falls casually. If your hair is very short and you wish to wear a fall, first attach a hairpiece and use that as a base for the fall.

K. PROFESSIONAL HAIR CARE

There is a sad, familiar pattern to the life of a Black woman's hair. We are born with strong, healthy hair that, if treated gently, grows thick and long until we are about ten or eleven years of age. Within the next ten years, by the time we reach our mid-twenties most of us complain about thinning hair, dry or brittle hair, hair that is falling out, or hair that *just will not grow.* What happens in those crucial years to make our hair fail? Not enough research is being done to determine the exact causes, but I believe it may be partially due to a physiological maturation process on the one hand, compounded by harsh treatment on the other as a young girl starts to experiment with hairstyles and treatments. Often this transition from normal, healthy hair to hair that requires medical attention is so gradual and imperceptible that we are carelessly continuing damaging treatments up until the hair is ruined. Black women must never forget that our hair is more fragile in grade and texture than any other kind and must be treated very kindly.

Because amateur, at-home hair care causes more damage than any other kind of treatment, I counsel every woman to avoid doing anything at home other than grooming, washing, and conditioning. There are two types of professional qualified to touch your hair:

The Dermatologist

At the first sign of severely damaged or diseased hair, you must consult a medical doctor or dermatologist, who is a physician with a special interest in skin and hair. Do not let anyone who does not have a medical degree and license treat damaged hair. In the past few years, all women and Black women especially have been exposed to the advertising of self-appointed "trichonologists" who claim expertise in the science of hair. One need pass no exams nor carry any license in order to call oneself a "trichonologist," and we should be wary of these and any other similar-sounding "hair experts." If you are in doubt as to a particular person's credentials, you can always call a local medical institution (college or hospital) and inquire as to whether that particular title requires a medical degree. If not, steer clear. If such an "expert" damages your hair, you have absolutely no recourse, no professional body to complain to.

The Hairdresser

A competent, conscientious hairdresser can sustain and perhaps increase the health of the hair but should not attempt to "cure" damaged hair—that is a job for a physician. While researching this chapter, I found a very disturbing complaint common to almost all the Black women that I interviewed. They were adamantly opposed to the general level of care and competence found in Black hairdressing salons and always compared them unfavorably with "White" salons, not only in the area of competency but also politeness. My own experiences in some instances confirm this opinion, although sprinkled across the country are Black hairdressers whose talents and professionality outrank any others I have met. These are women and men who care for their profession, travel across the globe for new ideas, and take genuine pride in the importance of what they do. Too often, however, they serve to exemplify just how bad the run-of-the-mill Black hairdresser is, who cares little for the health of the customer's hair, treats her with no dignity, and has little time for the amenities of life. Some of us are to blame, of course, as customers. We encourage a lack of consideration and court accidents by not making proper appointments, arriving late, and rushing the operator. If we act as professional customers, we will, perforce, create professional operators.

To Choose and Work with a Hairdresser

1) Do not assume that the whole fate of your hair is in your hairdresser's hands and that you have no responsibility for it. An operator can aid and guide you in creating and keeping healthy, good-looking hair, but an operator cannot constantly correct your errors or make up for your ignorance. The more you know about Black women's hair and your own hair in particular, the easier it will be for you and your hairdresser.

2) Go to a hairdresser recommended by someone who has used them satisfactorily over a fairly long period of time.

3) On the first visit, the operator should ask you about any unusual conditions you have or have had that might affect your hair. Mention allergies or previous damaging treatments, if any.

4) You, in turn, should volunteer everything you know about your hair, its texture, the relative dryness of your hair or scalp, and how often you wash and condition it.

5) Before the hairdresser begins, ask exactly what is going to be done to your hair. Something is wrong if the operator prevaricates. There are no "hair secrets" that the customer must not know.

6) Be aware of how the hairdresser shampoos. If the scalp is not vigorously massaged, if the hair is rinsed poorly, if the hairline and the nape of the neck are ignored or only given cursory attention, then your operator may be just as careless about other things—such as a chemical treatment—that could permanently damage your hair.

7) Women who shop around and change their hairdresser often, and in between rely on themselves or a relative to give treatments, run the grave risk of not noticing the encroachment of a serious problem. If you find a pleasant, competent operator, stick with him or her; be faithful. This will encourage the whole trade.

8) Remember that a typical operator works a long, hard day and often does not have time to keep up with new ideas, problems, or products. Do not be afraid to discuss what you have read here or elsewhere. Knowledge shared in this way can only help your hair.

ONE WARNING: Do not attempt to self-diagnose a serious problem of your hair and scalp. What may suggest to you one treatment (i.e., frequent washing) may, in fact, require an abstinence from any wetness. In the long run it is cheaper to see a dermatologist and have you hair and scalp professionally diagnosed and treated. Although the dermatologist will charge a consultation fee, the treatment and medication may be less expensive than your endless trips to the beauty parlor and drugstore in an attempt to restore your problem hair.

L. EMERGENCY TREATMENT

The hair is very inflammable and our hair, containing as it does many tiny air pockets, may be even more inflammable than other types. If your hair catches fire, do not try to find water if this will mean giving the hair a longer time to burn. Without oxygen the hair cannot burn, so smother the head with a towel, blanket, or article of clothing and keep it tight around the scalp. Then drench with water.

Chapter IV

OUR HANDS AND NAILS

━━━━━◆━━━━━

The Hand

With the face, the hands are the most constantly exposed part of our body. They are always at work and in motion, subject to not only the elements of weather but the many harsh chemicals found in the products we handle daily. Our hands have less fatty tissue than is normally found elsewhere on the body, and the palms of the hands, like the soles of the feet, contain absolutely no oil glands. (These are linked with hair growth; thus, no hair on the palms of the hands.) Our palms do contain sweat glands, however, and perspiration is one of the most common problems of the hands, together with rashes and callouses. Historically, smooth, beautiful hands have always been considered desirable and as Black women we know that for the same reasons that our faces tend to age benignly, so do our hands—although, of course, our often strenuous and laborious activities may contribute to premature aging of the hands if they are not properly cared for.

CARE OF THE HANDS

In sixteenth-century England, women of means purchased from their perfumers gloves made of chicken skin which they would fill with cream, almond paste, ox gall, and egg yolk and wear while they slept in an attempt to preserve the beauty of their hands. Our hands withstand wrinkling better than those of Caucasian women, but because the hands contain a limited number of oil-secreting glands and are frequently in and out of water, all women alike should take precautions against rashes and scaling which are not only unsightly but most unhealthy.

For basic hand care I eschew all preparations supposedly created just for the hands, especially those that purport to contain secret ingredients. Your regular moisturizing cream or lotion functions as well, if not better, than all the expensive products put together. Keep a supply of moisturizer at home and at work and always with you when traveling. Apply it liberally and frequently, especially after the hands have been exposed to water and soaps, both of which dry out the skin.

In cold weather and when working with the hands at such chores as washing dishes or gardening, you must wear gloves. When working, unlined rubber gloves are worse than useless since they encourage perspiration, soften the nails, and may irritate the skin. Always wear plastic or cotton gloves that are lined. Too often unlined gloves will stick to the hands and pull at the nails when being removed.

A callous is a natural barrier of skin developed to protect underlying tissue in an area that receives continuous pressure or friction. When I used to model, I would have tiny callouses on my palms from carrying my heavy make-up bags; now I have a callous on my second finger from the pressure of my pen while writing. These are healthy callouses and are no cause for alarm. I have three suggestions for their removal, which will also keep your hands fresh and supple:

1) Each day while bathing, rub calloused skin gently with a wet pumice stone.

2) Once a week, apply a gentle abrasive formula before bathing while the hands are dry. Pretty Feet is the only such abrasive that I recommend wholeheartedly since although it is manufactured primarily for the feet, it contains no alcohol and is not gritty or greasy and is gentle enough for the hands.

3) Once a month I mix the following concoction:

2½ tablespoons of table sugar

1 teaspoon of honey

juice and pulp of one whole lemon.

This forms a thick paste which I massage into every part of the hands from fingertips to the wrist using a wringing motion of the thumb and forefinger. I rub the palms together vigorously and leave the paste on for five minutes. Then I rinse off and apply a facial mask to my hands for temporary smoothness and rinse that off with cool water. Salt may be substituted for the sugar; it is only the abrasive action that is required.

Prominent veins plague many women who feel that they are a sign of aging hands. When I began modeling at the age of seventeen, my hands were so heavily veined that I kept my arms raised before posing in the hopes of making the veins less noticeable. Although I am now older, the veins on my hands are hardly visible. If you are particularly concerned about bulging veins in your hands, it does help temporarily to hold your arms up over the head for three minutes, then rinse in cold water and apply a facial mask.

If your hands perspire inordinately, you should see a physician since it may be an indication of an ailment not localized in the hands themselves. As a temporary measure, mix a weak solution of aluminum chloride and water and apply to the palms with a cotton pad.

Fingernails

The nails are simply specialized parts of the skin and are made of the same elements as skin. Like hair, nails do not "breathe" or have an active existence other than growth at root level. Blood is supplied by the body to the cells that form the nails but not to the nails themselves. They are composed primarily of keratin and protein as well as small quantities of calcium and phosphorous. Nails enable us to use our fingers more efficiently and they protect the fingerbone and increase touch sensitivity in the fingertips. They are not purposeless ornaments. Often the visible change in the condition of the nails will indicate change in the body metabolism as a whole such as disease, infection, or nutritional deficiency. Any condition that can harm or help the skin will have the same negative or beneficial effect upon the nails.

STRUCTURE OF THE NAIL

The nail itself is a hard shiny plate originating in the nail *matrix* and ending usually with a whitish edge at the outer limits of the finger. The matrix is

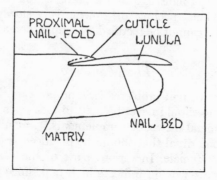

located at the base of the nail and is the site of nail growth. If the matrix is damaged, the nail growth will be distorted. That part of the matrix that is visible is called the *lunula*, a light, crescent shape at the base of the nail. The lunula is not obviously visible in all the nails to the same extent. A myth still believed by some doctors is that Black women and men have visible lunula only on the thumbnails. Like many other such theories, this is based not on fact but fiction. The nail rests on the nail bed, an area of soft tissue that contains the blood cells that nourish the matrix. At the base of the nail, the *cuticle* screens out dirt and germs and protects the growing nail. It is an opaque fold of skin.

RATE OF NAIL GROWTH

Not our race, but our health and occupation can affect nail growth. Generally speaking, growth is fastest up until the age of twenty-five, then gradually declines to half-speed in later years. At the same time, the nails may become thicker and the growth haphazard. Growth is directly related to exercise and activity, and thus the right-hand nails of right-handed women grow faster than the left, and typists and pianists experience a faster rate of nail growth than normal. Pregnancy can increase rate of growth and illness can retard nail growth. Nails grow faster in summer than in winter; a completely new nail may take from three to five months.

DIET AND THE FINGERNAILS

There is no conclusive evidence that the ingestion of gelatin, calcium, vitamin supplements, seaweed, or any such commercial preparation can nourish and harden the nails. A healthy nail will grow $\frac{1}{32}$ of an inch each week. Nails do require an adequate intake of the nutrient keratin for growth, but the intake of excessive amounts of such nutrients will not influence rate of growth or strength of nails. If you are eating a well-balanced diet and still experience nails cracking, peeling, or growing very slowly, the reason is not dietary deficiency and cannot be rectified by simple food additives.

The Manicure

The primary cause of nail problems is improper care. Nails are sturdy but they are not tools and should never be used to pick open containers or otherwise substitute for metal or wooden implements. A manicure is no more and no less than a hygiene ritual that should be practiced regularly by all individuals, male as well as female. In various parts of the world today, as in the past, lengthy nails on a woman indicate high rank since it is not possible for her to engage in any work. We still cannot alter the fact that the length of our nails must be determined by our occupation. Those of us who can afford lives of utter leisure and who never have to cook, clean, or work in an office or factory may be able to cultivate very long nails, but for most of us they are a positive drawback if they are too long and I believe that well-cared-for nails of moderate length are just as pleasing as painted talons.

When practicing nail care you must remember that the less cutting that is done the better. Most doctors agree that the cuticle should never be cut, only soaked in warm oil and gently trained back with a hindstone or an orange stick tipped with damp cotton. Only use an emery board to file the nails, not a metal file. The nail is layered like an onion and your filing motion must be in one direction only or the results will be ragged and uneven. If you seesaw back and forth when filing, you simply open up extra layers that will be able to peel more easily. Because the sides of the nail support the center, it is not healthy to file away too much of the sides and make the nails very narrow; this weakens the whole structure. Keep them fairly straight across, either slightly rounded or squared. If you have a problem nail that is split or peeling, always cut it square across to help it grow back quickly and strongly. The nails should never be pointed; not only does this make of them a dangerous weapon (most likely the victim will be yourself), but it severely weakens the structure and growth pattern of the nails.

My instructions for home manicure follow. This should be done twice per month and it is well worth your while to find the time to learn how to do it properly. If your nails are well cared for, strong and shapely, you will avoid many inconveniences that add up to a lot of lost time.

TOOLS

> Emery boards
> Moisturizing cream or lotion
> Warm (not hot) oil such as vegetable oil, castor oil, or baby oil
> Hindstone
> Orange sticks
> Petroleum jelly
> Pumice stone
> Soft child's toothbrush
> Nail whitener (pencil or cream)
> Nail buffer
> Nail buffer cream
> Oily nail polish remover
> Nail base
> Nail polish (clear or colored)
> Top coat or sealer

STEPS

a) Prepare a solution of warm cream or oil for soaking. Three quarters of a cup is enough; heat but do not boil.

b) With cotton pads and oily nail polish remover, taker off all old polish.

c) Do not scrub or soak nails before filing.

d) Shape each nail with an emery board by stroking from the side to the center. Start underneath the nail and remember not to saw back and forth.

e) Apply petroleum jelly to all the cuticles.

f) Pat moisturizing lotion on the nails, hands, and arms to the elbows.

g) Soak just the fingertips of each hand in the warm cream or oil solution for five minutes.

h) With the soft toothbrush, gently remove debris from beneath the nails. Do not scrub nail tops or cuticles.

i) Massage the nails, hands, and arms while rinsing under warm running water.

j) Dry hands thoroughly.

k) First with fingertips and towel and then with blunt end of hindstone or orange stick, train back the cuticle.

l) Remove all traces of oil and dry hands again.

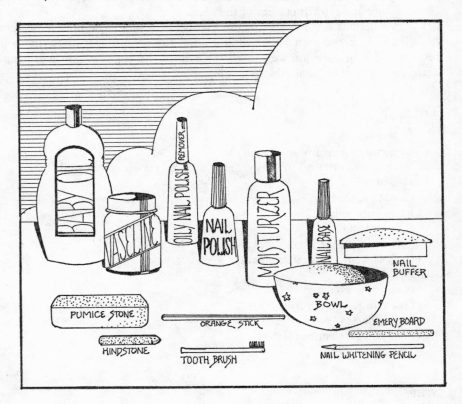

To Apply Nail Polish

Wait at least five minutes after the preceding instructions. When brushing on base, polish, or sealer, do it in three strokes for each nail, each stroke from the base to the nail end. The first stroke should always be down the center of the nail and then two successive strokes on either side of the first one.

a) Apply base. Let dry for five minutes and apply again.

b) Roll nail polish bottle in the palm of your hands (do not shake it). Open and gently dip the brush in and out in one movement, enough to gather sufficient polish to complete the three strokes on each nail. Let dry for ten minutes.

c) Repeat application of polish for second coat on each nail. Dry for ten minutes.

d) If your nails are well ridged, you may need a third coat of polish. Be patient and let each coat dry for the full amount of time.

e) Apply final coat of sealer in the same manner as the base and polish and let dry for thirty minutes.

Do's

Apply base, polish, and sealer beneath the nail as well as on top.

Use an orange stick with a moistened cotton tip to remove excess polish from the sides of the nails and the cuticles.

After manicure, buff the nails in one direction with nail buffer and cream. Soft chamois or cheesecloth is just as effective as a special buffer and this helps circulation and prevents cracking. Make the white tip of the nail appear longer and thicker with cream or pencil whitener. Use sparingly and do not press hard on the pencil. Buffing and whitening in this manner are alternatives to the application of polish; do not try to do both. Buff gently and stop as soon as the nails or fingertips feel warm. Cream whiteners are safer than pencil whiteners and are now widely available.

Remove particles from beneath nails by first running them over a soft damp cake of soap to collect soap shreds under the nails, then soaking in warm water and brushing with child's toothbrush. Never dig with an implement.

Don't's

Never remove polish by hand. Scratching in this manner will remove layers of the nail plate itself.

Never use nail polish remover more than once a week. It contains acetone-derived chemicals that can remove the cementing ingredients of the nail plate. Touch up the polish between manicures rather than frequently removing polish with chemicals.

Avoid nail hardeners. These often contain formaldehyde and formalin and can cause severe allergic reactions. Bleeding and discoloration can result. For the same reason, all preformed artificial nails are to be used with caution since many women, including myself, have experienced uncomfortable reactions to the glues used in these products. If false nails are worn for more than a couple of days at a time, moisture can collect under the false nail and soften the real nail.

Never remove cuticles with scissors.

Avoid "cuticle-removing" creams. These contain harsh, abrasive chemicals that will dry out the cuticle and the nail.

Never soak hands in warm soapy water before a manicure—this will dry and soften the nails and make them very hard to shape.

Avoid nail polish sprays; they run and "bubble," do not dry any faster than brush polish, and are much more difficult to control.

Never use stiff nail brushes, only very soft-bristle products such as children's toothbrushes, and only use beneath the nails—never on top of the nail or the cuticle.

AFTER MANICURE AND POLISH

You may have as many as five layers of polish, base, and sealer on your nails that will take twenty-four hours to dry effectively enough to protect the nails and last two or three weeks. During that drying period you should avoid immersing the nails in water of any kind, even with gloves on. This includes no baths and showers and shampoo and dishwater for at least twelve hours after the final application. At this time you should also avoid routine activities involving the nails. Dial the telephone with a pencil, not your finger, for example. Use the balls of the fingers for picking up objects, not the tips. Be very careful when putting on or removing pantyhose and girdles and manipulate light switches with the knuckles. You will keep your manicure and polish longer if you massage moisturizer around each nail and cuticle at nighttime after bathing and ease back the cuticle with a soft towel (not your fingernails). Apply one coat of sealer every two days on top and underneath the nails to keep them glossy and reduce the possibility of chipping.

If you experience an allergic reaction to a nail polish, it may not be the color but the ingredient of the polish itself rather than the dye. Change brands, and if it persists, see a doctor. Any stains on the fingers from smoking or household chemicals should be quickly removed with lemon juice.

"NATURAL LOOK" NAILS

After manicuring the nails, dry well and buff lightly (always buff in one direction only) with buffing paste or moisturizer. Gently whiten nail with pencil or cream whitener, then apply coat of clear nail polish.

NAIL PATCHING

A "nail patch kit" is inexpensive and available in most drugstores. This method is excellent for treating nails that are chipped or peeling and will last for up to five days. You are provided with thick clear polish, tissues, and a small stick. The polish should be applied to the nail in minute quantities and to the tissue. With the help of the stick, place the tissue around and over the nail with ⅛ inch extending beyond the nail; wrap this around the end of the nail. Smooth the tissue on the nail with the stick and trim so that it neatly matches the nail. Polish, clear or colored, can now be applied over the patch. Nails do not have to be long for this treatment to be effective.

PRESERVING THE NAILS

If you are going to be engaged in a sport or activity that will require constant tapping of the fingers, wrap masking tape or adhesive tape around the fingertips to protect the nails from breaking.

Nail Injuries and Diseases

Hangnail is a very common problem and consists of a ragged, often triangular flap of skin at the nail base. If allowed to remain, it can catch and rip deeper into the matrix. Unless the area is inflamed (in which case a physician should be seen), simply cut the skin swiftly and cleanly with a very clean pair of small scissors.

Onycholysis is the separation of the nail plate from the finger and this is a gradual process (unless due to sudden injury) that may be caused by disease or infection from false fingernails or nail-hardening products. The undernail may discolor to yellow, then black, and finally green. If you notice this change, consult a doctor. This condition can be remedied.

Paronychia can be caused by nail biting, splinters, or bacterial infection, and consists of a painful swelling of the soft tissue surrounding the nail. Treatment is simple but requires professional attention.

Following pregnancy, a woman may experience a very temporary drop in the quality of her nails. They may be brittle and chip easily. This is caused by hormonal change and quickly reverses itself.

Nail biting itself is not a disease but it can be caused by emotional imbalance. Manicurists claim that it is one of the most common problems they encounter. In addition to the removal of nail plate by chewing, other undesirable conditions can result from acids in the saliva retarding new nail growth and causing bacterial infection. My advice is that no matter how miserably small and bitten your nails are, it is never too late to begin a nail-care regimen. Follow my instructions in this chapter even if you have only very short nails. Apply nail polish and manicure frequently. You must get into the habit of regarding your nails as necessary and not expendable. Spend a lot of time on your nails, no matter how bad they are, and this alone will deter you from destroying that work by biting. Accustom yourself to holding, relaxing, and showing your hands in attractive positions—not clenched or palms upward to avoid showing the nails. If you can keep your nails unchipped and unbitten for just a few days, you will develop a firm pride in the appearance of your hands that you should be loath to destroy.

Professional Hand and Nail Care

MEDICAL

Like the hair and the skin, the nails mirror the internal condition of the body, and before a physical checkup you should note the condition of your nails and remove all preparations and polish so that the doctor can examine them. Mention any recent discoloration, ridging, brittleness, or pain in the nails. The specialist that deals with problems of the nails is the same person that treats the skin—a dermatologist.

COSMETIC

Manicurists are trained to clean and beautify the nails. They should do no more than I have outlined under home manicure and definitely should not be permitted to cut the cuticles. Pay attention to what the manicurist is doing to your nails and ask her to avoid the use of metal implements.

Emergency Treatment

Injuries to the nails are most frequently caused by forceful blows such as that of a hammer or car door. The area beneath the nail will bleed and the pressure of the bleeding causes acute pain. If the blow is not severe, the blood will coagulate and quickly stop, and the black marks on the nail will grow out in a few weeks. If the pain is severe, a doctor should be seen. In either case: Apply cold compresses immediately to the injured finger, and elevate the hand to reduce the accumulation of blood near the nail.

Chapter V

OUR FEET AND LEGS

A. STRUCTURE

Each of our feet contains twenty-six delicate, small bones held in place by 112 ligaments and activated by twenty muscles. Twenty-five per cent of all the bones in the body are in the feet. Like the hands, the feet have less fatty tissue than is normally found elsewhere on the body and there are no oil

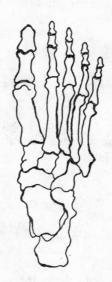

glands on the soles of the foot. It is impossible to manipulate the foot without using the muscles of the lower leg. Standing, walking, running, jumping, and dancing are all made possible by the harmonious interplay between the conjoined bones and muscles of both the feet and the legs. The feet cannot function independently of the calves.

There is absolutely no difference in the anatomy, average shape, or average size of Black women's feet and the American norm. If we appear to have a greater number of foot problems than the white American woman, it is because of such environmental causes as poor health care, bad posture, and the constant wearing of improper shoes. A woman's feet are as unique to her as her fingerprints and no two pairs of feet are alike. Unfortunately, the foot is the most neglected part of the human body, although it is vital for our mobility. Until we experience a serious foot problem we tend to ignore our feet altogether or else occupy ourselves only with beautifying the most superficial aspects of them. Because of this neglect, most of us possess feet that are far from being healthy, attractive, and problem-free. Our feet were designed to support and carry the body on natural surfaces such as grass, sand, and earth. These are pliant and yielding and offer both a firm yet soft surface for the foot to stand, walk, and run upon. Most of our days are spent on surfaces that are far from natural. Our homes and work areas have floors of tile, hardwood, or concrete and the streets are unresilient and solid. Such surfaces are designed to carry great weights and to endure for many years; they are not designed to support our naked feet. It is unwise and unsafe to habitually walk barefoot on such surfaces. Hard, flat, smooth floors do not yield to the tread of the foot. Each step taken jars the feet and legs and then the spinal column. Even when the feet are shod correctly these surfaces subject the body to constant stress.

B. CARE OF THE FEET

Although the feet are capable of adapting to almost any function, we generally assume that they can continue to perform excellently without special care and attention. This is simply not so.

Washing the Feet

The feet should be washed daily with warm water, mild soap, and a washcloth. Do not neglect to thoroughly soap between the toes. After washing, dry thoroughly with a terry cloth towel, again concentrating upon the areas between the toes. Rub the entire surface of the feet and lower legs with moisturizing lotion or cream, paying special attention to the dry skin of your heels and toes. Let the moisturizer absorb naturally. If your feet perspire heavily, powder them lightly and occasionally shake a small amount of powder into your shoes. If you do not have a perspiration problem, avoid powdering the feet because this can dry them out excessively. Remember, too much powder in the shoes and on the feet will only make a mess.

Maintaining the Feet

Change your shoes and hose frequently and keep your shoes always in good repair. Hose should be fresh and clean every day. If your feet perspire, change your hose twice per day. Clip the toenails straight across with a standard toenail clipper; this will prevent ingrown toenails. Practice good posture and when walking or standing, hold the body erect with the weight distributed evenly on both feet.

Home Pedicure

Because we will wear fashionable shoes that are not good for our feet and we will not always observe the best foot-hygiene practices, it is necessary for us to devote extra time to the feet in the form of a pedicure every two or three weeks. This care and cleaning should be practiced whether or not you paint your toenails. You need the following items:

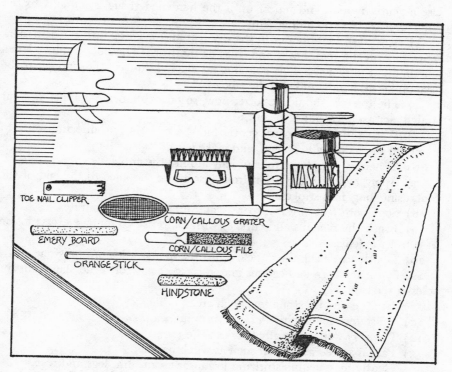

Toenail clippers
Emery board
Orange stick or hindstone
Moisturizing lotion (for very dry skin use petroleum jelly)
Corn and callous file
Corn and callous grater
Pumice stone
Soft-bristle nailbrush
Warm water
Mild soap
Terry cloth towel.

These are necessary if you want to apply make-up:

Oily nail polish remover
Nail polish "base" or "top coat" or "sealer"
Large cotton pads or large paper tissues
Extremely mild foot abraser.

Procedure

1) Make sure your feet are clean and very dry.

2) Draw corn and callous file across rough patches in one direction only. Use a gentle motion and repeat until the hardened tissue is reduced to the same level as the surrounding skin.

3) Apply the foot abraser to the dry feet and massage into the skin, concentrating on the toes, heels, and soles of the feet. (The only product I recommend is Pretty Feet. This contains no alcohol and is mild enough to be used on knees, hands, and also the elbows.)

4) The toenails should be softer now, so take the toenail clipper and cut straight across; never curve the cut.

5) With the emery board, gently file the nails in one direction only to round off the nails, reduce snags, and make even.

6) Generously apply petroleum jelly around the cuticles.

7) Apply moisturizing lotion from just above the knee to the end of the foot, using long, firm strokes.

8) Soak both feet in warm soapy water for at least ten minutes.

9) Brush the toenails and cuticles with nailbrush to remove excess lotion or petroleum jelly.

10) Gently ease back the cuticles with the orange stick or hindstone.

11) With the corn and callous grater, scrape away soft dead skin from the soles of the feet.

12) Use the pumice stone for rough areas.

13) Rinse feet thoroughly in clean, running water.

14) Dry very well, especially between the toes.

15) Pat on a mild astringent such as witch hazel.

16) Gently massage moisturizing lotion or cream into legs and feet.

To Apply and Remove Toenail Polish

REMOVAL

Always use oily remover, follow instructions carefully, and remove polish before pedicure.

APPLICATION

Wait five minutes after pedicure or foot bathing.

Separate toes with generous pads of cotton or paper tissue. Cotton balls are too small for this purpose.

Apply one coat of thin "base" polish. (This is sometimes called the "sealer" or "top coat.") Let this dry for ten minutes.

Apply one coat of nail polish (color). Wrap small piece of cotton around the end of an orange stick to remove excess polish from the cuticle.

If nail color is not strong enough with one coat it is because some of our dark nails require more than one coat, especially if the color used is light. Apply a second coat and wait another ten minutes to dry. Finally apply one more coat of "base" to seal the color and add a gloss. Let this dry a full ten minutes.

If you do not wait the required amount of time for drying, the result will be a sticky mess. After the varnish is completely dry, apply moisturizer to the feet and nails. Ensure that the nails are completely dry before wearing hose and shoes.

Foot-Care Warnings

Much damage is done to the feet by self-administered "bathroom surgery." If you have any problem that requires tools or attention more elaborate than that which I have mentioned, you must consult your doctor or a podiatrist.

NO   toenail *nippers*.

NO   metal nail files.

NO   scissors for cuticle cutting. (Cuticles should be trained, not cut.)

NO   chemical cuticle removers. The harsh ingredients can dry out cuticle and nail and severely irritate the foot.

NO   razors or corn and callous *trimmers*. Both can cause severe bleeding and infection.

NO   strong foot, corn, or callous abrasives or soaps. Many contain salicylic acid that can burn the skin and lead to infection.

NO   hard-bristle brushes.

NO   metal instruments for cuticle; they tear both nail and skin.

NO   strong deodorant sprays. If daily bathing does not deter odor, the problem requires a doctor.

NO   medication, oral or otherwise, that claims to stop feet from perspiring.

NO   commercial preparations in the form of plastic, liquid, cream, ointment, powder, or liniment to cure conditions that require medical attention. In most cases these will just aggravate the condition.

NO   unnecessary exposure of feet or legs to cold and damp.

NO   excessive use of hot-water bottles or electric blankets that can burn the skin and dehydrate the feet and cause circulatory problems.

C. THE FEET AND EXERCISE

The best possible exercise for the feet is walking correctly in shoes and hose that are properly fitted. When you walk, the toes must point forward and the heel should touch the ground just before the ball of the foot. As you complete this movement, roll the weight forward onto the toes. Your imaginary footprints should be placed on either side of a very thin, straight line. Comfortable shoes are essential for exercise that will benefit the feet. In this regard it is obvious that a flat or low heel is much better than a high heel. While sitting, do not keep your knees crossed for long periods of time. This will reduce circulation in the feet and lower legs. This will also occur if you wear garters or constrictive elastic hose.

One of the simplest foot-strengthening exercises is to walk or jog barefoot on a slightly yielding surface such as sand or turf. Any sport is beneficial for the feet if you wear appropriate shoes and hose. You can sprain, break, and severely damage the foot by attempting almost any exercise or sports event while wearing shoes designed only for street or evening wear.

Quick Daily Exercises for the Feet

1) For thirty seconds, firmly massage each foot manually, paying special attention to the toes.

2) Rotate each foot from the ankle in a clockwise manner (30 seconds) and then counterclockwise (30 seconds).

3) Stand flat on the floor and rise to the toes. Repeat ten times.

These three activities will strengthen the ankles and calves as well as the arches. They will help the legs and thighs also. Unless your doctor prescribes other exercises, avoid any that are more elaborate than I have described.

If after a very tiring day your feet are painful, soak them in warm water for ten to fifteen minutes. Rinse them in cool water and then apply a mild astringent. Lie on the floor or on the bed and elevate the feet on a pillow. This will return to the body the blood that has been concentrated in the legs and feet.

D. FOOTWEAR

Despite the fact that our technology is capable of providing us with inexpensive footwear designed to absorb shock and protect the feet from the resistant surfaces we walk upon, almost all footwear is both manufactured and sold on the basis of style rather than function. As a leading podiatrist wryly observed to me, in this country one requires a license to shoe a horse but absolutely no experience or credentials are necessary for those who shoe human beings. We should be thankful, though, that good leather shoes can be mass-produced and are widely available. This might not be the case today were it not for the invention of a brilliant Black genius named Jan Ernst Matzeliger who was originally from Dutch Guiana and in 1883 patented a machine of his own invention that revolutionized the shoe industry. He created a mechanical last that virtually put a shoe together in one minute. He died in Massachusetts without realizing the vast profits that this invention later made for others. In our time, few shoes are made to conform to the feet. Styles that incorporate pointed or square-toe features expect the foot to conform to the style. This inevitably leads to abuse of the skin, bones, and muscles of the foot. The foot resists all styles of footwear that do not take into consideration the natural form and function of the foot. Since few do this, we must face the fact that improper footwear accounts for the vast majority of common foot problems. As Black women, we are given to spending considerable sums of money on fancy dress shoes that ruin our feet and economizing by buying cheap work shoes that we wear for longer periods of time and also ruin our feet. The price of a shoe is absolutely no indication of its ability to treat the foot well or badly, and some of the best shoes for the feet are quite inexpensive while many of the most expensive shoes are virtual torture chambers.

Most shoes are made on standard-size shoe lasts, although, as we know, no two pairs of feet are the same. It is not necessary to wear custom-made or orthopedic shoes to save your feet from disaster, but you must bear in mind that the fit of a shoe is very important no matter what the style. If the shoe is too tight, you will damage veins in the feet and legs and constrict circulation throughout the lower body. If the shoe is too loose (clogs are almost always too loose), you will acquire corns, callouses, and a tendency for fallen arches and sprained ankles. "Correct" footwear is designed to protect your feet according to the task required. For this reason the shoes you wear to work should be bought with the most care and attention. The Women's Bureau of the United States Department of Labor states: "The shoes that women wear at work have a greater effect on their comfort, safety, and efficiency than any other item of clothing." No matter what you are doing—office work, housework, shop work, factory work, sports, or just relaxing—you will immeasurably increase your comfort and abilities if you choose well an appropriate pair of shoes. This task should not be attempted during a hurried lunch hour.

The "Ideal" Working Shoe

The classic though conservative style of the "Oxford" shoe exemplifies what we should look for when choosing shoes in which we will spend our working days. The toes should be more or less rounded, the sole must be hard (rubber or leather), and the heel less than two inches high and quite broad. It must be securely held to the foot with laces, a buckle, or straps. The insole and the uppers should also be made of a material that can breathe such as leather or rubber and the foot should feel well supported by the shoe. (Shoes such as high heels, backless, platforms, clogs, sandals, loafers, tennis shoes, and boots should not be worn continuously throughout busy days but really only worn for special occasions, brief periods, and when relaxing.) The upper part of the shoe should not constrain the foot but simply hold it neatly. The sole must be thick enough to absorb the repeated shock of the impact of your body weight against the concrete sidewalk. All of your shoes should have a metal shank in the sole that acts as a shock absorber. This is a strip of metal ½ inch wide and three to five inches in length that prevents the foot and thus the body from constantly vibrating as you walk on very hard surfaces. Your everyday shoe should give you permanent firm support; it must neither pinch nor flap but provide a cushioned grip.

How to Buy Your Shoes

Never buy footwear in a hurry. You will regret it every minute of every day spent walking in those uncomfortable shoes that looked so great in the window and which you did not try on properly. Your shoe size is measured by the length, indicated numerically, and the width, indicated alphabetically.

1) Never tell a shoe salesperson your size. Always have your feet measured each time you buy shoes. Not only do your measurements fluctuate according to climate and time of day, but different brands and styles of shoe may require varying sizes.

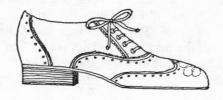

2) Make sure your feet are measured both while sitting and while standing —this can make as much as half-an-inch difference.

3) Ask what the shoe is made of, both sole and upper. Feel the upper for softness and pliability.

4) Gently bend the sole (not the instep) of the shoe to test the flexibility of the shank. This does not apply to certain types of sports or fancy shoes that have no shank.

5) Fit the shoe on the foot and test for a snug grip at the heel and instep. The toes must be able to extend fully at the front. Too big is as bad as too small.

6) Find a noncarpeted area of the store to walk on. Many stores encourage you to test the shoe only on carpet, which gives a false feeling of comfort and does not tell you how the foot and shoe work together on hard surfaces.

7) You may have one foot slightly larger than the other. Try on both shoes together. You may need a split pair, each shoe a different size.

8) Always shop alone for shoes. Your family and friends will try to persuade you to buy only according to the styles they themselves prefer with no consideration for the comfort or health of your feet. Take your time.

9) Do not let yourself be intimidated by a rude or opinionated salesperson. If you are being given a hard sell that you dislike, ask to see the manager.

If your feet have unusually extreme variances such as short toes, high instep, very wide or very long, there are many manufacturers who will accommodate any style to your custom fit and even orthopedic shoes can be made in fashionable styles. It is worth the extra cost if it saves you from crippling foot problems that always catch up, often later in life when your mobility is a precious asset.

Making the Most of Your Shoes

A good shoe that fits well and shelters and supports the foot must be treated with the same care you would give to your best clothes. Unfortunately, we never clean the *insides* of our shoes and that may be why fungus infections are so common. At least a woman should clean and maintain the exterior of her shoes and always keep them in good repair. Although they may seem comfortable, an old broken pair of shoes are in fact warping your feet and probably altering your posture for the worse. All shoes need frequent doses of polish. Use a neutral (colorless) liquid, cream, or paste and buff lightly. This will protect them from the weather and daily wear and tear. Suede shoes require brisk brushing with a stiff wire brush. Patent leather shoes can be shined with a soft damp cloth and they last longer if they are given occasional buffings with special patent cleaner. Do not try to clean fabric shoes yourself or any shoe that has an exotic material. Take them to a good shoe-repair store.

Stockings

In recent years hose have developed from silk to nylon stockings to the now widely popular pantyhose. One change that most consumers have disregarded is that although socks and stockings are sold according to feet measurements, pantyhose are manufactured according to leg and hip sizes. This means that the all-important foot-fit in pantyhose is often ignored. Your hose must fit loosely over the toes. If the fit is tight, especially when you are standing, it will be tighter still when you sit and quite capable of producing significant discomfort in time. When shopping for pantyhose, spend some time to experiment and find the brand and size that give you the most comfortable fit and stay with that brand. Always keep these items scrupulously clean, for they are capable of harboring and spreading bacterial infection. After each wearing, wash out in mild, soapy water.

E. FOOT AILMENTS

Americans spend two billion dollars each year on preparations manufactured to ease or cure foot problems. Nine out of ten of us will experience in our lifetime a foot ailment that requires special attention and treatment. I deal here with the most common of these and their causes; more complex conditions must be brought to the attention of a doctor.

Ingrown Toenails

The toenail is primarily a shield for the toe, designed to protect the nerves and bones. Most problems involving toenails stem from hose and shoes being too short or narrow, improper nailcutting, and fungus infection. Some toenail diseases are caused by congenital malformations, tissue stress (overweight), and illnesses such as diabetes and sickle-cell anemia. Ingrown toenails occur when the lateral edge or edges of the nail penetrate the skin and cut into the flesh of the toe. Treatment is not painful but must be done by a professional. This condition should not occur if you wear well-fitting footwear and keep the skin around the nails moist and lubricated (see Foot Care) and use an emery board to keep the skin supple.

Raised Toenails

These are most common in women over sixty and may also be shiny, fluted, and crumbling. The cause of this condition is usually a circulatory or coronary ailment.

Club Nails

These are overgrown nails that may become extremely hard and curl under the toes. This condition can be rectified painlessly by a doctor. Direct injury to the nail can result in thickening, discoloration, and elongation.

Fungus Toenail

This is caused by ringworm encouraged by the bacteria inside shoes. The nails appear dry and lusterless with gray, yellow, or brownish coloration. Treatment is simple but requires a doctor.

Corns

These are the most common foot ailment. They appear as soft or hard bumps of horny skin, usually surrounded by an inflamed area and often found on the tops of the toes. Corns are caused by constant alternating friction and pressure created by ill-fitting footwear. Some corns can also result from arthritis or bursitis. Corns can be surgically removed or displaced by chemical means. You should see a doctor before attempting either method at home. Never use a regular razor but obtain a correct corn and callous trimmer. First soften the area in hot water and pare the skin very lightly and gently. Do not try to take off too much at one time. This is only a temporary measure to be attempted when there is no possibility of professional medical help.

Bunions

The junction between skin and bones is lubricated by a *bursa*, a sac of fluid. When this becomes infected or inflamed it is called bursitis and when it occurs in the feet, especially at the joint of the big toe, we get what we term a bunion. Treatment is not painful but must be administered by a doctor. Do not let the condition worsen and increase.

Hammertoe

This is a deformity that may be congenital but is sometimes caused by consistently wearing narrow, tight shoes. One or more toes becomes permanently raised and overlaps another. Only a foot surgeon should attempt to remedy this condition.

Callous

This is simply a thickened mass of skin formed often on the sides or soles of the feet because of normal friction and constant movement. A home or professional pedicure should decrease most callous formations. If they persist, see a doctor.

Athlete's Foot

This popular expression is a misnomer for tineapodis, or fungus of the foot. This state creates hot, itching feet, often with peeling and cracking of the skin between the toes. It may be caused by a variety of factors including allergic reaction to drugs, dyes, perspiration, and certain chemicals found in soaps. If the cracking and peeling are extensive, consult a doctor who will be able to determine the cause of the allergy.

Foot Odor (Bromodrosis)

Although neither painful nor infectious, this is one of the most annoying foot problems. If my foot-hygiene regimen does not control your odor problem, do not waste time and money on fancy sprays and concoctions but consult a doctor who will trace the cause. It may not be localized in the foot itself but emanate from a disorder elsewhere in the body.

Fallen Arches

This condition is also known as "flat feet" and is characterized by a re-alignment of the bones in the feet including the anterior metatarsal arch. The heel bone rolls inward, the ankle drops, the shinbone protrudes and often the big toe and the little toe rise. Although this ailment can be inherited, it is often the result of obesity combined with ill-fitting shoes and an occupation that requires constant motion and prolonged strain on the feet. The back muscles attempt to compensate for the weakness of the foot muscles and low back pain frequently accompanies weak arches. The legs may also swell and appear puffy. Because shoes are difficult to fit with this condition, one is also prone to bunions, corns, and callouses. Weak arches, if not treated, can lead to arthritis of the feet, a most painful condition. Weak arches can be the result of injury, infection, or malnutrition. Weak arches in infants and children can be corrected with special treatment that is applied while the foot is still forming. Weak arches in an adult cannot be cured, but the condition can be effectively relieved. Do not buy artificial foot arches without a podiatrist's advice. They cannot match your foot exactly and may increase the misalignment of the bones. You must consult a podiatrist and be measured and fitted with a foot-molded support that is uniquely designed for your foot. Do not wear unsupported shoes for long periods of time such as clogs, high heels, and shoes that are backless or have a narrow instep. Sandals and platforms that leave most of the foot exposed and unsupported can gravely increase the discomfort of weak arches. The ideal shoe for this condition is an Oxford fitted with a personalized support. Inflammation that can arise from this condition can be relieved at home by elevating the feet and applying moist warm towels on the feet and legs; however, avoid heat lamps and the excessive use of hot-water bottles.

F. PROFESSIONAL FOOT CARE

In 1912 podiatry was established as a specific branch of medicine that deals with the diagnosis and treatment of foot ailments. At first these doctors called themselves *chiropodists* (chiro: hand; pod: foot) because originally these doctors specialized in both feet and hands, and both names are still in use, although "podiatrist" is more popular. Such a specialist is a qualified doctor of medicine, not to be confused with a *pedicurist*, who is merely a beautician who specializes in the feet but has no medical qualifications whatsoever. Many minor foot problems can be handled by a family doctor or a clinic doctor, and you should make sure that your feet are thoroughly examined when you have your annual checkup. If the problem requires special attention, it will be recommended that you consult a podiatrist. Unfortunately for our feet, too many of us rely on gadgets, patent medicines, and the advice of relatives to take care of foot problems. All of these amateur activities can lead to serious reactions such as dermatitis and permanent damage to the foot. Some attempt is being made to protect the consumer from fraudulent or dangerous foot medications sold over the counter, but many still contain as much as 60 per cent strength salicylic acid, although most doctors use at the very most a 40 per cent solution. Most often, self-treatment is not final and the problem will keep recurring in increasing severity until a doctor must be consulted and then the treatment may be arduous and expensive. You should see a doctor or podiatrist at the first trace of foot disease or malfunction and have the problem fully and professionally taken care of.

Professional Foot Examination

Remember that a podiatrist is not qualified to examine any part of your body other than the feet and lower legs. The following should be part of your examination:

1) Discussion regarding full medical history, including personal and family foot ailments in the past.

2) Physical examination of bare feet while standing, seated, and lying down.

3) The podiatrist may take measurements and X-rays to determine bone displacement.

4) Minor nonsurgical treatment may be performed in the office after the doctor has thoroughly acquainted you with the nature of your problem and recommended treatment. If the doctor suggests any immediate surgical procedure in the office, you have the right to decline and seek a second opinion—perhaps by talking to your regular doctor for reassurance.

Professional Pedicure

This should involve no more than I have outlined for a home pedicure. Do not allow a pedicurist to cut anywhere on the foot except the toenails, and then only straight across. Serious infection can result from inept handling by such beauticians of corns, callouses, bunions, etc.

G. OUR LEGS

Most authorities agree that because of increasing progress in nutrition and early correction of defects, we have better legs now than ever before. Black women often complain that their calves and ankles are too thin. I can only answer that I am proud of this and regard it not at all as a racial shortcoming but an elegant, distinctive characteristic that we should be proud of. Despite this tendency, however, four out of five of us experience increasing heaviness and flabbiness about the knees and thighs from our early twenties well into our thirties. The only way to counteract this tendency is by practicing good nutrition and exercise. Often ignored as a factor of exercise in this regard is the wearing of correct shoes and the necessity to alter the heel height throughout the day. This makes different sets of muscles get regular exercise, which does not happen when one wears flat shoes all the time or high heels all the time.

Varicose Veins

This complaint may be hereditary but often is caused by environmental factors such as occupation and lack of exercise. Avoid elastic hose and sitting for extended periods of time with legs crossed at the knees. It is most important to revive and maintain good circulation in the legs and feet. Ask your doctor's advice before purchasing support hose. Many systemic diseases first manifest themselves in the feet and at the forefront of podiatric diagnosis and care is an electronic device called a photoplethysmograph. This is used primarily on patients over forty with a history of circulatory complaints. The index fingers and all ten toes are wired to this machine, which can isolate possibly abnormal circulatory patterns.

Emergency Treatment for Feet and Leg Injury

BROKEN BONES

Keep the patient warm, loosen the clothes. If there is extensive bleeding, stem with clean linen but do not bind. If bone is protruding, do not attempt to push into place. Make no attempt to clean the wound but call for an ambulance.

PUNCTURE WOUNDS

With clean hands, squeeze the wound to encourage bleeding and remove foreign objects. Clean area with soap and warm water. Loosely cover the wound with sterile dressing and an icebag, if necessary, to relieve swelling. Take the patient to a doctor or emergency facility for examination of the wound and protection against tetanus.

SPRAINS

Elevate the injured joint to a comfortable position. Apply an icebag or cold compress over the sprain area to reduce pain and swelling. Severe sprains should be examined by a doctor for possible bone fracture.

Chapter VI

THE VISIBLE BODY

The physique is our most obvious attribute, certainly the one that is most immediately apprehended by others. The body's form can be either a source of great pride or constant embarrassment. No matter how stimulating and intelligent our conversation might be, we are almost always prejudged by both men and women according to the relative size, shape, and general aspect of our bodies. Nowadays it is fashionable to dismiss such judgment as sexist and superficial. I firmly believe that when a man or a woman, Black or white, is judged *only* according to his or her external, physical qualities, the conclusions drawn are worse than useless; but, as a very obvious and primary segment of our entire character (albeit a less important segment than, say, compassion or intelligence), the external body simply cannot be totally disregarded. The relative attractiveness of our physique does predispose others toward or against us no matter how vehemently they might deny it. Furthermore, our outward appearance, shape, and odor are frequently reflections of our internal order. The condition of the mind, the skeleton, and the internal organs is often mirrored in the external visage of a woman and the balance of her body condition as a complete whole is declared by the condition of the surface. We will examine the optimum appearance for the flesh and muscle and ligaments and discuss how we can effect changes that will be permanent.

A. EXERCISE

A woman cannot change her height. A woman cannot alter her build. If you are stocky, you will never be narrow, and if the size and structure of your bones are large, then you cannot make yourself small. As we strive for some perfection in our bodies, we must keep a firm grasp upon what is unalterable. We will only create enormous frustration with the futility of attempting to change the unchangeable. Such factors as are determined genetically—

height, build, and in some women the tendency to be underweight or over-weight—must be faced squarely and honestly and understood as absolutes. These are "givens" that we must work with, not against.

Most of us are brainwashed at an early age to believe that our bodies, although essentially weaker and more fragile than those of men, are capable of formidable and miraculous changes of shape. This is far from the truth. Because of certain antibodies and a substance called cortin that are found only in the female, we are actually less prone to certain diseases than men and thus constitutionally stronger. Women trained for sports such as track and swimming are rapidly proving to be men's physical equals. There are biological differences that very definitely affect our capacity to change our profiles. We have almost 40 per cent more fatty tissue than men and although judicious dieting can reduce that fatty tissue, we may not necessarily be able to diminish or increase the circumference of our wrist, or the measurements of our bust, thighs, and calves. Grotesque deformities aside, I do not believe that any specific body type is inherently more pleasing or beautiful than any other. Fashion changes with the calendar and although this country has been to date dominated by a concept of idealized female form rooted in Anglo-Saxon European culture, the constant contact between peoples of all ethnic backgrounds, which seems to be the hallmark of the second half of this twentieth century, is responsible for a much broader definition of what, in a woman, is beauty.

Every woman can realize her full potential for her physique by creating and maintaining a balance between the caloric value of the food she eats and the energy she uses. This balance cannot be accomplished by diet alone since we actually require only very, very few calories for minimum activity survival and consequently we all need some forms of exercise to work off excess calories. The purpose of exercise is multifold. It is a physiological fact that living matter that is not used simply atrophies. Present-day living reduces to a minimum the use of certain muscles. Automobiles and other labor- and time-saving devices rob us of the opportunity to put our bodies to the uses from which they evolved. The result is that vital muscles deteriorate and this contributes to a flabby, if not fat, appearance. Not only does controlled, regular exercise help us to reduce, gain, or maintain weight, but it markedly improves the functioning of such internal organs as the kidneys and the lungs and has a very definite effect on the large external organ, the skin itself. Exercise not only improves our looks but increases our stamina, zest, and self-confidence. Exercise improves the quality of one's sleep and helps to prevent many of the degenerative diseases of the heart and blood vessels that start to occur in middle life. Activity alone, however, will not reduce the figure. In order to work off just one pound of body fat requires twenty-two hours of laundering or 131 hours of sewing or eleven days of office work. If the only exercise one gets is mental, it would take 2,160 hours of strenuous thinking to "melt away" that one pound of fat! So everyday exercise is not the way to reduce.

However, regulated and regular exercise, combined with the nutritional necessities outlined in the next chapter, will trim the body to its appropriate weight and, most important of all, assist in the distribution of body tissue in an organized, healthy, attractive manner. Those of us who work and expend considerable energy in that work falsely hold the notion that we get sufficient exercise from this kind of effort. In fact, we may well be overworking some muscles at the expense of others. Random effort is not exercise and is absolutely no substitute for a personal program regularly adhered to.

Women who can afford to avoid strenuous work are usually unwilling to indulge in regular exercise, although they may need it the most. While perhaps keeping slim by undereating they are nevertheless potential hospital patients as their bodies gradually decay. Women who cannot afford to avoid physical labor must realize that proper exercise is absolutely essential to maintain the stamina required for the job and retrain the muscles. For years Black women simply could not afford to take care of their bodies, and we have inherited an attitude of neglecting exercise that derives from the days when our great-grandmothers worked so hard and so long that there was absolutely no time and no energy to exercise. We cannot lose sight of the fact that one extra slice of bread per day adds up to ten extra pounds at the end of the year and if we are not prepared to gain that weight, but insist on eating the bread, we must develop methods to use up those calories. Although exercise cannot correct the structural dimensions of our bodies that we are born with, it can make significant changes occur in the functional dimensions that are controlled by overeating, bad posture, and lack of activity. Correct exercise creates a strong, well-functioning nervous system and the nervous system, because it controls the cardiovascular systems, is the master of the body.

What Is "Correct Exercise"?

Much emphasis is placed on the efficacy of repeated daily exercise aimed at a particular section of the body. My studies and personal experience have led me to the conclusion that such "spot reducing" activity is of very limited value. The body loses and gains weight generally, not specifically. This action occurs as the delicate balance between food intake and energy dispersal is altered in favor of one or the other. Pounding away relentlessly at an offending waistline has little effect on this balance. Fat cells are not similar in all parts of the body and have varied loss patterns. Rhythmic exercise of just one muscle group will not necessarily burn up sufficient calories to make any substantial effect on that particular location. The *only* way to exercise yourself to total fitness is by indulging in those activities that actually cause hard breathing and a feeling of fatigue. If your exercising does this, you may well be on the road to fitness. Sustained activity that uses all the muscles of the body naturally and in unison with one another is the best possible form of exercise. Some organized sports, especially tennis, come into this category, as do many of the simplest, most economical and available activities such as hard walking, swimming, running, and jogging.

These must be enjoined vigorously with an honest attempt to work hard and expend significant effort. One's goal in pursuing these activities is to build up the capacity to assume a physical burden without draining the entire system of recuperative powers. In an emergency we are all able to sustain great efforts, physical or mental, but sometimes the damage to our system is irreparable. If, with regular, over-all exercise, we train our bodies to deal with excessive expenditures of energy without reducing our reserves, we not only use up all those extra calories but, more importantly, we will always be able to recuperate very quickly, often instantaneously, from all kinds of mental or physical stress situations. If you have made your body accustomed to swimming eighty laps per day, having a baby (a physical stress situation) will not throw the body into panic. If you are used to jogging nonstop for two or three miles per day, emotional problems (mental stress) are not so likely to produce physical debility. Making this kind of regular exercise effort will turn a fatigued, irritable, light sleeper into a sound, heavy, refreshed sleeper. The system must be taxed; there are no short cuts. When we wash the dishes, that energy expenditure keeps the heart beating at a normal 78–90 pulses per minute. Productive exercise is not achieved until that heart rate is moved up to 130 beats per minute. That is hard to do with yoga, isometrics, or spot-reducing exercises. Only when the lungs begin to strain and the breath becomes rapid does the system really come alive and work. Simple running in place with knees and arms swinging until you feel really out of breath, and for two minutes beyond that point, constitutes a form of gross motor activity that services every part of the body most beneficially and just cannot be bettered for over-all improvement.

There is no instant route to physical fitness, but your exercise regimen will be much simpler, more fun, and certainly more beneficial if you concentrate on gross motor activity and avoid the limb-twisting, eye-crossing gymnastic diagrams that appear in so many magazines. I expended a lot of energy as a model, constantly on the move, mostly by foot, in and out of the studio. When I ceased doing that as a major activity I continued to take in the same amount of food as before but because I was altering my personal energy-out/food-in balance, I naturally started to gain weight since sitting behind the desk in my office spends far less energy than modeling. I decided to counter the first signs of weight gain by faithfully following a set of standing, lying, and sitting exercises that I did with precision each morning, but with decreasing enthusiasm, ending, finally, with very little in the way of tangible results. Then I tried a form of exercise which I knew I would enjoy—swimming—and found that it is ideal as a gross motor activity. I swim hard for an hour every day in a local pool and not only is it very pleasant but I quickly went back to my normal weight. Instead of feeling stretched, strained, and dissatisfied after ten minutes of bending that seemed like ten hours, I am now fighting fit and invigorated after an hour of swimming that seems like ten minutes. No relaxing in the water or diving or dithering in the shallow end will do any good. You must work hard and nonstop. Find your own pace, whether swimming, walking, jogging, or running. Fast or slow does not matter, but duration does. You must really feel it in your muscles after the first day, and if you persist with the activity, that discomfort will very soon pass. Keep at it doggedly and, above all, teach yourself to breathe properly. That is the secret of sustaining these great forms of exercise. Never hold your breath. Be very conscious of this because many of us do it without really being aware of the fact. Never worry about inhaling; that takes care of itself. Think only of forcefully and rhythmically exhaling. Do it in audible gasps at first so you can actually feel and hear it. Expel all the air from the lungs each time you exhale. When running or jogging, this should be done every three or four steps. In order to realize the maximum effectiveness of your cardiorespiratory system you must expose the entire surface of the lungs to as much new air as possible; this means breathing deeply and quickly.

When to Exercise

Every day is ideal, but regularity is more important than frequency. If your schedule does not give you the time to exercise every day, then two or three times per week or even just once per week will produce results if you make an unbreakable appointment with yourself. You must work at it hard. The best time of day for exercising is when you can best find the time—morning, noon, or night. Always wait one hour after eating. It is a popular belief that exercise before meals is counterproductive for weight loss since the appetite is stimulated. This is not true. Appetite is likely to be reduced after exercise when the stomach, after having undergone a stress situation, will only tackle as much work (digesting food) as is absolutely essential.

Where to Exercise

Access to the sea, a lake, or a pool is of course essential for swimming. Running, jogging, and hard walking can be accomplished anywhere, although rural and suburban areas lend themselves more willing to these pursuits than the urban environment where, even if safe, the streets may be unsuitable. Since a lot of us are in the latter position I have devised an indoor regimen.

Exercise at Home

This series was designed by me to substitute for outdoor gross motor activity (sports, swimming, jogging, etc.) at times or in areas where such activity is impossible. In order for these exercises to be effective, they must be followed *every day.* No one has any excuse for avoiding them since they only take FIVE MINUTES!

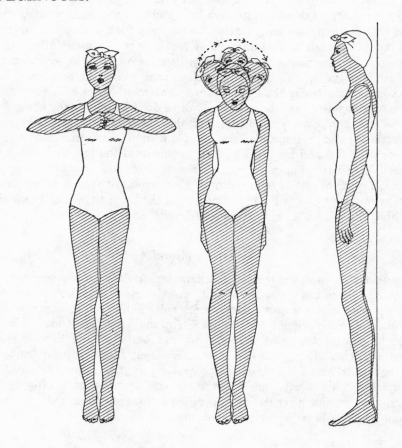

ARM PULL

With bent elbows, grip hands together across the chest. Breathe in deeply, pull hard, hold, relax, and breathe out all the way with force. This helps the whole upper torso including the shoulders and arms and also firms the bust.

10 Arm pulls   10 seconds

HEAD ROTATION

Drop the chin as far forward as possible. Draw head to the right shoulder, then let it drop back and around left shoulder to the front. Keep the shoulders down. This relaxes the upper back and the spine, areas particularly susceptible to nervous tension.

> 10 Head rotations clockwise   20 seconds
> 10 Head rotations counterclockwise   20 seconds

HEAD NOD

Throw the head back as far as possible, then let it flop easily and loosely forward so that your chin touches your chest.

> 5 Head nods   10 seconds

STANDING BACK PRESS

Stand with back against a flat wall. Make sure that heels, buttocks, shoulders, and head are all touching the wall. Breathe deeply in and lift the diaphragm while pressing the small of the back into the wall. Release and exhale hard. This exercise is invaluable for implementing good posture, aligning the internal organs, and firming the abdominal area.

> 10 Standing back presses   30 seconds

SEATED FORWARD PRESS

Sit on the floor with legs straight and spread. Grip ankles or calves with hands while keeping back flat, not curved. Press forward as if trying to touch chin to floor. This helps the waistline, strengthens the lower torso and the inside thigh.

> 10 Seated forward presses   30 seconds

PRONE BODY RAISE AND STRETCH

Lie flat on floor face down with arms extended straight ahead and legs straight behind. Stretch forward and try to raise the top half of the body off the ground. Keep legs firmly on the floor. Reverse motion and lift legs while

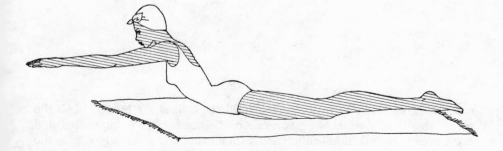

keeping top flat to the floor. Finally, stretch whole body and raise both arms and legs so that only the stomach is resting on the floor. This series of movements increases the flexibility of the whole body, keeps the spine supple and the chest, buttocks, back, thighs, and bust are straightened and tightened.

3 Prone body raises (Upper)　　　10 seconds
3 Prone body raises (Lower)　　　10 seconds
3 Prone body raises (Upper and lower)　　　10 seconds

JOGGING IN PLACE

While doing this, maintain a fairly rapid rhythm and breathe deep and hard, exhaling noisily. Lift the knee as high as possible and swing the arms so

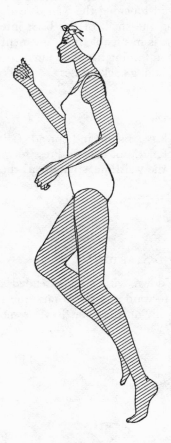

that the hands reach up to the ceiling and back behind the body. This is the most valuable all-over exercise you can do. Every muscle is implicated and every muscle is worked in conjunction with all the others. Keep going for the full amount of time without pause and increase your effort and speed when you begin to flag. As a daily practice, this is essential to benefit your entire health cycle.

Jogging in place   2½ minutes

REMEMBER: the total time for all these is only five minutes.

EXERCISE DO'S

Wear as few clothes as possible and never any shoes. Belts and girdles should be disregarded along with anything else that is tight and restricting. Take it slowly and easily at first, especially if you have not been used to exercise. Start with a limited program and work up to a full schedule. If you are doing my exercises, you must do them every day. If you begin to miss two and three days in a row, you are risking the loss of all that you built up. For an exercise to be effective it must be repeated regularly.

EXERCISE DON'T'S

Don't believe that furious bouts of violent exercise will get rid of many pounds. Exercising is to keep the figure trim and firm and reduce the possibility of cardiovascular and respiratory illnesses. Exercise has to be sensibly combined with limited food intake in order to aid and sustain weight loss.

Don't buy inflatable pants, girdles, or any other such contraptions that promise instant figure remodeling. They are sheer gimmickry.

Don't rely on a machine to do the work for you. Gymnasium-type equipment is not necessary for an optimum exercise regimen. If you do use, or want to use, any form of equipment, first understand completely what it does and how it should be handled. Serious injury can result unless use is preceded by demonstration and supervision. This applies to special tables, cycles, weights, and similar paraphernalia.

EXERCISE TIPS

Be wary of push-ups, sit-ups, toe-touching. These exercises can put undue and dangerous stress on the spinal column and will aggravate rather than correct back problems. Instead of touching toes straight-legged from a standing position, bend the knees and touch the palms flat to the floor. Likewise, if you do sit-ups, bend the knees and this will center the activity on your stomach muscles, not the fragile small of the back. When in a lying position, never snap up and down but always curl slowly, feeling each section of the body come off the floor. No matter what type of exercise program you are following, be sure to see a doctor as soon as you experience any abnormal pain. Aches and strain are perfectly normal at the start, but a persistent angry pain may indicate either you are doing an exercise incorrectly or that you have an existing condition that might preclude such exercise. Whatever exercise you take, effort is more important than duration; this cannot be stressed enough. After fifteen or twenty repetitions of any exercise, you are not doing any more good by going on to one hundred repetitions. Keeping fit is not a matter of endurance but regularity and effort.

Facial Exercises

Our faces consist of more than two dozen separate muscles, some of which are very rarely used. Facial exercises may be beneficial in improving the blood circulation in the face and to overcome certain types of facial ache, but facial exercises are often undeservedly praised as benefiting the shape of the face, eradicating wrinkles, and generally creating or maintaining beauty. I am very skeptical of these claims. Large noses, double chins, crow's-feet, and puffy eyes cannot be massaged or exercised away. To try to do so is folly. Elderly beauties who attribute their smooth and flawless skins to massage and exercise are also blessed with strong genetic tendencies that have preserved the skin, and for every such claim there are hundreds of very disappointed women whose daily hours of facial exercise have yielded no results at all. I will not deny that facial muscles can be firmed and tightened by exercise but loose skin will simply stay loose. If the appearance of your face alters when you overeat, you have to cut your food intake and indulge in gross motor activity in order to reduce. It is nonsense to talk of losing weight only in the face by means of facial exercise. In order for it to show in your face it must be part of an over-all adjustment. Short of surgery, you cannot alter the basic features of the face and the only way to make the face thinner or fuller is to adopt my rules for weight loss or weight gain. This means body exercise, proper nutrition, and sufficient sleep.

Exercise and "Cellulite"

"Cellulite" is an overused word that the diet industry has recently picked up to scare more women into buying more expensive products. Because fat cells are deposited differently in various areas of the body, and skin tissue also varies, we are often prone to accumulations of lumps or bulges that are very persistent despite all usual methods of weight reduction. These gel-like deposits of fats, water, and waste are given the grand name "cellulite." Now there is a panoply of gadgets and drugs and special programs to eradicate this "cellulite" scourge that is, of course, as old as time. The principal cause for these uneven deposits, aside from the body's propensity to accumulate fat in some areas and not others, is the modern woman's tendency to try many cures at different times and stick to none regularly. It is not at all surprising that we suffer from "lumps" when we move from diet to diet, drug to drug, yoga to isometrics. As I have mentioned, spot-reducing has negligible results, so no wonder there are bulges! In order to deal with "cellulite" you must take to heart my monotonous litany of correct nutrition, gross motor activity, and sound sleep. No one crash diet, novel exercise, or concoction can remove flab from the waist, shoulders, or thighs, but I know that my complete regimen can do this if you are willing to persist and look for permanent results in three months—not three weeks or three days—and if you are willing to *always* eat well, exercise, and take care of your body my way.

B. BODY SAUNA AND MASSAGE

Sauna treatments for the body consist of subjecting the naked body to dry heat, usually created by heating rocks with electricity or boiling water. This causes one to perspire profusely and it is difficult not to equate this with losing weight. In fact, although you do lose water in this way and the scales may register a lower reading immediately after a sauna, this is false loss and will result in no visible change: Your dress size will stay the same. Since taking a sauna is a completely passive activity and it has weight-loss connotations, some women use saunas or steambaths as a substitute for exercise. This is useless and can be dangerous since prolonged exposure to these forms of heat can evacuate too much moisture from the body. When first trying a sauna, never stay longer than a few minutes and leave as soon as you feel uncomfortable.

Massage has absolutely no capacity to rid the body of excess weight, whether performed by an amateur or a professional. It must never be considered as a viable alternative to exercise. A thorough massage can be most beneficial as a mind soother and a body relaxer, but fatty tissue cannot be removed by massage.

C. POSTURE

We are much maligned for the size and prominence of our behinds. Although there is some evidence to suggest that a deep pelvis is more common among us than white women, the principal cause of our protruding buttocks is bad posture. Most cases of bad posture are not due to inherited conditions but to environmental factors. Children wearing ill-fitting, worn-out, cheap footwear invariably develop bad posture. Teen-aged girls who are growing fast and by adolescence are quite tall often stoop with a rounded back and this position can remain through their lives. Although preadult conditions create bad posture, laziness is the only reason for its persisting later in life. Correct posture is not simply a matter of elegance. Knowing how to stand, sit, and lie correctly not only combats fatigue and relaxes the body but

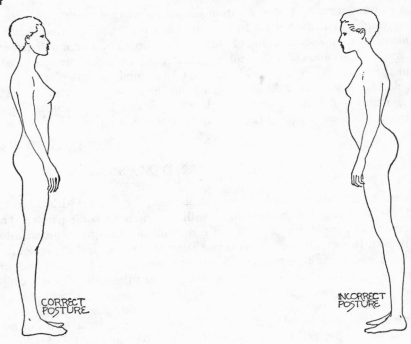

CORRECT POSTURE

INCORRECT POSTURE

preserves the internal order of all the vital organs. The back is perfectly capable of supporting the framework of the body if the weight is evenly distributed. Bad posture creates agonizing backaches. Posture is basically the way in which all the body parts relate while in motion or at rest.

By slouching and slumping we relax many of the back muscles and terribly overburden the rest. Good posture creates the most efficient, least stressful alignment of the body.

Standing

Stand flat with both feet firmly on the ground. Your weight should be slightly forward, not back on the heels. First, think of just the head and the pelvis. Pull your head up, keeping the chin tucked in. The top of your head must be at its farthest possible point from the ground. Now move your pelvis forward as far as it will go. Your spine is now perfectly aligned and your weight evenly distributed throughout the body. The spine should not be rigid like a rod but slightly, naturally curved. The shoulders are flat and level and your stomach should feel as if you are wearing a girdle. The diaphragm is relaxed and your breathing is steady and easy. Of course, not being used to it, the first time you lock into this position you will feel a strain, but after a few minutes your normal aches and pains should disappear. This stance is the basis of good posture and illustrates the least fatiguing use of all the muscles. When excess strain is placed on the small of the back, a swayback occurs, the buttocks then protrude to counterbalance and our rotund behinds come to dominate our figures. Not only is this unsightly but unnatural as well. Given sufficient years, this posture will cause serious back problems. If your occupation requires you to stand for long periods of time, you will be much more comfortable and incur far less strain if you adopt the good posture I have outlined and alternate resting one foot at a time on a low stool, box, or ledge six to twelve inches off the floor.

Walking

Start with the basic standing posture. Head up and pelvis forward. Proceed with the toes pointing directly ahead. The heel must touch the ground just before the ball of the foot. Roll the foot forward in one smooth movement onto the toes. Imagine that you are following a thin straight line and your imaginary footprints should just touch either side of it. Keep your thighs together and the head always erect.

Sitting

Do not lounge back into sofas and chairs but place the small of your back snugly against the backseat. Keep the feet flat on the floor and the body lean should be very slightly forward rather than back. At work or at rest, this position can be maintained for hours without strain.

Lying Down

The best bed posture is to lie on your back. Sleeping on the stomach encourages curvature of the spine and minor aches and misalignments. Next to sleeping on the back, the best posture is on one side with the knees half-bent.

There is a "better" way to sit, walk, stand, and lie. This is not based on propriety but upon the natural balance of the body as it has evolved over many hundreds of thousands of years. It is incidental that correct posture is also the most becoming to our eyes.

D. BODY SURGERY

There are two types of surgery, the purpose of which are to alter the surface appearance of the body. The first is called reconstructive surgery and the second, cosmetic surgery.

Reconstructive Surgery

This is performed as a consequence of accident where it is vital to rebuild part of the anatomy that has been destroyed or gravely altered. In such cases, of course, the paramount concern is the survival of the victim with the fewest possible permanent scars. I must say now that for the Black woman I believe this to be the only kind of body surgery she should submit to, i.e., when there is literally no alternative.

Cosmetic Surgery

This, as the name implies, is performed to "correct" a host of anatomical details that the patient wishes altered for purely beautification reasons. All over the world, from Latin America to Japan, this is becoming increasingly popular for women who seem to be trying to alter themselves in such a way as to imitate a wide-eyed, fine-boned, ample-chested ideal of Anglo-Saxon European beauty. The Black woman is the possessor of a body and set of features so wonderfully unique that her attempt to artificially mold herself into that ideal is nothing less than a travesty. Another serious objection I have to the Black woman casually contemplating cosmetic surgery is that our skin's delicate pigmentation and tendency to form keloids make any kind of surgery far riskier than for our white counterpart. In fact, many plastic surgeons will not operate on Black women because they are afraid that keloids, hypertrophic scars, or heavy scar tissue will produce a net result that is far from a cosmetic improvement. These considerations are the same, of course, in reconstructive surgery, but in those cases the odds weigh in favor of necessity whereas there is no medical necessity for cosmetic surgery. All doctors agree that the ears, chest, and back are particularly keloid-prone and many acknowledge that even with second surgery to remove keloids, coupled with X-ray therapy, one in four Black patients will continue to have an unsightly keloid problem.

It is quite normal in these instances for the patient to be asked to sign a release stating that the dangers of the operation have been explained to her and not to expect 100 per cent success. New techniques are being developed that may eliminate scarring problems for the Black woman, chief among them being intradermal suturing. This avoids large cuts in the skin surface and any stitching is buried deep in the skin, left longer than usual, and is removed gradually.

Before I delineate the various types of cosmetic surgery that are commonly performed, there are two types of body surgery that should be mentioned that fall between reconstructive and cosmetic.

Congenital Defects

Surgery to correct defects such as a cleft palate, cup ears, and severe birthmarks is definitely to be considered, despite the possibilities of keloid formation. Bear in mind that the best time for such surgery is not at birth but often later in the growing process when the child is better able to stand surgery.

Reductive Surgery

Obese individuals often experience *intertrigo* which is the chafing and breaking of two skin areas that are continuously abutting one another and rubbing. This can occur beneath the breasts and between the thighs. The rash can be persistent and painful. Surgical removal of skin tissue can reduce the discomfort considerably even though there is a risk of permanent scarring. This is not a measure to sculpt the body into a leaner or more alluring condition but simply a medical necessity to avoid great discomfort.

Despite the fact that medical necessity should be the only reason for body surgery, increasing numbers of Black women are becoming willing candidates for the surgeon's knife. They see it often as a potential miracle worker. In an effort to discourage this trend, I will itemize those surgical procedures that Black women are asking for most and discuss the merits and dangers of each.

Nose Shaping

Called rhinoplasty, this procedure for the Black woman usually consists of removing tissue from the nostrils and adding bone to the nose in order to change a broad, flat nose into a more aquiline shape. One of the drawbacks is that in a flat nose there is usually not enough cartilage upon which to base a new shape. The illusion of change can be created by transplanting a small piece of bone from the hip area and burying it in the nose. Silicone injections are used to build the nose in certain cases, but frequently the silicone can become infected or extrude. Since silicone is a sand-and-carbon compound, it can be made to assume a consistency that will vary from liquid to oil to gelatinous to spongy to rubbery. As a molding substance it is therefore very malleable, but in the nose it is least likely to be successful. Even though you may feel that your nose is the one bad feature on your face and if corrected would lead to greater beauty, remember that there is an underlying balance and cast to the face that when altered by surgery can lead to a very peculiar-looking imbalance.

Face Lifting

We are well aware that our skin ages much more benignly than that of Caucasian women and it should hardly be necessary for any of us to surgically eliminate wrinkles in order to appear more youthful. However, we must be aware of this procedure. The medical term for it is rhytidectomy or meloplasty and it consists quite literally of cutting out wrinkles. The scalp is usually shaved and then the surgeon makes an incision at the temple just behind the hairline. This is carried down in front of the ear lobe and back up to the hairline at the nape of the neck. The facial skin is separated and pulled up and back toward the ears. Excess skin is cut and then the incision closed with stitches that extend, of course, all around the scalp so that if keloids develop they will be impossible to hide at all points. Women who experience changes of weight in the body that reflect in the face should only have this operation performed when their weight is at its lowest.

Eye Shaping

The most frequent form of blepharoplasty (as eye shaping is called) for Black women is the removal of the fatty tissue above and below the eye that gives the eyes a puffy or baggy appearance. We have a tendency to exhibit this condition, as do people from the Mediterranean countries. Pea-sized globules of fat, three in the lower lid and one or two in the upper, are removed through very delicate incisions. If the incision is carelessly made or heals incorrectly, the eye can become distorted and its ability to close impaired.

Lip Thinning

This is called cheilotomy. An incision is made inside the lip and certain musculature and mucous membrane are removed. The lips are very carefully constructed and have many purposes so that this kind of alteration can cause changes in the voice, speech, and permanent drooling.

Breast Shaping

Augmentation mammaplasty is a procedure for small breasts that may consist of inserting silicone or fatty tissue taken from elsewhere in the body. The silicone for such operations is now subject to strict governmental regulation because in the early years of this operation many women found that it would not remain in the designated area but would travel to parts of the body not in need of enlargement.

Reduction mammaplasty involves the removal of tissue from breasts that are considered to be too large. When this is done, it is also possible to relocate the nipples so that a semblance of normal appearance is retained. Sagging breasts are corrected in much the same way as the face is when lifted. Although keloid formation on or near the nipples and lower breast is rare, it is very common on the upper chest.

Lower Body Surgery

This can take place on virtually any part of the body but often consists of surgical lifts, tucks, and "darts" on the thighs, buttocks, hips, and abdomen. Large flaps of skin are cut and resewn. The Black woman can never tell what part of her body may develop keloids or hypertrophic scars, so this kind of random shaping should be avoided.

Before Body Surgery

All surgery is very expensive and cosmetic surgery can be among the most expensive. You pay for surgeons, doctors, nurses, and hospital. If you are considering any form of body surgery, do not listen to friends' or relatives' advice —only to your own real needs and wishes. The most important decision is that of choice of doctor and this is where most women make their first major mistake. In most states after just four years of medical school and no experience, the student can take a state examination and procure a license that allows him or her to practice both medicine and surgery including all forms of reconstructive and corrective surgery. Many, many unscrupulous individuals who are interested only in a quick profit thus set themselves up as "plastic surgeons" and even advertise themselves as such in neighborhood newspapers. If you value your appearance, avoid these people at all costs. I cannot stress this enough. In order to keep out of these rascals' avaricious hands, demand that your surgeon be "board-certified," meaning that he has passed the exams of the American Board of Plastic Surgeons and also is permitted the letters "FACS" after his name, which indicate he is a Fellow (member) of the American College of Surgeons. In order to find such a doctor, inquire of your own physician (who should always be the first person to speak to about this kind of surgery), and if that is not possible, write or call your county medical society which will provide you with three names of doctors qualified to help you. There are two kinds of plastic surgeons. *Primary* surgeons number about 1,500 and are qualified in all phases of body surgery. In addition to these, there are 22,000 *regional specialists* who are particularly qualified to deal with one or another area of the body: noses, hands, eyes, etc. Of this total of 23,500 plastic surgeons, fewer than fifty are female and none of these are Black. Compared to the many thousands who can legally practice surgery but may not be at all experienced or qualified, this small number demonstrates how easy it is to make a mistake and choose the wrong doctor. This mistake is especially easy for the Black woman to make since there are only a handful of qualified Black male plastic surgeons in the entire country and many white surgeons will not risk keloid formation and simply refuse to perform purely cosmetic surgery on Black women. Into that gap will step any number of charlatans. If you are determined to have cosmetic surgery and have found a board-certified surgeon who is an FACS, the following activity should precede any hospitalization.

The doctor should show you photographs of similar operations, before and after, and discuss honestly with you the limitations of the procedure. He must be told in depth by you of all previous medical history including allergies and family sicknesses. The doctor must give you a very thorough and complete physical examination including laboratory studies. You must feel comfortable with the doctor and since so much depends on what he will do, you have to establish a good honest rapport with him. It is best to see two doctors before making a final decision. No surgery is ever minor and no decisions should be taken lightly.

Chemosurgery

This is related to body surgery but usually does not involve incisions in the skin. Chemosurgery can be applied to any part of the body, but the face is most frequently affected. The procedure was developed to remove acne scars and has been extended to correct wrinkling and any kind of skin surface abnormality. Sometimes a wire brush is used to abrade the anaesthetized outer layer of skin. This is termed *dermabrasion* and with exfoliation (literally, the chemical peeling off of the outer skin) is the most common form of chemosurgery. Neither is to be particularly recommended to Black women because of the relatively final nature of the treatments and the delicate pigmentation in our skin that can so easily be upset. As with body surgery, it is most important to check carefully the credentials of anyone offering these services.

E. BODY HAIR

Hair has a strong tendency to grow heavily where it is not considered attractive and lightly or not at all where it is needed. For centuries women and men in every part of the world have been removing their hair in a wide variety of ways for many reasons, ranging from the dictates of health to the fashions of society to religious beliefs and even for vengeful relief from emotional trauma. Nowadays most of us remove hair because we believe it improves our appearance.

The causes of excessive body hair on a woman may be hereditary or hormonal. Endocrine imbalance brought on by pregnancy, oral contraception, and menopause can often result in accelerated hair growth. One of the oldest methods of hair removal—invented in Africa and still in practice today—consists of applying and removing a paste mixture of quicklime and starch.

The question of what hair is removed is primarily one for fashion, not health. Some women feel that all body hair is unsightly and others have quite the opposite opinion. I believe that all women should remove the hair from under their arms since perspiration gathers in this part of the body, mixes in the hair with bacteria and contributes to a pungent, disagreeable body odor quite different from that of "honest sweat." In "Our Face" we saw how the eyebrows should be treated. In this chapter we will enumerate the methods of removing hair from the face (lips, cheeks, chin), underarms, legs, and pubic areas. Black women's body hair can vary from delicate and invisible to coarse and visible. Other than underarms, which should not exhibit hair, hair removal is purely a matter of personal choice and comfort.

Depilatories

The hair can be removed in many ways. Some ways are better for certain parts of the body and some for certain types of hair. Whatever method you seek to use, always try it out first on a small, inconspicuous area and wait at least twenty-four hours. It may take this long for discoloration or irritation to develop. Experiment with a number of different methods before settling on the one that is just right for your hair and body area. This will save you much future time and grief. Never try to remove hair in a hurry or when emotionally upset. Contrary to belief, different methods of hair removal do not stimulate heavier or thicker growth. When hair is removed at skin level, the shorter hair that then grows appears to be thicker and stiffer but that is only because it is short and growing. When full grown it is exactly the same as the hair that preceded it. Our dark hair appears larger in circumference when very short and because it is dark looks coarser, but is in fact no thicker than before.

Shaving

Although this is the least permanent method of hair removal, it is the easiest and surest, especially if done while bathing. Let the water naturally soften the hair. Do not put a razor anywhere near the face or the vaginal area. All other areas can be successfully shaved using a woman's safety razor and shaving cream. Women who complain that shaving is difficult are usually found to be using a man's old discarded razor and ordinary soap. There is a reason for the size of a woman's razor—to get at the problem areas around knees, shins, and ankles. Proper shaving lather will soften and prepare the skin and hair for the razor. When shaving underarms, do not shave too close or you will remove the uppermost protective skin layer. When shaving the legs, avoid cuts by gliding from knee to ankle—down, not upward. Immediately after shaving, rinse very well and pat the area dry, never rub. If you have a delicate skin, pat on cold water or witch hazel and apply a body lotion.

BLEACHING

Strictly speaking this is not the removal but the disguise of unwanted hair. It is a temporary procedure possible when hair is fine but individual hairs quite numerous. Because bleach also dyes the skin as well as the hair, unless your skin is quite light in color the result may be an ugly yellowish tinge that emphasizes body hair. The chemical ingredients in hair bleaches are strong and can damage our skin. It is especially necessary to experiment on a small patch before using bleach extensively. At first it will sting and cause reddening. Be careful to keep well away from the eyes; when using near the face always cover the eyes with tissue and dab bleach on carefully. Always follow the manufacturer's instructions.

Bleach can be used successfully on the very light "fuzz" above and around the mouth and on the cheeks if you leave it on for at least one minute *less* than recommended to avoid yellowing. Wash off well with hot and cold water and then pat dry and apply witch hazel. Avoid using bleach near the abdominal region.

PLUCKING

This is not permanent because one does not destroy the hair follicle, although the mouth of the follicle is usually removed. Other than for the eyebrows, I only suggest plucking for isolated individual hair growth, not for removing abundant hairs like those that grow on the legs. Constant tweezing may create minute scarring. Never pluck hairs from moles because damage to a mole may have far-reaching consequences. For removal of scattered chin hairs by plucking, first soften with petroleum jelly and apply a steaming hot cloth for one minute. Then pluck, using clean tweezers.

WAXING

Warm wax in the form of a paste is applied to the hair surface, allowed to solidify, then stripped off, taking with it the hair. This method does not destroy the follicle but leaves a very clean, smooth skin surface because removal is very close to the root. For best results, waxing requires that the hair be fairly long, not just a stubble, and that it be stripped off in the direction of hair growth. Although this method can be applied at home, it is painful, and if the stripping is slowed because of pain, the waxing is much less effective. Waxing is particularly good for legs and for best results should be done by a professional in a salon. Before waxing, make sure the area is free from body oils, perfumes, talcum powders, and all cosmetics; it should be as dry as possible. After waxing, the skin will be sore for about ten or fifteen minutes.

ABRASIVES

Hair can be removed by the friction of pumice or sandpaper but this method is tedious, time-consuming, and invariably damages the skin. Our skins can be darkened by this action and it should be avoided.

CHEMICAL DEPILATORIES

These can come in cream, paste, foam, or liquid form. Because hair contains the same substances as skin, anything that can dissolve hair will also have a potentially negative action on skin. Chemical depilatories are beneficial for some women who claim that hair regrowth is slower with these methods than many others, but for us Black women the delicate pigmentation of our skin is such that these products should be approached with great caution and tested on small areas first. Never use on the face and always remove sooner than the directions indicate. Formerly these products had an unpleasant but characteristic odor, but now manufacturers are producing scented chemical depilatories. Use just before bath or shower so that all traces of the chemical can be removed.

X-RAY

For the treatment of certain skin disorders it is sometimes necessary to employ X-rays in such a way as to permanently destroy the hair follicle, but this method should never be used for purely cosmetic purposes.

ELECTROLYSIS

This method can be permanent but it is very time-consuming and requires a painstaking, fully trained professional. An electric needle is introduced into each hair follicle and the follicle is destroyed by a negative galvanic electric current. If done by an inexperienced operator, scarring can occur and less than half the hair follicles may be actually dead. Even a very good operator will have a 20 per cent regrowth rate, and few women realize that only a few hairs can be treated at a time so that many visits are required and so, of course, the method is not cheap. Because this hair removal does involve the

destruction of the hair root (papilla) by electrical means, it is not worth risking faulty procedures; so I firmly suggest that you never try this at home
because even if the home equipment is safe, you are not an expert. When
looking for an electrolysis operator, only use either a doctor of dermatology
or a person recommended by such a doctor. Your physician or any university-
affiliated hospital should be able to help you.

Chemical depilatories should not be used more frequently than every three
weeks, waxing can be effective for up to six weeks. Personally, I prefer a combination of shaving and waxing, depending upon the time of year and my
needs and activities.

Hair Removal Problems

If a rash or any form of irritation develops and does not cease after three
days, consult a doctor. When shaving, never let the hair grow longer than
one-half inch or the hair will pull and irritate the skin. If your hair is longer
than this, cut it first to that length. Because of the curly nature of our hair,
we are prone to ingrown hairs which can be encouraged by shaving very close.

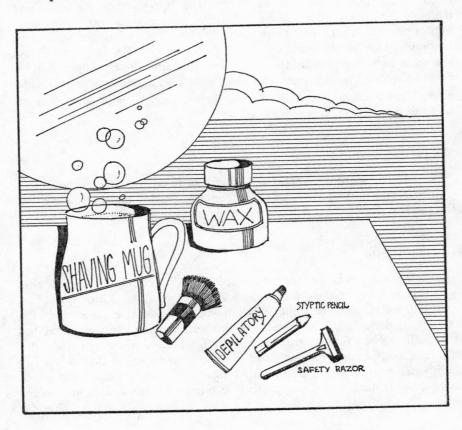

If the hair is ingrown, never try to remove it by plucking since infection can result. Waxing may remove it, or see your doctor.

Hair Removal Accessories

When shaving, there are two items commonly found in men's bathroom cabinets that we would do well to adopt. The first is a preshave conditioner that softens the hair, increases the effectiveness of the lather, and protects the skin. The other item we should not be without is a *styptic pencil*. This is inexpensive, long-lasting, and very easy to use. It is a bar of aluminum sulphate that is used to seal up nicks and cuts and immediately stop the bleeding. Just wet and apply. If you use a razor, you should own a styptic pencil.

Hair Removal from Sensitive Areas

PUBIC HAIR

The entrance to the vagina is protected by hair for a reason: to prevent bacteria from infecting that delicate part. Complete hair removal from the vagina can cause great discomfort, itching, swelling, and ingrown hairs, and the process of removing hair from that area is very tricky. It should only be done by qualified medical personnel. I do approve of the removal of hair from the inside of the upper thigh, which facilitates the wearing of brief swimwear. A so-called "bikini shave" can be accomplished standing in the shower with legs spread. Use a generous amount of shaving lotion and cut the hairs first if they are long. Shave very gently and always with a clean razor, never one that has been used elsewhere on the body. The safest method to remove hair from the inside upper thighs is by professional waxing. Do not use chemical depilatories, bleaches, abrasives, or electrolysis on this part of the body.

BREAST HAIR

It is quite normal for light hair to grow near the nipples, especially during pregnancy or when taking oral contraceptives. The only safe way to deal with this is to ask your doctor to make a referral. Do not try to remove it yourself. If it does not bother you, it is nothing to worry about, so just leave it.

F. BODY ODOR

In a recent article in the New York *Times*, discussing the dispensing of government grants to fund little-known projects, Dr. Laurence E. Karp, a professor of obstetrics and gynaecology at the University of Washington, mentioned that a study is in progress to investigate the smell of perspiration in Australian aborigines. Dr. Karp indicated how important this might be to our understanding of both race prejudice and the olfactory mechanism and continued:

> We've all heard at one time or another the complaint, usually made in a racist way, that "Negroes smell bad." And this is not a one-way street. In Stella Benson's short story, "Story Coldly Told," published in 1936, the native chief Rak Mandi says in disgust to his white captive: "Leave me. . . . You smell."

In fact, as early as 1903 it was established that quite separate racial scents existed for the Negroid, Mongoloid, and Caucasian races. This is further divided by climatic and nutritional differences. One of the largest body odor divisions is sexual in nature, separating women and men.

Although we tend to confuse body odor with perspiration, the latter has no odor when emanating from the profusely distributed eccrine glands. Offensive body odor occurs when this perspiration combines with the bacteria that is constantly forming on the surface of the skin. If this bacteria is not regularly removed, the smell is pungent and abnormal. On the other hand, our individual, sexual, racial smell is furnished by the apocrine glands that are located in the armpits, the anus, the nipples, the genitals, and the navel. These secrete a white, milky substance that carries our characteristic personal odor. Perspiration regulates the temperature of the body and should not be interfered with. If you sweat very heavily or not at all, you should see a physician. Disagreeable body odor is caused by lack of personal hygiene or an internal disorder. Avoid any medication for "preventing body odor" that has not been approved by your doctor. It may interfere with your perspiration and upset your body's metabolism. Body odor not caused by medical problems can be relieved by washing the body well and often with soap and warm water and by keeping one's clothes clean and fresh. Too often we fail to realize that although we are clean, our clothing has collected and retained bacteria and odors. The only place that deodorants or antiperspirants are needed is under the arms, and removing the hair from the armpits reduces the odor by a large degree. In Chapter VIII we examine feminine hygiene in detail, but it is important to note here that it is *not true* that bathing should be avoided by menstruating or pregnant women. In fact, more bathing is needed at these times and any increase in body odor during these periods is largely due to a belief in the old wives' tale and a lack of bathing, pure and simple. How frequently you bathe to remove odor-causing bacteria will vary according to your skin, the climate, and your occupation. Soap itself is a disinfectant, so germicidal soaps and deodorant soaps represent overkill; some of the "extra ingredients" may also irritate the skin.

Antiperspirants

These are products in cream, spray, liquid, or stick form that contain chemicals designed to prevent perspiration from reaching the skin's surface and, in effect, dry it up before it appears.

Deodorants

These are packaged in much the same way as antiperspirants but only disguise or counteract the odor caused when the perspiration reaches the skin's surface and mixes with bacteria.

Many products combine an antiperspirant with a deodorant. Try several before settling on the one for your skin. If used on the armpits just after shaving, a deodorant will sting because there are many invisible abrasions on the skin. Remember that you can become immune to one product after long use, so vary your purchases and always read the label carefully. If your skin is easily irritated, use a hypoallergenic deodorant. However, never believe that a body odor product is an alternative to careful and frequent washing.

Aluminum Chloride

Because I was brought up—as are most Americans—with cleanliness fever and body odor fetish and for years experienced the causes and effects of perspiration in the world of modeling, under hot lights and in crowded dressing rooms, I do not use a commercial antiperspirant or deodorant product but buy a liquid solution of 25 per cent aluminum chloride. This is the active ingredient in commercial deodorant products and is not only much less expensive when bought alone but it has no perfumed scent to interfere with the perfume of your choice or the body's own scent. Apply it with cotton under the arms and wait for it to dry before putting on clothes. For sensitive skin, dilute the cotton pad with water. Of course, discontinue use if a rash develops.

Fragrances—Toilet Water, Cologne, and Perfume

The ideal fragrance has immediate impact, diffusion, lasting properties, and individuality. Our ancestors, the ancient Egyptians, pioneered the use of perfumes, creating aromatic oils and unguents that were later adopted by the Greeks and Romans. The priests of the temples of Isis were particularly adept at creating scents from gums and wood. They were the first to learn what every woman must realize before she spends a fortune on advertised fragrances: a scent changes according to the wearer. No two women will ever smell alike wearing the same perfume. On one it may be heavy and disperse rapidly and on another be very light and last forever. In general, our Black

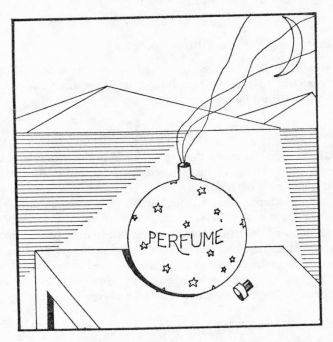

skins absorb scent heavily and diffuse it less. A personal refreshing scent is like a second skin after bathing. I use fragrance constantly throughout the day, changing with the seasons. If you stay with just one fragrance all the time, your nose may eventually fail to smell it at full strength, so you might be applying much more than you need. Check this and vary your fragrances. When shopping for fragrance, always shop alone; do not be influenced by someone else's taste and nose. If you know you are going out to buy perfume, wear none so that you can judge a fragrance well. Only try at most three per shopping trip. When testing, apply to the pulse at the wrist and *wait*. The alcohol must evaporate before the scent comes through. Sniff gently a few inches from the wrist. Keep away from clothing. The smell from the bottle itself is absolutely no indication of the true scent of the perfume or cologne. When buying, it is often a temptation to buy your favorite in toilet water or cologne and seemingly get more or less, but actually the perfume is a better investment and used sparingly will last much longer, being so much stronger.

Where to Wear Fragrance

After bathing apply in spots, just tiny dabs, to the warmest parts of the body where it will be encouraged to develop and rise. I place my perfume below the ear, at the throat, between the breasts, over the heart, inside the elbow, at the wrists, in the navel, behind the knees, and inside the ankle. Just before leaving the house I apply it to the temples and the nape of the neck.

Chapter VII

THE INVISIBLE BODY

———◆·◆———

We never feel or see what lies beneath our skin until our health is impaired. Our principal organs, the heart, the lungs, the stomach, the brain, the liver, and the kidneys, work unceasingly and are slaves to whatever rewards we give them or whatever punishments we inflict upon them. Sometimes unrelenting hard work is a reward for those organs that thrive on constant exercise. By the same token, to indulge in relaxation and pleasurable pursuits will punish the heart and the stomach that may be required to work overtime and irregularly without proper nourishment. We have to learn how to care for our organs and to maintain them for maximum survival. Since they are all dependent upon the food we eat, I shall begin with nutrition. As there is a direct link between health and beauty, so is there a strong and permanent bond between nutrition and health. We become what we eat.

A. FOOD

In this decade very few of our fellow Black Americans will die from starvation, but this does not mean that as a people we are properly fed. Once we could blame our state of malnutrition on circumstances virtually beyond our control; we ate only what we were allowed to eat. Now it is true that poverty and escalating food prices retard our ability to achieve a balanced diet, but the majority of us in all income groups consistently negate the goal of a balanced diet by injudicious shopping practices and a desire for prepackaged convenience foods that are sorely lacking in nutritional value. This is a desire we share with Americans of all colors, of both sexes, and from all walks of life. Most of us know that we are indulging in unhealthy foods and offer to make amends to our bodies by wasting money on useless food supplements or devastating our already ravaged systems with crank crash diets. To combat these aberrations, I have a very practical but firm approach.

Basic Nutrition

Who needs a balanced diet anyway? Did anybody die from an unbalanced diet? So long as the doctor knows what cholesterol is, why should I care? Flippant questions but all too common. Just one example might answer all of them. There are many Black women who after menopause become very susceptible to cholesterol build-up. This is one of three basic fats found in the body and derives from eggs, some seafood (especially shellfish), and butter-

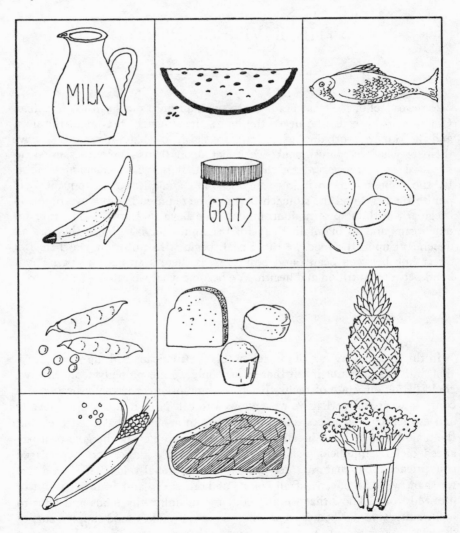

fat, among other common foods. Older women who become overweight often die at an early age from a stroke or heart attack, and the cause is hardened arteries, and the cause of hardened arteries is cholesterol. Everyone needs a balanced diet. Not only must you create out of your body a stronghold capable of repelling disease, but adequate nourishment builds healthy new tissue and makes the body resilient to the relatively minor but highly discomforting disorders of the urinary-digestive system such as flatulence, constipation, diarrhea, and all manner of stomach complaints. If certain essential vitamins and minerals are absent from your food, the condition of your skin, hair, teeth, and gums will deteriorate. Lack of calcium causes scurvy, and we must have some fatty acids to prevent the skin from scaling. If the damage to our pocketbook is severe at the supermarket check-out counter, we assume that we must be well fed. Not true. We can spend a lot of money on food and still be deprived of basic necessities. As Black women, we are getting sufficient nutrients, but our intake of high-calorie carbohydrates is too high and our diets are deficient in minerals such as iron and certain vitamins, especially vitamin A.

NUTRIENTS

These are the three major nutrients and examples of the foods in which they predominate:

Protein. Essential for the body's growth and repair: lean meat, poultry, fish, eggs, nuts, milk, and cheese.

Carbohydrates. Create specialized forms of energy for organs such as the brain, and contain vitamin B and iron: enriched bread, enriched cereals, flour, corn meal, grits, brown rice, macaroni, and spaghetti.

Fats. Are required for concentrated forms of energy and vitamins A, D, E, and K: corn oil, safflower oil, dairy products, beef, and pork.

Most foods consist of varying proportions of proteins, carbohydrates, fats, vitamins, and minerals. We must have moderate amounts of all on a very regular basis. This means eating a fairly wide variety of foods. It is common to think of proteins as "good" and fats and carbohydrates as "bad." All three are required and inherently positive. Abuse results from overindulging in certain nutrients to the exclusion of others.

Eating Habits

Our most ingrained prejudices are our food propensities and it would be a waste of space for me to fill these pages with nutrition charts and fictitious weekly menus that are unrealistic and unrelated to our eating habits. I can only point out what foods must be consumed on a regular basis. There is bound to be an important item like fish that you probably never cook at home and always assumed you did not like. If you make the effort just once a week to prepare and enjoy a fish dish, you will find that it makes a very appetizing yet economical addition to your menu and at the same time does not subvert a lifetime of eating habits. If you try out a new food by ordering it in a restaurant, you may simply confirm your dislike of it. On the other hand, if you shop for it, clean it, and cook it yourself, you will learn much more about that food, and this always increases the enjoyment. We must not forget also that as much as most of us enjoy "soul food," it developed out of exigency and as a steady diet is nutritionally deprived. It began as compromise cooking by our ancestors in this country but has little in common with the wide variety of indigenous gastronomic delights created by our Black sisters and brothers around the world. Our affection for soul food, its good taste, and symbolic meaning should not lead us to dismiss all other kinds of foods and cooking as "white." To do this would be to make the same mistake as millions of Americans who annually punish their bodies by consuming mountains of marbled steaks and greasy french fries and who then proceed to justify this self-inflicted damage-diet with the credo that any meal that cannot be found on lunch-counter menus is fancy or foreign and therefore unwholesome. We must all strive to achieve a balanced diet by becoming aware of the four basic food groups and varying our meals to encompass them all in correct proportions. It means extra attention to shopping and perhaps trying out new cooking methods. It does not mean spending more money for food and it definitely does not require us to switch to a difficult regimen of bland, uninteresting meals.

Basic Food Groups

1) DAIRY

This group includes evaporated, dry, and skim milk as well as homogenized fluid whole milk. The equivalent of two cups a day is a must. At least one cup should be in milk form. The other could be a portion of yoghurt, a large helping of cottage cheese, a slice of hard cheese (Cheddar, for instance), or a couple of scoops of ice cream.

2) CEREAL

Whole-grain bread, enriched bread, breakfast cereals, spaghetti, noodles, macaroni, rice, grits, corn meal, cookies, crackers, cakes, muffins, waffles, pancakes. We must have each day three slices of bread or the equivalent which would be four ounces of cereal or three medium-sized muffins.

3) VEGETABLES AND FRUITS

   a) Dark green and yellow vegetables for vitamin A:

Kale	Escarole
Spinach	Chicory
Mustard Greens	Peas
Collards	Green snap beans
Turnip tops	Green peppers
Dandelion greens	Carrots
Yams	Sweet potato
Broccoli	Winter squash
Cantaloupe	Tomato
Pumpkin	Mango
Peach	Watermelon

   b) Vegetables and fruit for vitamin C:

Oranges	Melon
Lemons	Cauliflower
Tomatoes	Asparagus

   c) For additional minerals and vitamins:

Apples	Potatoes
Bananas	Corn
Beets	Lima Beans

We must have a minimum of one serving from each category and a fourth serving from either a or b.

4) MEAT AND FISH

Beef, veal, lamb, pork, chicken, liver, kidneys, brains, all fish. Vegetarians can substitute eggs, dried beans and peas, soybeans, lentils, and nuts. The minimum daily requirement is six ounces of meat or fish or the equivalent (for instance four eggs).

It is hardly possible for me to list every food in each category, but what is important is the recognition that each food type must be present in the appropriate quantity in our meals every day.

Shopping

If you shop intelligently, your meals should be inexpensive, balanced, and gastronomically interesting. The secret of intelligent shopping is to concentrate on fresh, unprepared foods and to shun precooked, prepackaged products. The latter appeal to us enormously because of the mouth-watering illustrations on the box and the instructions that promise five-minute cooking time. In fact, we all know that the reconstituted, colorless food inside bears no resemblance to the artist's rendering, and usually the "five minutes" refers to just the simmering time after at least thirty minutes of cooking. What all of us do not know is that for nutrition, flavor, and price per pound we are cheating our pocketbooks and our stomachs by buying so much packaged food. The portions are small and the preservatives added for increasing the shelf-life of the product rob us of nourishment and taste. We save nothing—not time, money, or health—by purchasing TV dinners, canned meats, and prepared frozen vegetables. If it costs us fifteen or thirty extra minutes in the kitchen to clean, slice, and cook fresh food, that may be the most worthwhile time spent each day. Cooking is only a chore when it involves repetition and monotony. Experimenting with different ways of preparing new foods livens up the kitchen. Unless we all learn or relearn how to cook, all our cooking will soon be done for us by food conglomerates in factories utilizing tons of chemical preservatives.

DAIRY SHOPPING

Buy the local brand of whole milk for economy and freshness. Powdered nonfat dry milk is every bit as nourishing as whole milk and much less expensive. Mix it with whole milk to stretch the quantity. Yoghurt is really just an expensive way to purchase whole or partly skimmed milk. Store-bought yoghurt is particularly expensive when garnished with fruit. Buy plain yoghurt and add your own jam or fresh fruit or, better still, learn to make yoghurt inexpensively at home. Polyunsaturated margarine from corn oil does not build cholesterol nearly as fast as butter and, of course, is cheaper. Use it to spread and for cooking. Cheese is an excellent way to furnish yourself with your milk requirements, but avoid the cheese spreads and process cheeses which are full of water and preservatives. Much better is cottage cheese, pot cheese, or a large slice of cracker-barrel or unwrapped store cheese.

CEREAL SHOPPING

Nonenriched fluffy white loaves are the equivalent in taste and nutrition of flavored wet paper. "Enriched" means that the bread contains certain vitamins and minerals suggested and approved by the Federal Drug Administration over twenty-five years ago. Rye and pumpernickel are very nourishing and add variety. Never buy white rice unless it is also labeled "enriched." As an alternative, use brown rice, wild rice, barley, buckwheat, or cracked wheat. Presweetened breakfast cereals are quite low in food value; plain oatmeal and cornflakes provide more sustenance and are less costly. Unless you want to throw away your money, avoid one-serving boxes of cereal. The largest box of cereal is usually per volume the least expensive.

Vegetable and Fruit Shopping

Fresh. Get to know your counterman and ask him what just arrived. Examine produce very carefully. There are more than twenty year-round vegetables and almost as many seasonal ones. Cabbage, eggplant, zucchini, and beets are among the most nourishing and least costly. Lettuce is not a very good food; it is low in minerals and vitamins. Substitute dark green leafy vegetables such as kale for making salads. If you must buy prefrozen vegetables, at least shun the elaborate "vegetable dishes" that claim to be Hawaiian or Bavarian but are in fact glutinous with artificial preservatives. Buy the plainest frozen vegetables, without butter.

When buying fruit, try to avoid the overripe and the underripe. Certain produce such as grapes simply do not ripen after they have been picked and if you see tiny flies near any fruit you can be sure it is overripe. Look for small holes, bruises, and soft spots. Oranges and grapefruits are best when thin-skinned and apples should be firm and smooth. Bananas are probably the best all-around fruit for taste, economy, and storage. These you can buy when they are green and let them ripen at home. Apricots, raisins, and other dried fruits are good buys and much more nourishing than any packaged candy. The irony is that those ingredients that attract us to expensive confectionery (factory-produced cakes and candy) are the same fruits and nuts such as almonds, apricots, and coconuts that are plentiful and fairly inexpensive in most supermarkets.

Meat and Fish Shopping

Meat. Try to get the butcher to cut and weigh it for you. Most supermarkets can manage this unless you shop at the end of the day. The butcher will want to weigh the meat before cutting but, if you pay attention, you can get good lean cuts and save. Prime-grade meat is often not as lean or as nutritious as Choice or Good grade, which of course are far cheaper. Meat on the bone is very costly because you are charged meat prices per pound for the weight of the bone, which is sometimes one third the weight of the meat. A good buy is well-aged roast. Pork loin is nourishing and inexpensive, but it must be cooked to 160 degrees to avoid trichinosis, a disease not uncommon among our families. Bacon is mostly fat and processed meats such as frankfurter and bologna are sometimes as much as 50 per cent nonmeat. The label "100 per cent Beef" refers only to the meat portion of the product, not the whole product itself. The other half of the frankfurter is often fat, cereal, and water. Liver is an excellent source of protein. It does not have to be costly calves' liver; pork and lamb liver are less expensive than calves' or beef liver, and the taste and food value are the same. Canned stews and hashes are mostly potato filling and no bargain. Chicken is always worthwhile for price and nutrition. You will always save by buying a whole bird and cutting it up at home. At some times of the year turkey is less expensive than most meats and very good food value.

Fish. We neglect this excellent source of vital nutrition. You may find cleaning a fresh fish too messy, so buy fresh fish fillets which are often less expensive per pound than whole fish. When choosing fresh fish, the flesh should be resilient to the touch and the eyes bright, with no slime around the gills. I often buy porgy, which is available all year and is very flavorful but inexpensive. Only buy frozen fish if it is rock hard and never attempt to refreeze. Avoid breaded fish products like fish sticks which have more cereal and fish by-products in them than fish meat. Canned pink salmon and dark tuna or bonita are always cheaper than canned red salmon and white tuna and just as good. Add canned mackerel and sardines to your shopping list and, with tuna fish, you have a store of excellent proteins and vitamins. Use your imagination for serving these products that mix with practically everything and are wasted if simply slapped into a sandwich.

Enormous food savings are possible if you can invest in a freezer. You can buy in quantity when the price is low, and freezing keeps food fresh for months without artificial preservatives. This includes meat, fish, fruit, and vegetables. When freezing these, first remove all original wrappings and seal in moisture in vaporproof bags. Vegetables must be cooked first, about five minutes less than normal. Then freeze and when needed just thaw and heat.

Cooking and Nutrition

Certain methods of cooking and some cooking ingredients create an imbalance in the diet by depriving the food of its mineral and vitamin strength or by overloading the meal with saturated fats, as happens when one constantly fries food in butter or lard. Our native southern cuisine, for instance, although tasty and stomach-satisfying, provides the body with little protein and far too much fat and carbohydrate.

Many Black women, especially those of us like myself with recent southern backgrounds, use the top of the range too much. We prefer to fry our chicken and meat and boil the vegetables for too long. It is a fact that almost everything can be satisfactorily broiled or baked and these methods decrease the amount of excess grease and fat and are better for retention of nutrients in the food cooked. Use a meat thermometer and sometimes roast your beef or chicken. Add the vegetables to the roast about thirty minutes before serving. This will provide a more nourishing meal, save time and not leave a mess. Because we rely on vegetables for precious minerals and vitamins, here are some tips for preserving all the goodness, including color, flavor, and texture, in vegetables.

DO   Prepare at time of cooking, not before.
Start cooking in a small amount of boiling water.
Cover pan while cooking.
Cook only until tender.
Use the liquid from canned and home-cooked vegetables.
Cook vegetables with the skins on whenever possible.

DON'T Wash vegetables until ready to cook.
Keep vegetables in a warm place.
Soak vegetables in water.
Stir vegetables while cooking.
Thaw frozen vegetables before cooking.

Every individual and by extension every family, develops an eating routine and favorite dishes. This routine is almost impossible to change. It can, however, be supplemented by occasional forays into dishes and side dishes that are absent from your menus only because of lack of initiative. You probably do not really dislike salads but just always thought they were a bore to prepare. So, you systematically deny yourself the iron that all premenopause women require in large quantities and is present in dark green, leafy vegetables. The next time you have five minutes, make a quick spinach salad and dress it up with some favorite like hard-boiled egg or tuna fish. If you have this once or twice a week at lunch or dinner, you will decrease your diet imbalance without sacrificing any favorite dishes.

If you always keep in mind the four basic food groups and the need for balance among, and variety within, them, you will go a long way to achieving fully nutritious eating habits.

Food Supplements

Certain additives, such as vitamin D in milk, were deemed by the FDA to be essential to basic nutritional needs and are included in the production of cereal, bread, and other staple foods. These products are labeled "enriched" and the additive is usually announced on the package. Make these enriched foods your first choice; they are no more expensive than nonenriched products.

Chemical preservatives and dyes are present in most of the frozen, pre-cooked, and prepackaged foods that we buy. The federal regulations governing these substances need to be strengthened immeasurably. It has not yet been proved that occasional consumption of these products is harmful, but years and years of ingesting nothing but synthetically flavored, synthetically colored, and artificially preserved "junk" convenience foods deteriorates the system, weakens our defenses against infection and disease, and undermines our recuperative powers. Our alternative is to buy fresh food. As consumers we must convince the manufacturers that, instead of their investing millions of dollars in facilities to process and precook, we would prefer that food be shipped quickly to our markets uncooked and nonprocessed. It is possible today to ship fresh meat, poultry, fish, vegetables, and fruit anywhere in the country, but we are at fault for making convenience foods so profitable. Hardsell advertising convinces us to waste hard-earned dollars on simulated food. A seemingly pure-of-heart movement in the opposite direction has developed, but the profit motive is not entirely absent. I am referring to socalled "health" foods. Since the terminology used in connection with these products is vague and confusing, these definitions will help.

"Health food" is virtually meaningless as a label and is the equivalent of saying "food food" or "food for the body." A food producer can refer to a product as "health food" without having to satisfy any specific regulations.

"Organic food" means that the product was made from grain grown without the use of chemical fertilizer. Meat and poultry can be "organic" if the animals were raised without the use of chemicals to fatten or flavor them. By the same token, then, almost all fish is "organic."

"Natural foods" are those that have not been treated with sprays or chemical preservatives. Since most of these foods have to be preserved somehow, salt and sugar are usually found in them in abundance. Some "natural" breakfast cereals are as much as 20 per cent sugar—much more than regular presweetened cereals. This high sugar content is of no real value to your system other than to add calories. "Natural" foods are often lower in vitamin and mineral content than enriched products. You can bypass the high cost of these products and reduce your chemical intake just as well by shopping for fresh food.

Vegetarianism

Many Black families are eschewing the use of meat for many reasons, some religious and others more personal. You need not suffer nutritionally on a vegetarian diet so long as heavy reliance is not placed on a single plant source such as cereal grain. Certain high-protein meat alternatives must be consumed at a rate of two servings a day of any of the following: dark green leafy vegetables, nuts, peanut butter, dairy products, eggs, fortified soybean milk.

Vitamins

If you eat a balanced diet, you have absolutely no need for extra vitamins in pill form. The most pleasant and easiest way to consume your daily vitamin requirement is by eating proper food. Although certain vitamins can be taken in large quantities with impunity (many people believe large doses of vitamin C cure the common cold), others, such as A and D, are definitely toxic if taken in excessive quantities. Vitamin addicts are forcing their systems to deal with an influx of potentially harmful substances that do nothing but interfere with the function of the body. Only take supplemental vitamins for medical reasons and as prescribed by a doctor. Because vitamins can be purchased in any quantity without a prescription does not mean they are harmless. Supplemental vitamins are usually required only during, and immediately after, certain illnesses.

Weight Loss and Weight Gain

Most women arrive at their correct weight in their early twenties and gain steadily into middle age. This is not inevitable and is certainly not healthy, as well as being unattractive. Our desire to miraculously shed those unwanted pounds costs us almost twelve billion dollars annually. This accounts for diet plans, pills, injections, hypnosis, lotions, and machinery that all present the same extravagant claims. The phenomenon of the diet industry suggests an interesting dilemma: If any or all of the weight-reduction methods actually worked, the industry would be in serious trouble because everyone could get thin in ten days, stay thin, and spend no additional money on weight loss.

The majority of diet plans are hopelessly unrealistic. Some are downright dangerous to the health. Few take into consideration that the greater the change that has to be made in the woman's present diet the less likely she is capable of sustaining that change over a period sufficiently long enough to experience even temporary weight loss. In most cases the novelty of the plan wears off, no miraculous weight loss is evident, and the old, bad eating habits are returned to with a vengeance as the pounds pile on at an even more rapid rate than before. My single aphorism for would-be dieters is this: "If the weight change is to be permanent, the diet must be permanent." There is no other way. Every year new diet theories are touted by doctors and journalists in books, magazines, and newspapers. Most of them seem to me to have been designed with one particular woman in mind—a wealthy, unmarried mathematician. I deduce that she can obviously afford delicate portions of salmon and avocado and definitely does not have to work, or else she simply would not have the time to lovingly prepare three splendid little meals for herself every day. She is decidedly not married. No family, even assuming every member wanted to lose weight, would eat her meals. If they did, the children would die of malnutrition from night after night of dinners consisting of clear consommé livened up with a sprig of fresh parsley. Finally, our diet-conscious lady must be a mathematician to be able to calculate the correct percentage of niacin and pantothenic acid in each portion while she adds and subtracts calories at the same time. Since I am not, and most likely neither are you, a rich spinster computer, I will address my remarks to the woman who works during the day, either at home or outside, who cooks for others as well as herself, and who sometimes eats out at restaurants and friends' homes (where I consider it impolite to count calories, loudly or silently), and who has not the patience—let alone the money—to shop for strange, exotic delicacies that "melt away fat."

Weight Loss

Do not rely on a height-age chart to find your ideal weight; they are notoriously inaccurate and so generalized as to be virtually useless. Your doctor is really the only person qualified to help you make the judgment. Too often women are overambitious and the reason they fall five pounds short and give up is that the body needs those five pounds and will put up a massive fight to keep them. Unfortunately, too many women take their cues from fashion illustrations, not their doctors, and, in the fight to lose too many pounds, become part of the "yo-yo syndrome," always fluctuating between weight gain and weight loss. Not only does this destroy the morale but encourages rapid cholesterol build-up in the arteries. Women who know or suspect they have any ailments related to the heart, kidneys, or liver should not attempt any form of weight loss without a doctor's opinion. This is true too for women who are pregnant or diabetic.

The advice that follows is for the woman who is prepared to make a serious, sustained effort to get rid of five to fifteen pounds and stay that way. If you are obese, you must see a physician. The least of your worries is how you look; you may very well be suffering from high blood pressure.

1) Remember that high-cholesterol-saturated fats predominate in eggs, butter, milk, shellfish, pork, liver, brains, kidney, and heart. When possible, consume only skimmed milk, polyunsaturated margarine, brown rice, wild rice, green leafy vegetables, fish, chicken, and lean meats such as veal. Black women must get more into the habit of trimming all fat from meat before cooking. We love to cook with it and eat it—sheer folly.

2) We consume far more than we need from the Cereal Group at the expense of the Vegetable and Fruit groups. You can correct this by occasionally substituting cooked or raw vegetables or an apple for bread or pancakes in the morning.

3) Always eat three times a day. Ardent dieters usually starve until the evening, then, dying of hunger, guiltily eat a huge but hurried meal and compound the error by sleeping on it—the very best way to convert any food into fat. These women always wonder why they cannot lose weight on only one meal a day. Never wait until you are hungry. A hearty breakfast is very important for the dieter. You will work off the calories during the day, refuel with a fairly substantial lunch, and by dinnertime your stomach will still be full and your will power less taxed to enable you to eat only a moderate

amount and skip dessert. A light dinner is a much more successful dieting device than no breakfast and no lunch, and much healthier.

4) Steer clear of fried foods heavy with batter. Cook with margarine, not butter or lard. No matter what or how little you cook, if you use lard you will never lose weight.

5) My only absolute NO's:

No carbonated sodas	No peanuts
No cakes	No pretzels
No popcorn	No candy AT ALL
No potato chips	No other junk foods

Snack on fresh fruit, which is tasty and filling and not at all fattening unless you eat five oranges in ten minutes. Refined products such as white flour, white rice, sugar, and salt are low in vitamins, minerals, and proteins and high in preservatives and, therefore, calories. Avoid them as much as possible. Unless you live in the tropics or perspire profusely for some other reason, you need no more salt than is naturally contained in the food you eat; the same is true for sugar. Table salt and sugar are bad habits.

6) Foods marked "dietetic" are misleading. Most were developed for diabetic persons and contain no sugar. This does not mean the food is low in calories. A sugar-free cookie is still very high in calories. Dietetic products can be low in salt or sugar and very fattening. They may also be low in vitamins and minerals vital for the dieter.

7) Yoghurt and complete meals in package or liquid form should be used only sparingly as substitutes for real meals. Never try to base your diet on these products. You do not get sufficient nourishment and the lack of hunger-satisfaction inevitably precipitates an eating binge.

8) Diet pills are very dangerous. While containing drugs to curb your appetite, they can be ruinous to the health and have been known to produce seriously debilitating side effects such as extreme fatigue, vomiting, headache, and dizziness.

9) Completely avoid diuretics and laxatives. Diuretics rid the body only of water, not fat. Laxatives work by irritating the intestinal tract. Food is rushed through the system without adequate digestion and the body is deprived of nutrients and essential minerals such as potassium.

10) How you eat is almost as important as how much and what you eat. If you eat three meals a day instead of gorging yourself when hungry, you will be able to eat slowly and thoughtfully. It takes seventy-two hours for food to pass through your body and twenty to thirty minutes before the stomach signals to you it has received the food you sent down. Never eat a meal in less time than that or you will just keep on eating up to the moment the stomach says it's full. Spin out your eating time by chewing slowly and thoroughly. Wait between bites and wait at least five minutes between courses. We pile too much onto the same plate at the same time. Split your meal into courses

and eat the various parts slowly and separately. Eat everything on your plate but at the same tempo as you might imagine a very thin woman who hates food would eat.

If you are eating alone, it helps if you read while you eat. This slows you down and occupies your mind with something other than just feeding. With company, talk between bites and don't be afraid to put your knife and fork down for a while. If your family or friends complain about your slowness, tell them you enjoy eating and want to give your food a chance to digest.

11) Eight glasses of water a day do not a diet make. Six of these will pass through your system with no effect at all. Two per day are sufficient and since so much of your food is water, additional intake may only bloat the body. Alcohol is extremely fattening in all forms but some less than others. A glass of dry white wine will not make a big difference to your diet, but a couple of scotch-and-sodas will.

12) Weigh yourself every forty-eight hours and if there are two extra pounds, immediately cut out snacks, bread, and potatoes, and reduce the size of your portions until those two pounds disappear.

13) Never shop on an empty stomach. You will buy more than you need and fill the house with dangerously tempting in-between foods that will haunt you when you are hungry again.

14) Tell no one you are trying to lose weight. Instead of concentrating on your own private battle with the scales, you will be fighting everyone else's opinion of your relative success and failure and be on the receiving end of a variety of useless information, more a hindrance than a help.

If You Are Underweight

1) Tissue is built with protein, not carbohydrates, so eating huge quantities of bread and potatoes will not necessarily help.

2) Eat three meals a day—normal, balanced meals. Increase the quantity of your intake in equal measure, bearing in mind the four basic food groups.

3) Weight-gain pills and other products can be as dangerous as weight-loss drugs. Avoid them.

If you have no diseases, are relatively free from serious emotional problems, avoid junk food, and stick to a balanced diet, your body will find its own right weight and realistically you should stay with that. No diet program can be efficacious without exercise.

B. SMOKING, DRINKING, AND DRUGS

Our vital organs are required to handle a number of substances other than food that for one reason or another we force into our bodies. With the exception of legally prescribed medication, all nonfood substances introduced into the body are poisons. Their short-term and long-term devastation to the body and mind far outweighs the transitory satisfaction they create. Some of these poisons are uninvited invaders, such as air pollution. We can only prevent the high incidence of air pollution in our cities by forcing legislators to regard it as a very major health priority. Most of the poisons in our bodies are self-administered. A complex matrix of stimuli contributes to the desire to smoke, drink, or take drugs. Trauma, stress, tension, and anxiety as well as the desire to appear sophisticated and to be accepted by a particular group all play a major role.

Smoking

Quite apart from the known links between smoking and cancer, the habit has many other directly prejudicial influences upon the body. Tobacco tars irritate the mouth, throat, and lungs; night vision is impaired; nicotine creates specific changes in the nervous system and the voice; the entire circulatory system including the heart is impaired and the body's oxygen supply is altered; the liver and the kidneys have to cope with the excretion of raw nicotine; the digestive organs and all endocrine functions are upset. The more you smoke, and the longer you smoke, you are risking the following: cancer of the mouth; cancer of the larynx; cancer of the esophagus; chronic bronchitis; pulmonary emphysema; cardiovascular dysfunction; peptic ulcers, and cirrhosis of the liver—as well as accidental death from fire related to cigarette smoking. A woman who smokes more than one pack a day is five times more likely than a nonsmoker to die from disease. Why, then, have women become such avid smokers? Almost 40 per cent of the female population of this country are smokers, a phenomenal increase over the 15 per cent calculated in the 1920s. We take up smoking at a faster rate than males and we smoke to excess more than males. We are less willing to drop the habit than males and more likely to return to it if we do stop. Every day hundreds of fine young Black women are beginning to smoke. My mother did not start smoking until she was thirty. Twenty-five years later, she died of cancer. I still smoke ten or twelve cigarettes a day. I am not at all proud of that. Neither am I proud of the fact that as a model I participated in a national cigarette-advertising campaign designed to convince young Black women that smoking was the chic, liberated thing to do. Tobacco companies realized that women were becoming heavy smokers and encouraged sales by saturating the media with specious suggestions that to smoke is to be free, to be modern, to be antiestablishment. In fact smoking is a prison, a trap, an early grave. There is no one reason why we smoke. It is not a true addiction; our bodies will not collapse without it. We survive without too much agony when in a subway, bus, or other transportation, where we are forbidden to smoke.

SMOKING AND SKIN

Nicotine contracts tiny blood vessels and in time this causes a deterioration in skin tissue. Research not yet complete points to a definite correlation between heavy smoking and premature wrinkling in all age groups. Further tests are being made to investigate the possible connection between heavy smoking and the prominent wrinkling that is sometimes the early warning sign of heart trouble.

SMOKING AND WEIGHT GAIN

Women are convinced that if they quit smoking the pounds will pile on. This is by no means true for all women, or even most. When we stop smoking, the body does not require as much oxygen as before and this may lead to temporary weight gain; but the body adjusts in a matter of months. Those for whom oral gratification has been a major factor in smoking will want to eat more if they smoke less. They should resist reaching for the cookies and the candies and instead chew sugarless gum, drink soda water, and snack on fruit, carrots, celery. When you stop smoking, increase your schedule and breathe deeply. Given the choice, I would rather be fat than dead.

> **Warning:** The Surgeon General Has Determined That Cigarette Smoking Is Dangerous to Your Health.

TO STOP SMOKING

All smoking has a negative effect, but more than five cigarettes a day drastically increases the damage. I never chain-smoked, but I was in the habit of smoking ritually as I performed various tasks. I always smoked after eating, while telephoning, and when traveling. Without announcing to myself or any acquaintances that I was trying to quit smoking altogether, I managed to first stop smoking when on the telephone. Since my business activities demand a lot of office work, this reduced my daily consumption by about 50 per cent. I still smoke after eating, but less when traveling. I wait as long as possible before lighting up and occasionally reach my destination cigarette-free. There are many different theories about stopping the habit. Certainly filter cigarettes are less harmful than nonfilters, but beware of "low tar and nicotine" products. Some authorities believe that because these cigarettes usually contain a low grade of tobacco that is actually stronger, there are no health benefits. Admonitions such as to smoke only the first half of the cigarette and not to inhale are based on fairly sound advice, but if you continue to smoke in large amounts, the effect will be negligible. There are no magic routes to nonsmoking since your will is the prime factor. You must be completely motivated and willing to try and try again. Even if you fail a few times, you are actually strengthening your ability to finally stop as you learn about the physical and mental obstacles that must be overcome. It is helpful to utilize forms of therapy with yourself, giving yourself rewards or punishments. Many women are finding strength in numbers and forming group therapy programs. A drug has been developed to aid the would-be nonsmoker, Lobeline. This is only available by prescription in full strength but one product that does contain effective amounts of Lobeline is Nikoban, in chewing gum or lozenge form. Nikoban is recommended by health authorities and results are encouraging. Withdrawal symptoms from smoking can be severe, such as vomiting, headaches, irritability, extreme impatience, agitation, and insomnia. The strength of the symptoms is not related entirely to the amount smoked. Some women have stopped after sixty cigarettes a day and experienced only minor symptoms while others who smoked less than one pack per day have had extreme nausea. In either case the adverse effects rarely last more than one month. Compared to the extreme pain suffered by cancer victims, they should not deter any woman from deciding to give up smoking. Your doctor can be a great help when you decide to stop. Since the Surgeon General's report on smoking and cancer in 1964, over 100,000 doctors have given up the habit. We must also sum up all our will power to withstand the insidious campaigns of the tobacco merchants. Smoking is not charming, it is filthy and polluting. With characteristic lack of subtlety, cigarette manufacturers sponsor sporting events to instill in our minds the notion that smoking is a fresh, outdoor, exercise-related activity. This is ludicrous. Smoking raises the blood pressure, quickens the pulse, drops the skin temperature, increases the heart rate, and contracts the peripheral blood vessels. That is all the exercise your body gets from smoking—exercise that kills.

Drinking

Alcohol is an anaesthetic drug capable of causing euphoria, sedation, unconsciousness, and death. Alcoholism occurs when an individual so loses control of drinking that it seriously compromises physical and mental health, family life, social activities, and employment. Proportionate to our percentage of the population, we account for fewer heavy drinkers than whites, but we are still plagued by alcoholism. This condition has received scant attention, compared to the efforts being made to educate the white middle class about problem drinking. Such a social oversight is rooted in behavior patterns created during the slave period. In his 1882 essay, "The Best Slaves Got Drunk," Frederick Douglass states:

> Not to be drunk during the holidays was disgraceful. . . . When the slave was drunk the slaveholder had no fear that he would plan an insurrection or that he would escape to the North.

This attitude, somewhat updated, is still rampant among the arbiters of health and welfare programs who adhere to the viewpoint that alcohol abuse among whites is a problem but among Blacks is normal behavior. Because of this attitude there are no firm statistics covering alcohol abuse by Black women, but we do know that although almost 40 per cent of us do not drink at all, 11 per cent are heavy drinkers compared to only 4 per cent of the white female population. Many factors contribute to this including our prolonged history of suppression, the intense struggle for mere survival, and the pressures many of us endure trying to raise families on our own. We do not know exactly how alcohol intoxicates or how alcohol addiction develops. Each individual presents a different set of problems and there is no consensus about what constitutes the responsible use of alcohol. Those of us who drink only occasionally do so to a particular level of tolerance with no ill effects and every woman has her own limitations. Few of us realize, however, that alcohol is not a stimulant but a depressant. Because it tends to remove psychological inhibitions and induce uncontrolled activity, we incorrectly assume that our system is being stimulated. Some of us consistently seek to exceed our level of tolerance not because we enjoy drinking but because it temporarily suspends us from the necessity to face seemingly insoluble problems. The only way to avoid the casual abuse of alcohol is by always being aware of the amount we drink and how often we demand alcohol. There is no "less alcoholic" beverage. A normal serving of gin, whiskey, wine, or beer contains almost the same amount of alcohol. Sometimes we are pressured into drinking by an influential peer group that appears to admire the woman who dares to drink a little bit more than others. Often she refuses to admit to herself, let alone to her doctor or close friends, that she is a problem drinker. If you do enjoy the occasional drink and want to avoid becoming an alcoholic:

1) Never let anyone convince you to drink more than you want.

2) Sip a beer slowly all evening; mix wine with soda water for a long, tall spritzer; order grenadine and tonic for a tangy, elegant nonalcoholic drink that does not sound like fruit juice.

3) If you have not eaten, drink a glass of milk or have some cheese and crackers before taking alcohol. You need a buffer.

4) Drink no more than one glass an hour.

5) Avoid drinking alone and don't drink every day.

Alcoholism can be cured if it is viewed as an illness and isolated and treated at an early stage. There is no specific amount of drinking or number of years of drinking that makes one an alcoholic. The disease is very subjective and self-diagnosis requires ruthless honesty. Alcohol has cumulatively a more damaging effect on the body than heroin and one of the most likely candidates for cancer is the heavy drinker who is often also a heavy smoker. Studies have even determined that alcohol ingestion may initiate the typical symptoms of sickle-cell anemia. Heavy drinking damages the liver and the kidneys and plays havoc with the digestive system. Nutrition is seriously impaired since alcohol only supplies thousands of needless "empty" calories and no protein, mineral, or vitamin value at all. Drinking frequently inhibits the desire to eat and a balanced diet is impossible. Blacks buy more alcohol per capita than any other group yet also include more teetotalers per capita than any other group. To the Black woman who does not drink: Stay that way. To the Black woman who does drink: Keep it in moderation. To the Black woman who drinks heavily: See your doctor or hospital outpatient department as you would for any other illness.

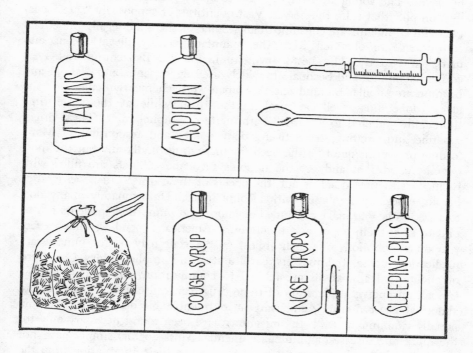

Drugs

All drugs, addictive or not, are potentially very dangerous. We are all aware of the social chaos caused by drug abuse and most of us are aware of the social and psychological conditions that breed drug abuse. Chronic injustice, poverty, and ignorance create the feelings of personal inadequacy, fear, and hopelessness that drive so many of our people to seek release in drug dependence. In drug abuse research and drug control programs there is a very strong male bias that not only prevents the female drug user from being identified but also reduces her chances of adequate treatment. It is generally conceded that there are more Black than white female drug abusers, but there are no national statistics available and this view may well reflect the racist attitude that pervades the opinion of the white establishment. What the drug-dependent Black woman must understand is that all forms of abuse produce rapid mental and physical deterioration which often constitutes protracted suicide.

LEGAL DRUGS

Our whole society is drug-dominated. The child is given a pill to stop a headache. The young adult takes a pill to stay awake and study. The adult lives on pills that calm the nerves. Vast quantities of supposedly "safe" sedatives and stimulants are consumed daily. Some of these are legally prescribed and others are obtained from the manufacturers by illegal means and marketed covertly. The best-known stimulants are Benzedrine and Dexedrine; Nembutal and Seconal are widely used depressants; and Valium and Librium are popular tranquilizers. A woman who vehemently denies that she takes "dope" may well be speaking the truth while at the same time thoroughly addicted to a "legal" barbiturate or amphetamine. These drugs, soporific and exciting, respectively, deny reality and responsibility. Many leading physicians question the need for these drugs under any but the most extreme conditions and yet the nation's medicine cabinets are filled with them. Legally prescribed or not, the effects of these drugs can be as fatal as heroin, especially combined with alcohol intake. Unfortunately, many doctors are too lazy to make a detailed diagnosis and pump their patients full of pills to keep them happy and functioning. Americans spend $5 billion every year on prescriptions of which almost 60 per cent may be for unnecessary medication such as tranquilizers, barbiturates, and amphetamines. One third of all hospital admissions are related to complications from drug therapy. Casual, unsupervised ingestion of these drugs can cause liver damage, create abnormal heart rhythms, and start uncontrollable bleeding. Even the supposedly vitamin-potent "B-12" injections have been found necessary only for the quite rare disease of pulmonary anemia. Most doctors simply have not the time to learn about new drugs, so they derive their information from the manufacturers who are naturally inclined to maximize the benefits and minimize the dangers of their product. If you suspect your doctor may be overeager to try out new pills on you and frequently prescribes combinations of drugs, then ask the following questions:

1) Will the drug react favorably with my blood chemistry?
2) If the drug is antibiotic, have you taken cultures?
3) What type of drug is this and how does it work?
4) How often and for how long should I take it?
5) Should I avoid any substances such as alcohol?
6) What possible side effects may occur?

Make sure that the doctor marks "label" on the prescription so that in case you experience complications you or another doctor will know the name of the drug and its strength. When filling the prescription, always ask the pharmacist to give you the insert, a leaflet explaining the properties of the medication. Check with the doctor when the period of medication is over and do not refill unless advised.

If you ignore the following, you may end up in a hospital with a severe drug reaction:

DON'T   forget to tell your doctor about every other medicine you are
              taking, even aspirin, vitamins, and antacid formulas.
DON'T   take drugs prescribed for someone else.
DON'T   take "old" drugs left over from a prior illness.

ETHICAL DRUGS

This term encompasses all the remedies that are available over the counter without a prescription. Many contain harmful drugs which when taken in excess are very dangerous. Always follow the directions carefully. Take such remedies only as the need arises and not from habit. It you receive no tangible results from such medication, discontinue its use and consult a doctor with your problem.

MARIJUANA

Marijuana is second only to alcohol in global use as an intoxicant. Very few countries permit the sale of marijuana and in some—for instance, Nigeria—the punishment for dealing in it is death. Proponents of the drug claim that it is harmless yet cannot deny that it loosens emotional and social restraints, creates temporal and spatial distortions, can produce mental confusion, anxiety, and paranoia, inflames the throat and bronchial tubes, and can lead to emphysema and chronic bronchitis. The fact that it may be no more harmful than smoking and drinking is a spurious argument since the latter can be very damaging, and their only very dubious merit is that they are sanctioned by society. Individual susceptibility to marijuana can vary widely and plant strength is quite unpredictable. What might be a very mild sensation for one woman could cause another to endure hours of mental anguish. There is a further danger in indulging in marijuana just for a casual thrill or experience and that is the increasingly popular custom of "spiking" marijuana by adding other drugs such as heroin, cocaine, or LSD.

HEROIN

The vicious cycle of heroin addiction can start at a very early age. The younger the girl is when she starts, the more difficult it will ever be for her to stop. Notwithstanding the fact that few can afford the cost of addiction without resorting to crimes such as theft and prostitution, many female addicts ignore the very real threat of hepatitis, syphilis, malaria, and tetanus present in each unsterilized needle they use. The female heroin addict becomes indifferent to food; appetite is lost and the consequences are malnutrition and total debilitation. The skin, the hair, and the teeth rot. Habitual use of heroin negates any euphoria that the new user experiences and the major stimulus for continued use is fear of the terrors of withdrawal. Some women are lucky enough to experience spontaneous withdrawal at the onset of middle age, but by then the damage to their bodies is quite unsalvageable. For many, addiction terminates in death or a lengthy jail term. Methadone is now being widely tried as a legally available alternative to heroin addiction, but for many it represents an equal evil. Now methadone addiction ranks second only to heroin as a major drug habit of Black women.

COCAINE

This drug, although very expensive, is becoming increasingly popular with some of our women. It is a fashionable and very potent stimulant that has gained ground, encouraged by the myth that it is not physically addictive and therefore can do no harm. A woman may have been taking cocaine for years or use it for the very first time and suddenly sustain direct paralysis of the breathing center in the brain. Death is instantaneous. The lucky woman may only undergo convulsions, tremors, and delirium.

If you have a drug problem, nobody can help unless you are motivated to make the first move. The impetus for treatment must come from you. If you have a doctor, she or he must be consulted to put you in touch with the most appropriate method of treatment. Most cities now have a telephone "hot line" that will immediately refer you to a group such as Synanon or a clinic that will provide help. Most hospitals are now equipped to deal with all kinds of drug emergencies. Go directly to the emergency room and insist on admission. You must be absolutely honest about what you have taken if you want help.

Combining Smoking, Drinking, and Drugs

Heavy drinkers are heavy smokers in most cases and the combination more than doubles the likelihood of cancer. Women who take drugs invariably smoke heavily to ease anxiety, and the smoking can be as harmful as the drug-taking. The combination of barbiturates and alcohol can be fatal even when only small amounts of each are ingested. In fact, combining any of these poisons simply multiplies enormously the damage they can do individually.

C. COMMON COMPLAINTS

Although we endure many minor aches and pains, three conditions are predominant among Black women and we cannot afford to ignore their persistence. These are fatigue, backache, and headache. They are not entirely unrelated and often spring from a common well of depression. Although they can cause acute discomfort, many of us are embarrassed to bring them to the attention of a doctor because we have been conditioned to consider them as very ordinary ailments that are part of womanhood. This attitude prevails strongly among our older sisters who frequently ignore these complaints for years while stoically tending the needs of their families and friends. Unfortunately, the complaints do not decrease with age but gradually worsen. They are seldom fatal but often indicate the presence of a serious illness among the aged. Do not take any of these minor pains for granted. In the majority of cases, their origin is emotional and the result manifests itself in very tangible pain.

Fatigue

All of us at some times in our lives go through periods of feeling sluggish, useless, completely worn out, and indifferent to our circumstances. We feel helpless and guilty. This fatigue may not necessarily strike after strenuous effort or intense work but can occur while on vacation or even after having relaxed. This makes it all the more puzzling and misunderstood. Fatigue is the result of the failure of the basic metabolism to adapt to stress. We are each born with a specific, different metabolism. This consists of all the biochemical changes that occur in the living cells of the body. The metabolism is regulated by the nervous system and the glandular system. These are genetically controlled and environment has little effect on them. Since we cannot suit our metabolism to our life style, we must, if we wish to avoid fatigue, suit our life style to our metabolism. Every woman is not the same. One might collapse each afternoon with no energy to go on, fiercely jealous of a neighbor apparently capable of working and playing nonstop into the night. Another woman might find the mornings to be the most catastrophic time of day when she cannot, for all the good will in the world, summon up the ability to be bright and cheerful and talkative. I know one woman who led an intensely hard, active life, working and single-handedly raising a large family with no real tinge of fatigue. After her children were grown and she could afford some leisure activities, she was beset by an awful lethargy. That may well have been a legacy from the years of hard work. Your stress threshold may be high or low, but it is fixed. Instead of feeling guilt-ridden about your lazy periods, try to predict when they happen and make allowances. If you follow a system of regular exercise and good nutrition, you will limit your attacks of fatigue. Try to vary your daily or weekly schedule. Fatigue is increased by monotony. The same breakfast, the same bus, the same faces, the same lunch all hasten sluggishness. Change your route to work if you can, or your system of shopping. If television is your main source of entertainment, read more or take up a nonenergetic hobby such as knitting or crocheting, as our grandmothers did. Proper rest is essential and if you are a woman who must have a quiet hour during the day in order to make it through the evening, then make no bones about taking it and do not let your family make you feel irresponsible. Beware, though, of oversleeping which often stimulates a pattern of fatigue and a cycle of eternal tiredness. Try to understand your personal metabolic pattern and adjust to it. Never let yourself be fooled into thinking that fatigue can be combatted by drugs or vitamins; these can only postpone the effects of fatigue which will inexorably build up. If you consult your doctor about fatigue, be very specific and tell her or him exactly when you get tired and for how long; express honestly what you feel it might be connected with.

BACKACHE

There are two major causes of backache. The first is sudden stress backache, as in lifting or pulling. This often causes the ligaments and spinal vertebrae of the back to move out of alignment. The second kind is caused by a pattern of inactivity that leads to persistent strain on the back and the result is a nonalignment of muscle, ligament, and vertebrae. Both kinds can result in what is commonly called a "slipped disk." This is a picturesque term that hardly conveys the correct situation. The jellylike substance (called disks) connecting the twenty-four detached vertebrae may leak in parts and press on a sensitive nerve ending; we call the result a slipped disk.

Sudden-stress backache. Can be avoided by NOT:

1) Leaning out and over as one does across a wide sill to open a window.
2) Lifting a heavy object while the body is twisted.
3) Bending straight-legged to pick up objects from the ground. Always bend the knees, crouch, and as you rise hold the object close to the body.

Inactivity backache. Has many complex and varied causes. The emotions play a major role and depression and tension often cause the back muscles to become hyperactive and tighten. The pain that results deepens our depression and a cycle has begun that may be hard to break.

Women who are overweight are most prone to back problems and sometimes the most effective treatment for back pain is not surgery but the shedding of a few pounds. The key support for the back is the stomach muscles, which must be strengthened by exercise to become effective. Correct footwear and posture reduce the possibility of back problems. Our natural instinct when suffering from throbbing back pain is to rest by sitting or lying down and generally treating the back as if it were made of glass for an hour or a day. This may be precisely the wrong thing to do. Of course all serious pain must be referred to a doctor, but most frequently the advice given is to increase your exercise, not diminish it. There is a very simple exercise that has often relieved my minor backaches; it can be done anywhere and in any clothes. Lie face down across a bed, table, or desk with your hips at the edge and your feet on the floor. Raise the legs horizontally and hold for as long as you can. Rest feet on the floor for a few seconds and repeat four or five times. Then lie across the same surface face up, and again raise the legs and hold. The very best antidote to back pain is regular exercise and one of its major causes is unpremeditated, sudden spurts of exercise that are irregular and infrequent. If you do develop chronic back pain, you must consult a physician. Definitely do not wear braces or corsets without a doctor's advice. If the doctor advises surgery, I suggest you get a second medical opinion since spinal surgery is not only very expensive but, with hysterectomies, accounts for the surgical procedure most often performed unnecessarily. Women who work in a seated position are very prone to backache, and if you are seated for most of the day, try to shift your position frequently and use supportive, straight-backed chairs. The majority of the furniture we buy—beds, chairs, and couches—are murderous for our backs. They may have a luxuriously soft, cloudlike appeal but without firm support your back will be ruined.

Headache

Headaches have many possible causes, including allergy, eyestrain, high or low blood pressure, kidney disease, digestive disturbance, brain-tumor neurosis, and hangover. If your headache is strong and frequent, do not try to diagnose and treat yourself, but see a doctor. There are two common forms of headache.

1) *Tight-band.* As the name implies, this is caused by muscle contraction and feels like a clamp on the skull exerting pressure usually on the sides of the head. Depression and fatigue often bring on this type of headache. Aspirin may dull the pain for a while but it cannot correct the source of the discomfort. Whenever possible, at the onset of this type of headache you should try to change your activity and pace. If you have been very busy, lie down. If you have been relaxing, get busy.

2) *Migraine.* One out of every ten Black women suffer from migraine

and although the pain can be excruciating, many of us attempt to ignore it. Little is yet known about the causes of migraine, but it is vascular in origin and confined to one side of the head. The blood vessels first become constricted and the pain occurs when they then dilate. Some doctors believe migraines are related to hormonal change since they are most common in women between the ages of twenty and forty and often disappear after menopause. There is substantial research to indicate that there are genetic factors involved and that the proclivity to migraine is inherited. There is no cure for this condition but it can be successfully treated. Too many women increase their acute discomfort by attempting to allay the pain of migraine by taking standard headache preparations such as analgesics and sedatives. These will have little or no results. You must see a physician. Strong medications have been developed for migraine sufferers that are only available from a doctor. The most commonly prescribed include drugs such as methysergide and propralol which have met with considerable success. Recent experiments with biofeedback and acupuncture have reported easing migraine pain, but not nearly enough research has yet been done in those areas.

D. MAJOR DISEASES

Life expectancy for the Black male is sixty years and for us, sixty-six. It was forty-five for Black women in 1920. More research is now being done in exclusively Black diseases and more information is available to us about others that we are particularly susceptible to. Other than certain genetic diseases such as sickle-cell anemia, most of our killers can be rendered harmless if detected soon enough and correct health-behavior patterns followed. I shall outline the main threats to our health other than those such as cancer of the cervix and cancer of the breast that are related to our reproductive systems and are discussed in Chapter X.

High Blood Pressure

The correct name for this condition is "hypertension," although that is a misleading appellation since to most people it implies a state of tension related to the nervous system. That is quite wrong. Hypertension, or high blood pressure, eventually manifests itself very tangibly and is responsible for a number of different types of fatalities. It is our number-one killer. It is by no means confined to the Black race, but the incidence of high blood pressure is far higher among Blacks than whites and far higher among Black women than any other group. It is a disease no Black woman can afford to ignore since at least 25 per cent of all American Black women suffer from it. No race-related factors have been isolated, but certain genetic tendencies are evident. If your mother or grandmother suffered from it, there is a very strong possibility you will also. It strikes hardest at lower-income groups (Black and white) and it is thought by most experts to be directly related to psychological stress and several contributing factors, some hormonal and others nutritional. Permanent high blood pressure can be caused by a mosaic of interlocking factors such as anxiety combined with an overweight condition, aggravated by excess salt in the diet and heavy smoking. One consolation for Black women is that somehow we are better able to cope with the disease and we are less likely than the male to die from high blood pressure. However, this does not mean that we are immune from its ravaging effects on the system and its ability to predispose us to contracting other fatal diseases. When the blood pressure exceeds what is considered to be normal, a number of chain reactions are set in motion that lead to heart attacks, strokes, arteriosclerosis, and kidney disease.

Heart attacks. These are caused by the heart being forced to pump harder as the walls of the blood-carrying arteries weaken. The eventual result is congestive failure.

Strokes. The arteries of the brain are more fragile than elsewhere and when they weaken sufficiently, hemorrhaging occurs in the brain. This is called a stroke and can cause partial paralysis or death.

Arteriosclerosis. High blood pressure increases the build-up of calcium and cholesterol in the arteries. This can thicken them and in time the blood supply is choked off from the brain and the heart.

Kidney disease. This is sometimes attributable to high blood pressure in cases where the blood supply to the kidneys becomes diminished and the filtration units in the kidneys that form urine are destroyed. Uremic poisoning is the result and this is often fatal.

The real insidiousness of high blood pressure is that there are no symptoms. Until you have a fatal or near-fatal stroke, you may not know you have the condition. There are no warning signs. Popular belief is that headaches and dizziness presage and herald high blood pressure. That is a dangerous myth. The only way to find out if you are suffering from high blood pressure is to have your pressure checked. This is a quick, absolutely painless procedure that only requires you to bare your upper arm. Half of our women with this condition do not know it. Of those who are aware, only one in five is receiving proper treatment. There are still a few doctors who are not enlightened to the absolute seriousness of high blood pressure (for many years it was thought to be a very minor condition attributable to age), which is why we must not remain in ignorance about it. It can be prevented or reduced. Specially formulated drugs such as Aldomet and Ismelin have been developed that are sometimes prescribed in conjunction with a diuretic to rid the body of excess salt. These drugs can have uncomfortable side effects, but an experienced physician can prescribe a personal formulation without untoward side effects. Because high blood pressure builds dangerously during the years between thirty and fifty, we must establish a pattern of protection that will reduce the likelihood of serious illness. All-round good health, exercise, and nutrition are the key elements in this. Since mental stress and obesity make a perfect match to spawn high blood pressure, we must stop smoking, lose weight if necessary, exercise regularly, and eat balanced meals. It sounds boringly familiar, but not only will that regimen keep you beautiful, it may well save your life. The most difficult cause of high blood pressure to eradicate is stress. As we struggle for a better life, beset by frustrations that produce fear and anger, an intolerable strain develops that is often compounded by a low salary and a poor education.

Systemic Lupus Erythematosis

Commonly known as SLE, this is an arthritic disease that takes its highest toll among Black women. The causes are still being investigated and there is no known cure, but at least nowadays it is being correctly diagnosed. In the past, white doctors often confused the symptoms with those for syphilis, with which SLE is not remotely connected. Such diagnostic prejudice is still quite common in certain areas where simply because of racial prejudice white physicians expect to find a high incidence of venereal disease among their Black female patients and will often ignore other, more likely explanations for some symptoms. Medication is now available that can ease the pain of SLE and sometimes prevent permanent damage. SLE is a breakdown of the natural defense systems of the body. Instead of manufacturing substances that ward off infection, the body seems to turn on itself and develop substances that attack the kidneys and the linings of the joints. Symptoms include fever, pain in the joints, extreme fatigue, kidney dysfunction, and often a butterfly-shaped skin rash on the face similar to chloasma. As with chloasma, exposure to the sun aggravates SLE. In some instances of this disease, significant hair loss has been recorded. Sometimes SLE can stop of its own accord and remissions are fairly common, although all sufferers must take constant medication and have frequent examinations. If the disease is allowed to progress unchecked, death can occur. The Arthritis Foundation is attempting to educate all of us about this disease and organize groups of victims who find that being able to share the burdens of SLE and discuss common problems help to alleviate the mental anguish.

Sarcoidosis

Sarcoidosis is a disease akin to tuberculosis that can debilitate any organ in the body and which primarily attacks American Blacks and especially women. It can be diagnosed and if detected soon enough can be controlled.

Sickle-Cell Anemia

Sickle-cell anemia receives the lion's share of attention as a "Black disease." It affects one Black person out of every five hundred. It can only be transferred genetically and cannot be "caught" as one would catch a cold. It is not infectious. One gene from each parent must be impaired in a specific manner to produce a child with sickle-cell anemia. The hemoglobin is abnormal and crescent-shaped (hence the name), and red blood cells are systematically destroyed. Many born with this do not live past the age of ten. Sickle-cell anemia is as common in Black men as Black women.

I have singled out those afflictions that Black women are particularly and often exclusively vulnerable to. We must remember also that we are not immune to other grave causes of death that reach all Americans. Cancer, diabetes, pneumonia, cirrhosis of the liver, and many diseases of the heart kill a lot of us every year. Few of these deaths are inevitable. The key to prevention is early diagnosis and treatment. The only way this can be done is by submitting to frequent voluntary checkups.

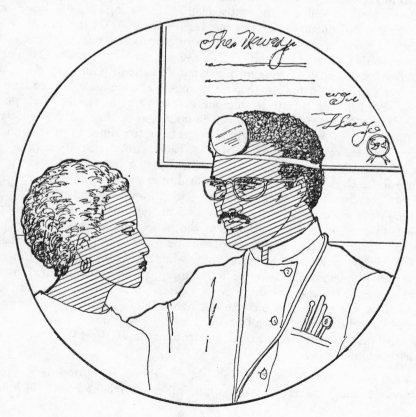

E. THE ANNUAL CHECKUP

We cannot be too young or too old to be excused from this absolutely essential life-saving practice. No history of blooming good health protects you from the crippling onslaught of a sudden, symptomless disease. Some of us have doctors whom we visit regularly. Unfortunately there are many, many Black women who have no private physician and the only time they see a medical facility is in an emergency. Often, this is too late. The overwhelming reason for this neglect is financial. Until our federal government is willing to spend as much of our taxes on health as it does on war, we will never aspire to that keystone of democracy whereby standard health care is provided equally for all citizens regardless of race or ability to pay. Even as we pressure our city, state, and national legislators to achieve this, we must survive under the present haphazard and elitist system of health care. Far too many doctors choose the lucrative fields of specialization, and the general practitioner of former years is a dying breed. Fortunately there are a number of internists trained in various branches of internal medicine who are prepared to work as family doctors and who are eminently qualified to do so. This still leaves us woefully short of doctors to service our vast population. Of the existing approximately 360,000 physicians in this country, only 2½ per cent are Black and of course only a tiny percentage of that 2½ per cent are female. Our goal should be Black female doctors for Black female patients. Currently those of us who can afford a doctor usually have to endure a white male. The rest who cannot afford or find private doctors are at the mercy of the hospitals and clinics. There are many excellent clinics in operation throughout the country, but there are also many fly-by-night organizations that operate in the inner cities purely for profit and provide totally inadequate service. Even in a responsible clinic the organization is more like that of a factory than a medical facility and each doctor may have a work load of anywhere from thirty to fifty patients per day. Under such conditions, it is impossible to establish any personal rapport essential to a doctor-patient relationship. One is lucky enough to get a doctor who recognizes the patient twice running. We are treated like cattle and emerge confused, humiliated, and abused. It is no small wonder that so many of us are loath to go voluntarily for a checkup. But no matter how embarrassing or uncomfortable it may be, we must fight for a checkup once every year at least. Our lives deserve it and our bodies must be strong if we are to fight to increase our rights. The following *must* be performed for a checkup to be at all worthwhile. No matter whether you go to an expensive private doctor or a hospital outpatient clinic, you have to demand these procedures.

1) On your first visit the doctor should take down your complete medical history, including any serious illnesses and minor complaints, and also infor-

mation regarding your occupation, diet and any current or recurring emotional problems. It is vital that you be absolutely candid with the doctor since these facts can be crucial to correct diagnosis and treatment. If it is not your first visit, the doctor should have consulted your file and become reacquainted with your history.

2) The doctor must conduct a complete and sound head-to-toe physical examination. This involves some prodding and pressing but it should not be painful or demeaning.

3) The doctor makes four vital laboratory studies:

    a) Blood pressure
    b) Blood examination
    c) Urinalysis
    d) Pap smear.

The last three involve taking samples which are then sent to a laboratory for examination and testing. These four procedures can detect almost every known disease, including potential cancer, heart trouble, diabetes, and tuberculosis.

4) The results of these tests may indicate to the doctor that further examination is necessary, perhaps with the aid of an X-ray machine or electrocardiogram.

The above procedures can hardly be performed in less than thirty minutes. Too many physicians get away with giving poor patients a ten-minute "quickie." They take the blood pressure, listen to the heart, touch the stomach, and take a urine specimen. This is a short cut to disaster and you must not allow it. It may not uncover serious illness. If you have a complete annual checkup, disease that otherwise might cripple or kill can be isolated, treated, and often cured. There is no short cut to this complete examination and you cannot give yourself a checkup. Remember also that the pharmacist is not a doctor. The pharmacist is not qualified to practice medicine, so to tempt the pharmacist to overstep the boundaries of competence by taking all your afflictions straight into the drugstore is seriously compromising your health. In an emergency, if you cannot reach a doctor, do not wait for one but call the police or fire department and ask to be taken to the emergency unit of a large hospital. If you have a choice, the nearest one that has a college affiliation will probably provide the best care. Doctors in training at university hospitals are both numerous and conscientious.

The right to basic health care, including regular preventive examinations, is as important as any other civil right. In these times it is a right enjoyed only by Black and white Americans who can afford the ever-increasing costs of private medical practice. Doctors are among the wealthiest of our citizens, and many hospitals are run as profit-making operations while millions of us must endure facilities that are solely crisis-oriented because they are so overcrowded and understaffed that the concept of preventive medicine is like a bitter joke. With services inadequate for the fatally ill, how can time and money be spent for the apparently healthy? But spent it must be. Few priorities are more urgent than health care and I urge every Black woman to bombard her local authorities and elected officials with demands for Health, without which we have no Welfare and certainly cannot enjoy any form of Education.

Emergency Treatment for Internal Disorders

CHOKING WHILE EATING

Lay victim on her side and give only one swift slap between the shoulder blades. Open the mouth and remove food with fingers. Use a spoon to hold down the tongue if necessary. An alternative method is to grasp the victim from behind with both hands just under the rib cage and with a sudden tug pull hard against her upper abdomen. This compresses the lungs and propels the food out of the windpipe.

POISONING

If you know that the substance is not a very strong acid (carbolic) or alkali (such as ammonia), induce vomiting in the victim and first give several glasses of water. If the poison is known to be a strong, damaging substance:

Acids	two teaspoons of baking soda in water
Alkalis	lemon juice or vinegar in water followed by milk
Gasoline	four or five glasses of water

STOMACH PAIN

If the pain is on or near the lower right side, suspect appendicitis. Do not give any food or laxatives and keep patient lying still. Give nothing to drink and contact a doctor.

HEART ATTACK

If you suspect this, call an ambulance immediately. Do not force the victim to lie down, but steer into a comfortable position and loosen all tight clothing. Give nothing to drink and above all try to keep the victim calm and reassured.

Heartbeat but no Breathing

Remove any obstructions from mouth and throat and prepare for mouth-to-mouth resuscitation.

1) Lay victim on her back. Place one hand under neck and tilt head back by raising neck.

2) Pinch nostrils shut with free hand and place mouth directly and entirely over victim's mouth and blow hard to make the chest rise. If the victim is a child, place your mouth over both her nose and mouth.

3) Repeat this at a rate of one vigorous breath every five seconds. If no air is being exhaled, check again for mouth and nose obstruction. If necessary, turn victim on her side and slap between the shoulder blades to remove matter from the throat. Keep up the resuscitation until the victim breathes alone.

No Heartbeat and No Breathing

Lay victim flat on her back and kneel at her side. Strike breastbone sharply with your fist. This may start the heart. If not:

1) Place one finger of your left hand on the cartilage located at the lower tip of the breastbone.

2) Move the heel of your right hand (never use the palm) against the finger. Place the left hand atop the right.

3) Push down with a firm thrust, using your back and body for leverage. Lift and press again. Keep this up indefinitely.

4) If you are alone, stop after every fifteen presses and administer mouth-to-mouth resuscitation (see above) at the rate of two breaths for every fifteen presses. If you have help, they should administer mouth-to-mouth resuscitation at the rate of one breath for every five presses.

Chapter VIII

THE REPRODUCTIVE SYSTEM

What distinguishes us so marvelously from the male is the incredible equipment we all possess that renders us capable of ensuring the continuity of our race. Most of our organs of reproduction are hidden within our bodies and far too many women live in total or partial ignorance concerning their functions. These organs play a major role in our development from childhood to old age, yet we know far more about the care of our hair and nails than we do about the care of that part of our body that is the cradle of life itself. We simply cannot allow the physician, in all likelihood a white male, to have total control over our childbearing faculties. That responsibility is unfair to us as women and Blacks and very unfair to the doctors who have to repair so much damage caused by sheer ignorance. As with any other part of the body, we must understand enough to know how we function as women, what the various parts are for, how to keep them clean and healthy, and how to spot any kind of abnormality before it becomes serious. It is impossible to do any of this if we persist in regarding our genitals as either "dirty" or embarrassing and therefore not fit for discussion or thought. There is nothing more immoral than a woman who allows her body to decay because she is too embarrassed to examine herself and too self-conscious to seek proper help.

A. ORGANS OF REPRODUCTION

We are all, of course, familiar with the *vagina*, but other than its location and partial functions, that is about all. In fact, the vagina is a short sleeve of muscular tissue lined with mucous membrane. The opening of the vagina is surrounded by the *labia* or lips. This opening, together with the labia and the clitoris, constitutes the *vulva*. The *clitoris* is a small, erectile organ equivalent in position to the male penis (just as the male has nipples) that is an important source of sexual gratification. The vagina leads directly to the *uterus* by way of the *cervix*. The cervix is simply the neck of the uterus, a pear-shaped

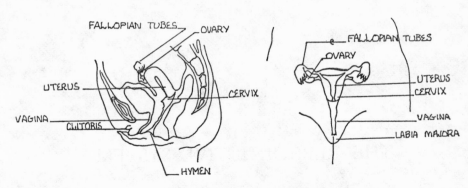

muscular organ about the size of your fist. The uterus is also known as the womb and is quite hollow, lined with endometrium, a blood-rich mucous membrane. From the uterus, one on either side, extend the *Fallopian tubes*. These are short, slender ducts the ends of which envelop the *ovaries*. We have two ovaries, each the size and shape of a large walnut. They and the uterus and the Fallopian tubes all lie in the pelvic cavity corresponding to the lower abdomen. The ovaries are really the "brain" of the reproductive system. They secrete two important hormones, estrogen and progesterone, that are vital for conducting the changes that occur as we pass from puberty to adulthood and then to menopause. The ovaries also produce ova (singular: ovum) which are literally the eggs that mature at the rate of one a month and cause the menstrual cycle unless, of course, one is fertilized and a fetus, or unborn child, develops.

The opening of the vulva may be partially closed by a mucous membrane called the *hymen*. The presence or absence of this tissue is often erroneously considered to be a determination of virginity. In fact, a woman's hymen may be absent from birth, accidentally ruptured, or removed for medical treatment. Conversely, women who have borne children have in some instances retained an apparently intact hymen.

Urinary-Digestive Tract

Our organs of reproduction are located in direct proximity to the urinary-digestive tract, which makes both doubly vulnerable to infection. For this reason we must be aware of three organs not unique to the female but which, because of their function and location, have strong bearing on the considerations of this chapter. The *bladder* is located between the pelvic bone and the uterus. It is a membranous, sacklike organ that serves as a receptacle for fluid and gas.

From the bladder to the exterior of the body extends the *urethra*, which is simply a membranous tube that carries waste liquid (urine). Because the urethra is relatively short and its mouth located in direct proximity to the vagina, the possibility of bacterial contamination from one to the other is always possible. Likewise the *rectum*, resting between the spine and the uterus, leads to the anus which is also very close to the vagina and through which waste solids are passed.

The Breasts

We tend to be very concerned about the size, shape, and relative firmness of our breasts and in doing so forget that their primary function is not decorative or as a source of sexual gratification. They are, in fact, extremely complex, functional glands and their main purpose is the production of milk. Men also have vestigial breasts, but in the male they are without anatomical

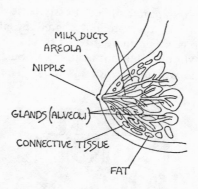

function. Each of our breasts contains seventeen *alveoli*. These are small, cell-like cavities that produce milk and each has a duct leading to the end of the nipple. The breast itself consists of fatty tissue that holds and protects the alveoli. This tissue also connects the breasts to the chest itself but in the breasts there are no muscles. Women can lead totally productive lives after breast removal, but that does not contradict the fact that the breasts are very important to the reproductive system. Do not be alarmed if you notice that one breast is slightly larger than the other. The left breast of most women is larger than the right because it is nearer the heart and receives a slightly increased supply of blood. Other minor abnormalities such as hair around the nipples, bumps, or dark spots on the nipples are no cause for alarm and may be caused by hereditary factors or hormonal changes. If they upset you, consult your doctor. Breasts contain no muscle tissue, so exercise cannot have any effect on the size or shape of the breast itself. There is muscle under the breasts, however, which can be developed to alter the apparent size and shape of the bosom. Weight gain and weight loss caused by dietary changes are often reflected in the size of the breasts. Excessive change in weight can cause permanent alterations in the size and appearance of the breasts because the skin is stretched or loosened and the result can be sagging or flabby breasts. As one matures, the skin loses its elasticity and the breasts will not take the strain of weight change easily. Some women believe that if their breasts developed at an early age they will lose their firmness also at a relatively early age. There is no factual basis for this supposition. Although the skin of your breasts and nipples is no more sensitive to the sun than the skin elsewhere on your body, care should always be taken when sunbathing to protect the entire body skin surface. (See Chapter I: "Our Skin.") No harm will be done the breasts by sleeping on them. If your breasts are large and you experience any discomfort at night, support them with a light brassiere.

B. GENERAL CARE AND THE NEED FOR SELF-EXAMINATION

As a Black woman, you are not subject to any basic conditions of puberty, pregnancy, and menopause that are not shared by all women. If certain diseases or malfunctions occur more frequently among Black women, the reasons are entirely environmental, not anatomical. Such problems, therefore, being socioeconomic in origin, are not insoluble. The first priority in this

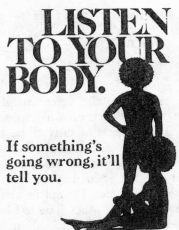

regard for all women should be an ability to examine oneself without fear and to do it regularly. This is by no means to replace professional medical examinations of the lower body, but unless you make self-examination a habit, you may not know that you need medical attention until the disorder is very severe. You should be the first to know if something is amiss with your body. That is impossible in this area unless, with a strong light and a mirror, you are prepared to check out your more intimate parts either in the bathroom or on the bed. This should be a routine, natural part of your health program, and there is absolutely nothing vulgar or embarrassing about becoming visually acquainted with what is part of your most treasured possession, your body.

Numerous women's groups across the country are spreading a new awareness of this aspect of practical home preventive medicine. Courses in anatomy, birth control, self-examination, and all phases of female health are becoming widely available for all women. I feel very strongly that no such knowledge is dangerous unless it seeks to completely replace the role of the professional doctor and institution. So that we are not taken advantage of by others, it is very vital that we are able to understand how our bodies work. Coupled with this is the ability to examine ourselves and be able to detect conditions that require attention. I do not believe, however, that we should attempt to become diagnosticians. All of the most minor irritations and infections must be brought to the attention of a qualified physician.

C. PERSONAL HYGIENE

You can never be free from vaginal infection, irritation, or objectionable odor unless you practice a conscientious ritual of personal hygiene. A bath or shower at least once a day is mandatory in this regard. Doctors are not agreed upon whether a bath is more effective than a shower or vice versa. Advocates of the bath suggest that the vaginal and anal areas receive a more thorough cleansing in the tub since they are completely immersed in water. Others feel that the constant flow of the shower is more hygienic. Your choice of either is not nearly as important as your activities therein. You must take a mild soap and with fairly hot water bathe the entire vulva, taking care to spread apart the labia and wash the numerous folds and creases that are ideal sites for the accumulation and growth of bacterial organisms. When feasible, it is very important that a woman bathe the vulva in the morning and after work. She should be especially aware of personal hygiene after sexual intercourse and bathe well.

Douching

This is a form of cleaning the vaginal cavity by introducing a solution under pressure which is squirted into the vagina through a tube. The solution is usually a commercial preparation in powder form that is mixed with warm water. The majority of the doctors that I have questioned regarding douching feel that it should not be used on a regular basis as part of the hygiene program. They feel that it should only be done on the recommendation of a physician for the specific treatment of certain problems. They state that constant douching can gradually weaken the natural defenses of the vagina and leave the outer genital area vulnerable to infection. Not only does the douche remove certain protective fluids from the vagina but some of the chemicals used in the douche solutions can be irritating to the very sensitive tissue of the vagina. The body secretes its own cleansing substances that protect inside the vagina and it is primarily the exterior area that must be frequently washed. Many women overestimate the potency of the douche and achieve a false sense of security by frequent douching. I seriously feel that if you do wish to douche, it should be only with the approval of a physician who advises you exactly how it is done and what products to use. Never force the nozzle of the douche into the vaginal cavity; this can cause inflammation of the lower abdomen. Although there is no danger of water entering the uterus via the vagina, it is possible for bacteria to enter, and any foreign object, even though it is ostensibly a cleansing device, should be kept away from this part of the body. Unless you are following a doctor's instructions you should never douche more than once a week and avoid it completely during menstruation and pregnancy. Douching is totally ineffective as a contraceptive even immediately after intercourse and is equally incapable of inducing abortion. Do not ever douche during the twenty-four hours immediately preceding an internal examination since vaginal secretions are necessary for correct diagnosis and the douching may temporarily disguise any internal problems you may have and make it very difficult for the physician to get a clear picture of your state of health.

Underwear and Hygiene

No amount of washing will counter infection unless you are prepared to wear a clean, comfortable pair of panties at all times. You are courting danger unless you wear a fresh pair every day. Today's synthetic fabrics may make more attractive panties, but cotton-knit panties are by far the most hygienic. The cotton is able to absorb perspiration and secretions from the body and also act as an excellent shield against bacteria and fungus infections. If you must wear a synthetic fabric, remember that a loose weave is much better in this regard than a very smooth surface. Pantyhose should never be worn without panties and panties must always be worn inside the pantyhose, next to the skin.

Feminine Hygiene Products

VAGINAL DEODORANT SUPPOSITORIES

These gel-like tablets are supposed to melt because of body heat after being inserted into the vagina and then coat the interior of the vagina with deodorant. In fact, most doctors feel that, like douching, more harm than good can come from the irritation and possible infection that can result from the chemicals used. The natural condition of the vagina is temporarily altered and temporarily made vulnerable to problems far more severe than odor. These deodorant suppositories cannot be effectively substituted for contraceptive devices; they have absolutely no ability to prevent conception.

DEODORANT SPRAYS AND POWDERS

These do not contribute at all to the cleanliness of the vulva and are basically no more than forms of perfume to temporarily mask odor. As the spray evaporates, a high concentration of irritants remains on the skin and these can easily stimulate allergic reactions. If you insist on using these products, never spray *into* the vagina itself; that is just asking for trouble. Such powders and sprays should not be used before intercourse or on sanitary napkins or tampons since these are all ways that the chemicals themselves can be introduced into the vaginal cavity.

Genital Odor

If frequent and thorough washing of the genital area does not prevent unpleasant odor, then you need a doctor's examination, not a deodorant product. Bear in mind, though, that some genital odor is absolutely normal and any attempts to completely eliminate it will at best be futile and at worst result in serious infection. If the odor is strong and quite intolerable, it is probably caused by either stale urine collecting and drying on pubic hair or the presence of bacteria thriving on accumulated vaginal or menstrual discharge. Very conscientious bathing will eliminate both causes of strong odor. If the odor persists after careful washing over a week-long period, then infection may be present and it is time to see the doctor. The urinary and anal tracts are perfect breeding grounds for bacteria and since they are so close to the vulva, great care should be taken to avoid the spread of such bacteria. A very simple practice will almost certainly prevent this from happening. After elimination, always wipe with toilet tissue from the front of the lower body to the rear, never from the rear toward the front. To avoid excessive genital odor during menstruation, you should change your sanitary napkins and tampons very frequently since these harbor the bacteria within the clotted blood and the sooner it is removed the better. During menstruation and pregnancy, hormonal activity causes the oil glands to become agitated and this causes a distinct odor. Hot water and mild soap, frequently, are the very best antidotes at these times. The entire body requires careful cleansing, especially the genital area.

D. MENSTRUATION

The first of three major stages in our body's development commences with the onset of puberty and is known as *menarche*. This is followed by the fertile years during which pregnancy is common, and the final change is menopause which marks the *climacteric* stage in our life. In most women, menstruation occurs with some regularity every twenty-eight days. We refer to the discharge of blood and dead-cell debris as *menses*, a name taken from the Latin for moon, the phases of which determine our calendar and thus the months during which we menstruate. It is quite common for the menstrual cycle (the time elapsing between the first signs of bleeding) to be as short as twenty-one days or as long as thirty-five; nor is an irregular cycle necessarily an indication of any abnormality. The timing of the cycle is determined by hormones in the ovaries and the pituitary gland. Once a month, one of the hundreds of thousands of ova (eggs) that we are born carrying is sent from the ovaries to the uterus where the lining, the endometrium, thickens with blood in preparation for the nourishment of the egg should it be fertilized with a male sperm. If this fertilization does not take place, the egg and the extra mucous membrane lining of the uterus are discharged through the vagina, a process that may take from four to seven days and which is accomplished by means of muscular contractions of the Fallopian tubes. A young woman's first menstruation normally occurs between the ages of eleven and fourteen. If it occurs a year or two earlier or later, nothing is wrong; but if a woman has not menstruated by the age of seventeen, a doctor should be consulted. Puberty commences about a year prior to the first menstruation. At this time the ovaries begin to produce hormones that accelerate and orchestrate sexual development. The adolescent girl experiences marked and sometimes frighteningly sudden body changes. Height increases, hair grows under the arms and around the vulva, hips broaden, and the breasts develop. Menstruation is a perfectly normal physiological process that should never interfere with routine activities or sound hygiene habits. Many factors can influence the menstrual cycle and create definite problems. As Black women, we may be particularly prone to some of these factors such as lack of proper nutrition, obesity, inadequate rest, and emotional turmoil. Those diseases that afflict us such as hypertension, diabetes, and sickle-cell anemia all cause abnormalities to occur in the menstrual cycle. For the healthy woman, diet is very important in maintaining a trouble-free cycle, and often women do not realize that much of their monthly discomfort may be traced to crash dieting and similar inadequate weight-loss programs.

The Discomforts of Menstruation

The most common discomfort is premenstrual tension. Five to ten days before any actual menstrual flow, we may experience pelvic congestion, a bloated feeling, general sluggishness, tender breasts, weight gain, and depression. If you experience these conditions frequently, do not be reluctant to mention them to your doctor. Medication can be prescribed for these disorders which are not to be considered a "curse" that must be stoically borne. The discomfort is very real and it must be treated seriously. Most doctors now recognize this and are prepared to understand the complaints as legitimate, treatable ailments—not, as was formerly the case, "a woman's lot," about which nothing could, or should, be done.

Menstrual Abnormalities

Endometriosis is quite common in women between thirty and forty and consists of the displacement of the thickened matrix of blood and tissue from the uterus to anywhere else. Sometimes it will be found growing near the ovaries, the cervix, the abdominal wall, or the bladder. This condition is usually accompanied by significant pain before or during menstruation. If there is no pain, the endometrial cyst is sometimes large enough to feel. In mild cases, little treatment is required, but all women suffering from this should be aware that it may cause infertility. Endometriosis disappears at menopause or with the removal of the ovaries, as by a hysterectomy.

Amenorrhea is the absence of menses and that is now not uncommonly found in women who stop using oral contraceptives. Sometimes menstruation does not return for as long as six months after a woman has stopped taking "the Pill." A number of conditions can cause amenorrhea, and although it is treatable, a woman must see a doctor if it persists more than three months.

Dysmenorrhea, or severe menstrual cramps, may be caused by physical or emotional problems. In the past the male-dominated medical profession often told a patient suffering from this that she would "outgrow" it or that it would cease after she had a child. We now know that is nonsense and if you have dysmenorrhea, see your doctor. It can be helped.

Irregular bleeding, such as between menstrual periods and occasional spotting with blood of the underclothes at times other than during menstruation, is abnormal and should be reported to a physician. The cause is usually hormonal and can be treated.

Shortened cycles are caused by the ovaries passing the egg (ovulation) prematurely, every three weeks or less instead of every four. If you are menstruating every twenty-one days or sooner, you should consult a physician.

Prolonged menses happens when the ovulation is delayed or the egg never leaves the ovary. Meanwhile, estrogen and progesterone are being released and the result may be highly irregular intervals of menstruation with frequent bleeding at different times. This condition must be reported to a doctor.

Dilation and Curettage

There are a number of surgical procedures connected with the treatment of menstrual problems but, by far, the most common is dilation and curettage usually referred to as "D. and C." Many people erroneously associate this solely with abortion procedure, but in fact it is a very common diagnostic procedure used to determine the cause of many menstrual difficulties. This is not a major operation; no incision is made. The doctor, using an instrument called a *curette*, takes a specimen from the uterus for laboratory examination. Most patients stay only overnight in the hospital, and although there may be slight bleeding for four or five days, after one week recovery is usually complete.

Menstruation and the Breasts

Between the ages of ten and fourteen, the first fatty deposits begin to accumulate in a young woman's breasts. The halo around the nipple (the areola) becomes strongly defined and the nipple itself becomes more prominent. In many young girls and full adult women, the period of menstruation is preceded by a special tenderness of the breasts that sometimes swell and accumulate water in the tissues. This is caused by the increased hormonal activity at these times, and if discomfort is severe, your physician can prescribe a mild medication.

Menstruation and Diet

Poor eating habits cause a great deal of menstrual discomfort. The nutrients that one normally requires are readily available in many foods. At menstruation, however, one does lose a considerable amount of blood and tissue and this loss must be rectified. Women who are dieting forget that, although under normal circumstances they can restrict the intake of certain substances, this can have uncomfortable consequences if combined with menstruation. During adolescence, iron is required in large doses as menses starts. This consumption should be continued in the years that follow. Foods rich in iron include liver, turkey, whole-wheat bread, oats, egg yolk, spinach, and seafood. If you remember to have one serving of liver and spinach after menstruation, you will make up for any losses. If you are on a low-fat diet, you must use some fats in your cooking the week prior to menstruation. There is a correlation between menstrual cramps and irritability in women who are on heavily fat-restricted diets. Calcium is lost in large quantities due to menstruation. The days preceding menses, the level of calcium in the blood falls and this can be a cause of nervous tension and uterine cramps. Milk and cheese are rich in calcium and must be taken at this time. Skim milk and nonfat powdered milk are excellent substitutes and provide as much calcium as whole milk. I am really speaking to the dieting woman. One of the purposes of good basic nutrition, as outlined in Chapter VII, is to avoid such complaints as menstrual discomfort. If you abide by the general principles outlined there, you will not need any special supplements. There is no need, for instance, of vitamins for the menstruating woman if she is consuming daily servings from each of the four basic food groups. Overreliance on vitamins for remedying menstrual cramps can lead to toxic poisoning.

Menstruation and Elimination

Many of us have a tendency to retain water and also become constipated during menstruation. Absolutely avoid diuretics and laxatives other than natural food sources. Chemical laxatives can upset your system at a time when it needs to be calm. Apples, grapefruit, oranges and, when possible, strawberries are excellent diuretics, and unpolished rice, green leafy vegetables, and unprocessed cereals provide the fiber and roughage to act as natural laxatives.

Menstruation, Drugs, and Alcohol

It is believed that persistent use of heroin, cocaine, and other drugs creates changes in the normal functioning of the pituitary gland, and the ovaries are thus influenced. Studies are not conclusive at the present time but the risk is too great to be taken lightly. Alcohol consumption poses a principal danger to the health of the liver and the liver is where many of the hormones governing our menstrual functions are metabolized.

Menstruation and Exercise

In recent years, since such information has been kept, women have won gold medals and broken Olympic records during all phases of the menstrual cycle. One American woman captured three gold medals and set a new world's record in swimming events in a recent Olympics while at the height of menstruation. Most doctors are now prepared to admit that, far from inhibiting trouble-free menstruation, exercise in fact encourages it. Women must realize that we can actually benefit from exercise during menstruation, especially those sports that exercise the whole body such as swimming. A recent study comparing swimmers with nonathletic students at a large university revealed that the swimmers had much less menstrual difficulty. Whatever exercise you choose, there is no medical reason to modify or stop activity during menstruation.

Menstruation and Posture

The major cause of menstrual pain is attributed to the uterine membrane stretching and an increased blood supply to that area. This specific pain cannot be eased by any particular posture even though you may have been cautioned not to lie in a fetal position in order to ease pain while menstruating. That has no scientific basis and should be ignored. Any position that increases comfort can be adopted except to lie on your stomach. This causes the spine to curve which presses on the rectum that in turn increases pressure on your already swollen uterus. Sleep on your side with knees drawn up or on your back. If you follow the rules for posture in Chapter VI, they will serve you in good stead during menstruation. Generally poor posture increases menstrual discomfort.

Menstruation and Clothing

No change in your clothes habits should be necessitated by menstruation. Obviously you will use sanitary napkins or tampons and should frequently change into freshly laundered, preferably cotton, panties. The only other item of clothing that should be suggested for some women at this time is the brassiere. If your breasts do swell—and this heaviness can stretch breast tissue and cause irritation—support is required. Unless you are a size 34A-cup or smaller, always wear at least a light brassiere for support while menstruating. If you have large breasts, a light bra worn around the clock will ease sagging and reduce the possibility of flabbiness that will probably increase during menstruation. Regardless of breast size, many women find that a light bra worn to bed helps to relieve soreness and tenderness.

Menstruation Products

Both sanitary napkins and tampons are perfectly safe to use; personal comfort should dictate your choice. Tampons may even be worn by women who have not had sexual intercourse, if their hymen is perforated.

E. PREGNANCY

A woman's reproductive, fertile period technically begins as soon as menstruation starts in puberty, but eighteen is generally considered to be the age at which normal pregnancies can safely begin to occur. Earlier than that a young woman may not be sufficiently developed in all parts of her body. Although many successful pregnancies have been enjoyed by women over the age of forty-five, that is usually mentioned as the age at which a woman begins to enter her climacteric stage.

Advocates of the Woman's Liberation Movement and population control are quite right to fight the widely held viewpoint that women are incapable of endeavors not related to the bearing and raising of children. While we should firmly resist such classification, we must realize that not only are we capable of achieving all the worthwhile goals usually associated with males (pre-eminence in the arts, business, politics, sports), but we are *also* able to have children as well.

Our abilities and capacity thus quite supersede the male. With the help of a fairly enlightened mate we can and should beget, bear, and raise children without sacrificing our ability to make significant material and spiritual contributions to society.

A healthy woman in her fertile stage ovulates once every month and, short of artificial insemination, must have sexual intercourse with a male in order for that ovum to be fertilized and become a fetus. We are not simply passive vessels waiting to be filled, but our frequent ovulation and the accompanying heightened sexual desire that often goes along with it are in every way as "aggressive" as is the male's expected courtship of the female. Unfortunately, fear and ignorance regarding pregnancy are rampant in many Black families. Sexual discrimination and taboos are widely practiced among devotees of religious sects that have gained popularity in Black America in recent years. I believe that my ability to reproduce makes me potentially superior, not inferior, to the male.

Ovulation and Conception

Many women are quite unaware of ovulation, but others may notice a slight increase in body temperature and, as I have mentioned, an increase in sexual desire. After the egg is released by the ovary, it lives in the Fallopian tubes for about four days. The male sperm also lives that long so that sexual intercourse before, during, and after ovulation greatly increases the possibility of conception. It is untrue, however, that there is any hour, day, or week in the menstrual cycle when it is absolutely impossible to conceive. There are times when conception is less likely, but pregnancy has resulted often from sexual intercourse even during the menstrual period. At intercourse, the male deposits literally millions of sperm in the vaginal cavity. Only one of these has to find its way past the cervix and into the uterus and from there to the egg in the Fallopian tube. When this happens, the sperm penetrates the membrane of the ovum and forms a single embryonic cell.

This usually occurs in the middle portion of one of the two Fallopian tubes. The now-fertilized ovum travels down to the uterus where it becomes embedded in the endometrium, the prepared lining of the uterus. Immediately, the embryo starts to grow. Although menstruation can occur after this has happened, it is unlikely, and normally a woman is first made aware of the possibility of pregnancy by a "missed period." The ovaries now cease to send monthly ova into the Fallopian tubes. Very soon the fertilized cell develops two separate parts. One is the embryo itself which will later be the child and the other is a life-support system attached by a network of blood vessels to the uterine lining. This *placenta* monitors all exchanges between mother and child. Very thin membraneous walls separate the blood of the mother from that of the child, but essential hormones, nutrients, and waste substances pass through these walls. The embryo develops within a bag of fluid and it floats in this bag, well protected from all but the most severe external traumas. In the first eight weeks of life, the embryo grows from the size of a dot no larger than the period at the end of this sentence to one inch and a half of recognizably human features.

When determining pregnancy, it is important to differentiate between *signs* of pregnancy and *symptoms*. Signs are evidence and there are only three: presence of fetal heartbeat, fetal movement, and X-ray showing fetal details.

Symptoms are not absolute but do aid early diagnosis. These include breast fullness and soreness, nausea and aversion to certain foods. A couple of weeks after a "missed period," frequent urination may commence and may be accompanied by constipation and fatigue. Not all of these symptoms occur in every pregnancy and many are totally absent. If you suspect you are pregnant, find out immediately by consulting a physician. The first two months of pregnancy often determine the health of the child, and if you are to have a strong child, you must immediately improve your own habits if they are flawed.

Pregnancy and Race

Since there are absolutely no physiological differences in ovulation, conception, pregnancy, and birth among the races of women, we have to face the fact that when twice as many newborn Black babies die as do white babies, the causes are environmental and therefore must be eradicated. Three per cent of our babies do not survive, a very high figure in this country. Much of this mortality is due to a lack of prenatal care. This can be the fault of the mother through laziness or ignorance, or the fault of a society that makes professional obstetrical attention a luxury only to be afforded by the relatively well-to-do. Many Black women simply do not have access to adequate prenatal advice, examination, and care. No matter whether you are having your first child or your fifth, the baby and you need proper prenatal ministration. The majority of healthy young pregnant Black women need fear no dangers or complications, but long before your pregnancy "starts showing," you should be under the care of a physician.

Pregnancy and Bodily Change

That remarkable, efficient factory, the placenta, produces large amounts of several different hormones that conduct the dramatic changes that the body undergoes during pregnancy. There are few parts of the body unaffected by the growth of the new life. The entire body must take on an increased amount of stress, and fine and detailed adjustments must be made so that the mother does not suffer. In a woman free from serious handicaps, this adjustment is made so perfectly that she can enjoy several pregnancies with little risk to herself. Pregnant women secrete extra quantities of cortin, that immunity hormone which effectively fights disease. If you are emotionally stable at this time, eat properly, and have regular examinations by a doctor, this can be the most healthy time of your life.

Varicose veins in the legs during pregnancy are caused by the increased pressure of blood in the veins of the lower body. The heart has to work an extra 25 per cent and this increased circulation can cause varicose veins. Women often have an inherited tendency for them, but the effects can be lessened if you avoid garters and elastic mid-calf stockings. Wear pantyhose or support stockings.

Nasal congestion sometimes accompanies pregnancy and the ears too can feel plugged up. Warm weather can increase your propensity for allergies and cold weather may bring on an inordinate number of colds. Nosebleeds are also common but not serious. If any of these conditions persist, by all means tell your doctor.

Vomiting, especially early in pregnancy, is normal and may be coupled with nausea, flatulence, and constipation. The stomach is slower to empty itself. Heartburn is common later in pregnancy and at all times avoid heavy, rich, spicy foods. All of these gastrointestinal problems should respond to a regular, well-balanced diet.

Urinary infections are frequent in pregnant women and are among the most common complications. The ureters connecting the kidneys and the bladder dilate during pregnancy and this predisposes the entire urinary tract to infection. To reduce the possibility of this, drink at least two quarts of fluid per day so as to clear the ureters frequently.

Pelvic discomfort and backache are common in the late stages of pregnancy, as the joints of the pelvis soften slightly to allow passage of the baby. If this becomes a problem, ask your doctor if you can wear a maternity girdle. Remember also that exercise will allay many such aches and pains.

Skin undergoes significant changes during pregnancy. Sometimes the nipples become darker, as do moles and other congenital markings. The cheeks and forehead of lighter-skinned women may suffer some blotchy discoloration called chloasma or "mask of pregnancy," but this is not permanent. Often a poor skin will improve and claims have been verified that acne has retreated and sometimes disappeared because of pregnancy. Stretch marks on the abdomen are caused by the skin actually stretching to accommodate the baby and enduring superficial separation. There are no sure-fire preventive measures that we can adopt to ensure that the skin tone and clarity of the abdomen will remain the same after pregnancy, but in the majority of cases the marks shrink rapidly after the birth. Black women suffer from stretch marks not because of any deficiency in the skin but because the pigment shows change more obviously than in whites. Caucasians are just as prone as we are to stretch marks but the progression of the mark is from bright red to pink to a gradual fade and near invisibility, whereas with us the marks are either lighter or darker than our skin. Extra care of the skin all during pregnancy can effectively reduce the incidence of stretch marks and they are less likely on women who exercise and have strong abdominal muscles. Observe my regimen for the skin outlined in Chapter I and keep it thoroughly lubricated at all times with body lotions. During my pregnancy I used a combination of "Mother's Friend" lotion (this also comes in cream form), cocoa butter, and baby oil. Lubricate the abdomen with such high-oil products twice a day, avoid excessive weight gain, and exercise properly. These should curb a tendency to form stretch marks.

Hair often grows more heavily during pregnancy, stimulated by the activity of the endocrine system. This can lead to increased hairiness all over the body or only in certain parts. This subsides after pregnancy and for many women present no problems. Hair may also become thinner at this time, for other reasons. If you do consult a professional, such as a dermatologist, for any such condition, do not fail to mention that you are pregnant since that will determine the nature of treatment. Many Black women enjoy a spurt of hair growth for the first time in years during pregnancy and we should consider it one of the advantages of child-bearing. Always remember to keep the hair clean and rinsed and conditioned during pregnancy. Wash frequently.

Teeth are part of a calcium myth that one often hears regarding pregnancy: that for every child the mother will lose a tooth because the baby needs her calcium. This is sheer superstition. It is true that the fetus needs calcium, which is why the mother should drink plenty of milk during pregnancy, but the fetus cannot take calcium away from the mother's own formed teeth. It is quite true that women find their teeth often in bad condition after pregnancy, and this is due to neglect. The mouth becomes a vulnerable area, especially if you are nauseous and frequently vomiting. Bacteria stays on the teeth and gums and dental caries will form unless brushing is even more frequent during pregnancy than at other times. Hormonal changes in the body increase the supply of blood to the oral region and for a while the gums may be sensitive and some bleeding is quite normal. Usually what occurs is that with the preoccupation with pregnancy, the woman neglects her teeth and over a year passes before she sees her dentist. The innocent baby is blamed for the condition of her teeth that the mother alone is responsible for. If you visit the dentist in the early stages of pregnancy, make sure that she or he is aware of your condition because the administration of nitrous oxide (laughing gas) or X-rays may be harmful to the fetus. If you are prone to morning sickness, remember to brush your teeth several times each day.

Pregnancy and the Breasts

As pregnancy progresses, the milk-duct system within each breast is stimulated and the breasts grow larger. The blood vessels in the breasts expand and the breasts can sometimes double in weight. After the third month, the breasts should not feel so tender and in the fourth month the mammary glands start to produce *colustrum,* which is a thick, yellowish fluid sometimes called foremilk that is secreted by the breasts immediately after birth. Within two or three days the action of the pituitary gland has created a decline in the levels of estrogen and progesterone in the system and the colustrum becomes milk. If you do not intend to nurse your child, the doctor can prescribe a drug to prevent lactation (the process of producing milk), but to be effective it must be administered immediately after birth. Some women who do not nurse prefer to remove the milk from their breasts with a suction device. Neither pregnancy nor nursing stretches the ligaments attaching the breasts to the chest wall and if they have been properly supported during pregnancy, they should return to their original size. Some women have even noted a decrease in the size of the breast after pregnancy. Stretch marks on the breasts cannot be prevented, although they do not occur to every woman. If they do show signs of emerging, treat with oils as you would the abdomen.

Breast Problems and Pregnancy

Flat or inverted nipples may present an obstacle to nursing if they cannot be manually drawn out. Your doctor will know if this is possible and advise you accordingly. Women who have had plastic surgery to increase the size of the breasts usually have no problems nursing, although if you are contemplating surgery to reduce the size of your breasts and you wish to nurse your children, this may not be possible.

Diseases of the Black Woman and Pregnancy

Our tendency to suffer from hypertension, diabetes, and kidney diseases accounts for a fairly high incidence of toxemias (blood poisonings) during pregnancy that can affect the fetus. If you suspect you are suffering from any such illness, you must make sure that your doctor keeps you under close observation during pregnancy. For reasons not yet fully understood, we are more likely than other women to develop fibroid tumors during pregnancy within or on the walls of the uterus. These fleshy growths are in most cases benign, but they can create delivery problems.

Common Complications in Pregnancy

A *miscarriage* occurs when unfavorable conditions are so severe that the fetus is prematurely ejected early in pregnancy. In many cases this indicates that the fetus would not have developed into a normal baby, but does not mean that future pregnancies cannot be perfectly normal. Miscarriages usually occur in the first three months and during those months special care must be taken to preserve the health of both mother and child. After that, your health and your baby's health grow stronger and safer each day.

German Measles and similar virus infections can injure the fetus during the first three months when the eyes, ears, brain, and heart are developing. Since a pregnant woman cannot be vaccinated against such viral diseases, make sure you have been protected by vaccination long before you entertain the idea of having a family.

Surgery and Childbirth

The most common surgery associated with delivery is episitomy and Cesarean section. Seventy-five per cent of all deliveries in the United States involve episitomy, which consists of an incision at the opening of the vagina just prior to birth. This is made to facilitate passage of the baby's head through the vagina. Immediately after delivery the incision is stitched and within two weeks the wound is healed. It is impossible to predict how painful this incision is going to be; some women find it negligible and others quite severe. Postnatal treatment including the use of a heat lamp often speeds healing. Cesarean section is a procedure used when for a variety of reasons it may be dangerous to have the baby emerge via the vaginal cavity. The mother's pelvis may be too narrow or the baby unusually large. An incision is made in the abdomen and the baby and the placenta are removed directly from the uterus. As with any abdominal surgery, there are dangers in this procedure, but it is far from rare and is not considered a particular hazard.

Pregnancy and Diet

There are many superstitions still rampant in all parts of the world regarding the diet of the pregnant woman. If we lived in Northern Rhodesia, for instance, both ourselves and our husbands would be forbidden to eat the flesh of the hartebeest, a staple meat. It is thought that because the young of the hartebeest are born blind, the same fate—but a permanent one—will befall the baby whose parents digest the meat. We may find that hard to believe, but in this country some women are still told by the medical profession to keep their weight even during pregnancy by limiting their food intake. That is just as erroneous as the hartebeest story although a lighter mother will deliver a smaller baby and trouble the doctor less at the time of delivery. Such babies, however, if they are underweight, are much more prone to illness in the early weeks of life than a large, well-fed baby. I am by no means suggesting that the pregnant woman can, and should, gorge herself, but she must be fully aware of the necessity for an adequate and nutritional diet. Control of your weight by following a proper diet is the most important single aspect of prenatal care for both the health of the child and the return of the mother's figure after delivery. The best preparation for this, of course, is to practice good nutritional habits whether pregnant or not, and it is very important to continue those habits following pregnancy. While pregnant you are eating for two, but you do not have to eat twice as much. The quality of your food is far more important than the quantity. Some women become ravenous when pregnant and eat constantly and carelessly. There are usually emotional problems contributing to this desire; it is not the fetus demanding constant nourishment. You should not have to snack between meals if your diet is carefully arranged. The ideal weight gain for the mother is a fairly steady half pound per week after the first few weeks. This increases in the final week as the fetus itself is growing at a rate of almost one ounce per day. You must be prepared to gain at least fifteen but no more than twenty pounds during pregnancy, assuming that you are neither emaciated nor obese. You will lose those pounds during delivery and in the days that follow.

There is no reason to accumulate weight while pregnant and retain it for the rest of your life. You can eat well and heartily and be back to your normal weight within two weeks of delivery. Consider that of the twenty pounds you acquire while pregnant, between six and nine will be the baby itself and the rest just about divided equally between the afterbirth that is lost in delivery and normal postpartum weight loss. If you gain more than twenty pounds, you do run the risk of putting on extra pounds that you will not shed so easily. It may be a struggle to keep the weight gain in pregnancy down to twenty pounds, but not if you weigh yourself frequently and follow my nutritional advice. Under no circumstances should you starve yourself or follow any diet program that is not specifically geared to the pregnant woman; if you do, you may be endangering two lives. If you enjoy counting calories, remember that you must never go below 1,500 per day while pregnant and preferably keep your intake between 2,000 and 2,500.

Basic Nutrition for Pregnant and Nursing Women

EVERY DAY:

1) Two 3- to 4-ounce servings of meat, fish, or fowl. At least once a week this should mean liver for protein, minerals, and vitamins.

2) One serving of a cooked green or yellow vegetable such as peas, beans, broccoli, cabbage, spinach, collard greens, turnips, kale, peppers, carrots.

3) One serving of any of the above raw.

4) One serving of fruit, especially oranges, grapefruit, tomatoes, pineapple, cantaloupe.

5) Bread, rice, spaghetti, potatoes, corn, squash, eggplant, sweet potatoes, and yams are high in calories and low in proteins, minerals, and vitamins. Limit to three or four servings *per week*.

6) One quart of milk (four 8-ounce glasses) is recommended but not mandatory. If you dislike milk, drink only two glasses and make up the difference with cheese or yoghurt.

7) One quart of liquid other than milk: water or fruit juice. Avoid carbonated beverages. On this diet you should not need diuretics or laxatives, but if you are constipated, only use products recommended or prescribed by your doctor.

Ways to Safely Curb Weight While Pregnant

1) Cut out salt after the fourth or fifth month. Salt encourages water retention and excessive water retention at this time not only adds to your weight but can endanger the fetus.

2) Substitute skim milk for whole milk. If you use low-fat dry milk, you need less than one quart per day because it is concentrated. Flavor with honey or chocolate to make palatable. Substitute cottage cheese for regular cheese.

3) Use vinegar and lemon juice instead of mayonnaise on salads.

4) Make open-faced sandwiches with just one very thin slice of bread.

5) Do not cook with lard, butter, or fatty oils.

6) Avoid cold cuts; these contain too much salt, water, and sugar.

7) When hungry between meals, drink a cup of hot bouillon soup.

8) Substitute low-salt Melba toast for bread.

9) Always satisfy sugar cravings with fruit rather than desserts.

10) Eat as much raw vegetable as you want.

11) Substitute fish for meat.

All pregnant women do not get a craving for exotic foods at 3 A.M. There is no medical basis for this widely believed myth. If you do change your eating habits, it may well be away from sharp, spicy foods to more bland fare.

Many of us Black women feel that pregnancy is an excuse to stop work and gain fifty pounds. Such behavior is inexcusable. If you are seeing a doctor once a month or more, you must keep working and keep your weight down. There is no reason for pregnancy to ravage your body and interrupt your ability to earn or to keep house. It is cruel to you and to your child to emerge from confinement fatter and poorer.

Pregnancy and Drugs

Other than doctor-prescribed medication, nothing should enter your system during pregnancy except nutrient food and liquids. *Vitamins* are quite unnecessary if your diet is adequate. No study has determined that vitamin supplements during pregnancy are advantageous to mother or child. *Appetite-suppressant* pills or liquids have limited effectiveness at any time and, for the pregnant woman, can be very harmful, encouraging nervousness, insomnia, and fatigue and lead to quite serious emotional disorders. Doctors often prescribe such medication to pregnant women, but I am strongly against it. *Drugs* from aspirin to heroin have no place in a pregnant woman's body. The symbiosis between mother and child is constant and even cough medicine or a nose-drop preparation are potentially dangerous. In the last decade, thousands of American and European women took thalidomide while pregnant; it was then widely available as a mild sedative. Many of their offspring were deformed. Check with your doctor before ingesting any such commercial preparation, no matter how apparently innocuous. If we are to endure and achieve as a race in this country in future generations, we must produce drug-free, strong, robust children. There is no need to abstain totally from *alcohol* while pregnant if you are used to an occasional drink. Heavy drinking, however, can damage the fetus directly and inevitably prevents the mother from following a proper pregnancy diet.

Pregnancy and Smoking

Smoking women give birth to more underweight babies than nonsmoking women. One theory for this is that smoking causes constriction of the arteries and less nourishment reaches the fetus. Women who smoke more than two packs a day have significantly more stillbirths than nonsmokers. Premature births and spontaneous abortions are twice as numerous among smokers. Unborn children of smoking mothers suffer from a lack of oxygen, impaired heart rate, and nicotine poisoning. Smoking mothers who nurse their babies are introducing them to traces of nicotine present in their milk. You are risking two lives if you smoke during pregnancy.

Pregnancy and Exercise

Delivery of the baby requires great muscular effort on the part of the mother. Far from avoiding exercise during pregnancy we should pay special attention to achieving and maintaining a state of body preparedness for this effort. This can only be done by constant exercise. A pregnant woman is the exact opposite of an invalid and should not be treated or treat herself as one. I sustained my normal eight-to-ten-hour work day throughout my pregnancy and until the eighth month swam eighty laps a day. Unless there is a serious overriding medical reason to avoid exercise, all pregnant women should continue and, if possible, increase their work and exercise schedules. All gross motor activity forms of exercise as outlined in Chapter VI are excellent for the pregnant woman—swimming, jogging, walking, running. However, obtain your doctor's permission before undertaking any of these. Team sports that might risk a direct blow to the abdomen should be discontinued after six months and your doctor should be consulted first. A study of women athletes and childbirth recently concluded that of seven hundred athletes researched, their average length of labor was 87 per cent shorter than that of nonathletes and they required 50 per cent fewer Cesarean sections. Olympic records in rowing and discus throwing have been won by women four and a half months pregnant and of the twenty-six Soviet women medal winners at the 1964 Melbourne Olympics, ten were pregnant when they won their medals! Properly supervised indoor exercises can be as effective as sports, but make sure your doctor approves the specific calisthenic or isometric positions. Group lessons for women wishing to practice drug-free natural childbirth are becoming available all over the country and of course vigorous exercise is very important for this activity. If your body is unaccustomed to strenuous activity, do not rush into it blindly at pregnancy but take it slowly and easily at first. All pregnant women should avoid straining the body during what would be their menstrual periods in the first three months of pregnancy. This allows the fertilized egg to become securely implanted in the lining of the uterus. Remember that the uterus is one of the most protected parts of your entire anatomy and the fetus floating in fluid is very secure.

Postnatal Exercise

Most women complain of flabby abdomens after childbirth and notice this getting worse with the number of pregnancies they enjoy. Few of us just snap back into shape. The only way to counter this natural tendency is by dogged, regular effort and exercise. Consult your doctor at first, especially if you are nursing, about what exercises you personally can sustain. The most important fact to keep in mind is that nothing is going to change in two weeks or even two months, but if you keep up a daily grind of exercise for three to four months after pregnancy, you will end up with a firmer, better shape than before. When you exercise, whether during or after delivery, you must also watch your diet carefully and always maintain your daily nutrient requirements.

Pregnancy and Posture

Obviously your changed body shape during pregnancy encourages the posture characteristics of this condition. It is important, however, that you maintain all the basics of normal good posture until it is absolutely no compromise. Do not become lazy and prematurely throw out the stomach, no matter how initially comfortable or satisfying you feel. This does not help the abdominal muscles and may increase your fatigue. At all times remember how to bend: never with the legs straight but always bent—deeply if necessary. Do not stretch out across wide surfaces as you might normally do to close a window or make up a bed.

Pregnancy and Clothes

Your most important item is your brassiere. Your breast size will increase and during the hormonal changes of the first and last three months always needs support. If you are a size 34B or larger, always wear a brassiere night and day. Smaller women may be able to do without one for the middle three months but otherwise should not neglect this garment if they want to preserve the size, shape, and firmness of their breasts. If you wish support for the abdominal area, there are girdles and foundation garments easily available, but seek your physician's advice and make sure they are not too tight. Avoid stocking supports that rely upon elastic. Garters are out; they will only encourage varicose veins. Wear pantyhose or a garter belt. Sensible shoes are most important for posture, comfort, and to avoid fatigue, especially later in pregnancy. Your feet will probably swell slightly because of water retention, so wait until the fourth or fifth month before buying a pair of enclosed, low-heel walking shoes. Sling-backs and clogs are no good. Maternity clothes present a particular problem for the woman who wants to keep looking smart without spending a fortune for clothes she will rarely wear. I refused to buy a maternity swimsuit; sixty dollars was just too much! The cheap maternity clothes are simply large-size children's clothes and the moderately priced dresses are very conservative, almost old-fashioned. One can buy very good-looking maternity clothes, but the prices are very high because manufacturing costs are high for fashions with such a limited market. I solved the problem by buying only two fairly expensive maternity dresses, one for day and one for evening wear. If you invest in just two such purchases, you can easily make up the rest of your maternity wardrobe by sewing yourself very simple smocks or buying the inexpensive African, Indian, and Mexican caftanlike garments now sold practically everywhere. I also wore large men's sweaters and shirts while pregnant and, although proud of my shape, I avoided clinging clothes and chose garments with a loose silhouette that nevertheless fitted snugly the shoulders, arms, and wrists.

F. MENOPAUSE

Between the ages of forty-five and fifty, most women gradually change from their reproductive stage to the *climacteric* stage. This is marked by menopause which simply means a completion of the menses. Often this is referred to, in a hushed or dramatic fashion, as the "change of life."

Signs of Menopause

The passage of menopause usually takes from six months to three years. A woman is considered to have entered this stage when she has ceased to menstruate for one year. The ovaries have stopped producing eggs and reduced their secretion of estrogen and progesterone. This change may be preceded by alternating hot flushes and chills. These are often the first signs of menopause and they gradually disappear when menstruation has ceased. These flushes and chills may be limited to the face and neck or extend to the entire body and can be so severe as to cause perspiration even in very cold weather. The hands and feet may occasionally become cold and headaches are common at this time. Other very common disorders of menopause include irritability, fatigue, depression, nausea, loss of appetite, dizziness, and a frequent desire to urinate. We may feel a tightening of the vagina and will certainly experience menstrual irregularity and spot bleeding prior to the complete cessation of menstrual activity. One may undergo aches in the bones from the slight softening that occurs at this stage.

Treatment of Menopause

It is very important for us to realize that, like menstruation and pregnancy, menopause is by no means an illness or disease, but a normal, stabilizing part of our life cycle. However, like menstruation, the discomforts of menopause can be very real and very disruptive. The medical profession is rapidly catching up with the necessity for adequate physiological and psychological counseling for women passing through the menopausal stage. If you take my advice, you should be making two regular visits to a doctor every year after the age of thirty-five. Mention to your doctor any signs you may interpret as indicating the onset of menopause and your physician and you can prepare to handle the change without fear or panic. Because some of the important changes are related to a decrease in the amount of estrogen in the ovaries, much research is being done in the possible use of estrogen therapy to relieve some of the more acute discomforts of menopause. This is a delicate and potentially dangerous hormone and estrogen should only be used if specifically prescribed by a doctor who is aware of your medical history. Self-prescribed and administered hormone therapy can have devastating results.

Menopause and the Breasts

The possible decrease in breast size for hormonal reasons is usually offset by a tendency to put on weight during and after menopause.

Abnormalities of Menopause

It is quite normal for menstruation to stop suddenly, then return for a few months, stop, and start again. If, however, you experience any kind of bleeding after menstruation has been absent for twelve consecutive months, you should see a doctor immediately. This bleeding may indicate a serious disorder.

Menopause and Surgery

The simplest and most common form of surgery related to menopause is the dilation and curettage (D. and C.) that I have described earlier in this chapter. This is usually considered a diagnostic procedure when performed during menopause to ensure that the patient is not suffering from any serious complications. Another frequently performed operation on the menopausal woman is the hysterectomy. Strictly speaking, this consists of removal of the uterus only, but it is now increasingly prevalent to remove the ovaries and the Fallopian tubes as well, whether they are healthy or not, to insure against the possibility of cancer. I share the opinion held by an increasing number of medical specialists that more unnecessary hysterectomies are performed than any other operation. Black women are often the victims of this expensive, needless surgery. Examination of the removed organs frequently reveals no malignant condition. Often the treatment is similar to that of arbitrarily removing aching teeth without first investigating the exact cause of the pain and trying less drastic methods of treatment. I am not suggesting that there is never any need for a hysterectomy. Many women's lives are saved by this procedure when it has been conclusively proved that the organs are cancerous or otherwise diseased. If your doctor recommends this operation without having you examined by a specialist, I strongly suggest you seek a second opinion, preferably that of a gynaecologist. Often Black women are prone in the menopausal stage to the development of tumors on the uterus wall. In many cases these are benign and noncancerous and require no surgery.

Because hysterectomy involves the removal of much or all of the organs of reproduction, it should be considered very carefully indeed if suggested to a woman still in her fertile, premenopausal stage and only agreed to if there is proof positive that life is endangered.

Menopause and Body Change

Hair often starts to grow more heavily after menopause because the endocrine function of the pituitary, thyroid, and adrenal glands has been limited. This is quite usual, as is a slight thinning of the hair. If either condition becomes disagreeable, consult a dermatologist. The same endocrine change can affect the *skin* which in most women becomes drier. Hormone skin creams will do very little in the way of stimulating your glands and you are better off practicing frequent use of normal moisturizing creams and lotions for the face and body. The idea that postmenopausal women require different cosmetics is a sales device and has absolutely no basis in fact. Other skin developments at this time are the possibility of mild growths and some women find their skin actually more oily than before.

Menopause and Diet

The recommended dietary requirements are no different for a postmenopausal (climacteric stage) woman than for a menstruating woman. If you read elsewhere that an older woman needs less nutrients, the amount less so described would be for survival only and has no practical, effective application. Some additional vitamins are helpful if taken in natural food sources, not pill form. One glass per day of fresh fruit or vegetable juice is wise. Never completely stop drinking milk, especially at this time, because your bones are prone to a slight softening (osteoporosis) and the calcium in milk or skimmed milk will help to rectify this condition. If you continue to eat a regular, balanced diet you have absolutely no need of patent formulas claiming to "perk up" the tired older woman. Be careful of taking any drugs, mild though they may be, for menopausal discomfort unless they are approved or prescribed by a physician. Alcohol in very limited quantities may help as a tranquilizer for some of the more severe symptoms, but since this is likely to be a time of emotional turbulence, the dangers of heavy drinking and alcoholism are rampant at this time. Smoking at any stage in life is very dangerous and since this is the age at which cancer often reveals itself and does the most damage, smoking should be given up if it has not been before. The idea that it is too late to give up, the damage is already done, is self-defeating and spurious. If you continue or increase your smoking during menopause, you may just tip the balance in favor of the coffin.

Menopause and Exercise

Your mental outlook and physical well-being can be especially enhanced by exercise through these years. You must keep the cardiovascular and respiratory systems vigorously mobile. Any form of energetic activity will combat depression and control fatigue and insomnia. If you have had no exercise regimen before menopause, consult your doctor about the safest kinds of exercise you can indulge in. If you have been used to any form of regular physical activity before menopause, there is absolutely no reason to curb that regimen during or after menopause. This is a good time to boost your exercise schedule if it has become irregular, because you should try to offset the tendency we have at that age to gain weight.

Menopause and Aging

Contemporary American society is preoccupied with youthfulness. It used to be that youth was a time for folly and maturity was defined by wisdom, but we frequently allow the printed word and electronic media to portray the opposite. Consequently, we women develop many forms of paranoia associated with the aging process. We are afraid that when we reach maturity we will no longer be desired or useful or considered attractive. We suffer relentless pressures, some subtle and others very blatant, to retain a youthful demeanor. As the years go by, we are expected to use our faces and bodies as canvases upon which to paint revised, corrected, up-to-date images of ourselves. No matter how sensible or stable we imagine ourselves, we cannot but associate the onset of menopause with decline, decay, old age, infirmity, cessation of sexual activity, and a host of similar images more obscene than pornography. We may be so full of fear of aging that when menopause does occur, the psychological trauma is far greater than the physical change. In fact, we completely misinterpret menopause. It is a neutral stage and signifies nothing other than the possible liberation of the woman from childbearing. Fertility is no more a woman's natural state than puberty or the climacteric stage. Arithmetically, we spend more of our lives being infertile than fertile. If we expect to live to a modest sixty-five, probably less than thirty of those years will be childbearing ones and almost forty of them barren. Unless we so demand it, there is no decrease of sexual desire or activity; in fact, sexual freedom is increased since no forms of contraception are necessary. While we envy the male who worries less about his age, and fret that younger women are tough competition, we must not forget that a man of forty-five who chases young women has a serious problem coming to grips with his own maturity and is no fit companion for an adult female. The advent of menopause should be viewed as the beginning of a new life experience, just as vital and potentially creative as the years behind, if not more so. Instead of bewailing a lost youth and despairing that life is almost over, the Black woman must take advantage of her maturity to perhaps loosen her family ties, as the children grow older, and get out of the house, go back to work, or get involved in community group endeavors. Fear keeps the mature woman at home, but often when she ventures out she may find she has more to say and more to do than women twenty years younger.

We must try to refute society's whispered myths about "that time of life" and a "dangerous age." Our health, mental and physical, demands that we take a positive, outgoing, liberated attitude to menopause. We must not be influenced by what happened to our mother, aunt, or best friend; this is no age for mourning the past. You may have forty free years ahead!

G. DISEASES OF THE REPRODUCTIVE SYSTEM

One of the best ways to protect your health is by learning to recognize the symptoms of the most common female disorders. At the first sign of trouble, see a physician. Never try to diagnose yourself because symptoms of quite minor ailments may also indicate to the trained doctor much more serious diseases. Early cognition of even the most serious illnesses is by far the most important factor in achieving total recovery.

Vaginal Diseases

1) VAGINAL DISCHARGE

This is a normal occurrence and is usually related to the menstrual cycle. A healthy woman is constantly secreting lubricating and cleansing fluids in the vagina. The force of gravity and natural movement draws some of these out. Usually the discharge is white, or colorless, and has no strong odor. This is quite normal and harmless. Many factors, including the use of certain medication, contraceptives, hormone pills, excessive douching, pregnancy, and illness, can change the nature of your vaginal discharge. If the quantity, coloring, and odor of this undergoes substantial change, your doctor should be informed.

2) VAGINITIS

This takes several forms and generally refers to any infection or inflammation of the vulva and vagina. Vaginitis is commonly recognized by severe itching, pain when urinating, and a heavy, malodorous discharge. Prompt treatment can quickly terminate these conditions, so any signs of vaginitis should be reported at once.

3) TRICHOMONIASIS

This long name describes an infection caused by a very small, one-celled parasite. It is generally believed that the rectum harbors the parasite which is common to both sexes but does not harm the male. When the parasite travels to the vagina (often this voyage is encouraged by lazy or improper hygiene habits after elimination), it can create a very unpleasant infection that causes burning and itching of the vulva and vagina and can lead to chronic inflammation of the cervix. Discharge is strong smelling and yellowish. This condition is easily treated with either vaginal suppositories or an oral medication. Because this infection can be sexually transmitted, your mate should be treated for it also.

4) MONILIASIS

Sometimes called candidiasis, this condition is caused by a yeastlike fungus that normally exists, as do many others, quite harmlessly in the body. This fungus is present on our skin and in our mouths and other orifices at all times. At times it can erupt into an angry infection that causes itching, swelling, and makes sexual intercourse quite painful. The discharge is whitish and smells very bad. With this infection, urination is painful but frequent. Once diagnosed, it can be treated with antifungicidal suppositories.

5) CERVICITIS

Most vaginal infections can also harm the cervix, which is vulnerable to injury during childbirth. Self-examination will not necessarily reveal such infection, which is why the suspicion of any such infection or inflammation must be brought to the attention of a doctor. Infected cervical tissue can be easily and painlessly removed with no loss of function. Because the cervix is so vulnerable to cancer, any minor complaint should be quickly taken care of.

6) ATROPHIS VAGINALIS

As the tissue of the vaginal area ages, infection increases and the older woman is prone to many minor vaginal disturbances which should be promptly seen by a doctor because they may indicate cancer. If there is no serious cause for such infections, they are usually treated with estrogen hormone suppositories.

TREATMENT OF VAGINAL DISEASES

Women who regard the slightest signs of discharge as indicative of disease often encourage infection by indulging in excessive astringent douching and vaginal cleansing in an effort to stop the discharge.

Such activity can destroy the natural acid balance within the vaginal cavity and this supports the spread of bacteria and increases the risk of infection. Fairly clear, slight discharge should be regarded as part of the body's own cleansing process, not as a danger sign. If the discharge alters in nature and is accompanied by any other distressing symptoms, you will only aggravate the situation and allow it to worsen if you delay seeing a doctor and try to treat it yourself. As Black women we may well think twice before taking such troubles to physicians, some of whom harbor innate prejudice that leads them to diagnose quickly any such internal disorder in a Black woman as venereal. I am sure many of us have had that experience, a particularly offensive and humiliating one. Nonetheless, if we arm ourselves with greater knowledge about our bodies and the variety of infections we are liable to incur, we can reduce the possibility of physician error through prejudice. One thing above all remember: You cannot treat these infections yourself. They will not go away unless treated by a professional and no matter how embarrassing the experience, that is more than made up for if you save your health, your capacity to reproduce, and perhaps your life.

The vagina is one of the most vulnerable areas of our body. Dark and moist, it is a perfect breeding ground for bacteria. For this reason the incidence of infection is very high and not a sign of uncleanliness or loose morals. It is very rare for any woman to go her entire life without at least one outbreak of vaginal infection. Be guided by these suggestions:

1) See a doctor at the first signs of infection.

2) Use the prescribed medication for the *full time* indicated. Often we stop when the discomfort ceases, but that may be long before the infection is cured.

3) Avoid excessive douching, suppositories, and vaginal deodorants.

4) Bathe and shower frequently.

5) Do not wear tight-fitting panties and panty girdles.

6) Wear cotton, not synthetic, panties.

7) If you suspect an infection or have had it confirmed and are being treated, you must first wash your undergarments in hot, soapy water, rinse well, then boil for twenty minutes. Machine washing will not kill bacteria; they must be boiled. This should include bathing suits and night garments. Also clean bathtub and shower areas very thoroughly.

Urinary Diseases

Cystitis, or inflammation of the bladder, may be indicated by abdominal pains, a burning sensation when urinating, frequent urination, pus or blood in the urine, and general discomfort in that area. Women are particularly prone to cystitis because the urethra leading from the bladder to the outside is short and very close to the vagina and rectum. If this is not draining properly, it can become a breeding ground for bacteria. Cystitis responds quickly to drug medication and the intake of large amounts of fluid. "Honeymoon cystitis" is so called because it is caused by the bruising and jostling sustained by the bladder and urethra during sexual intercourse, especially if after a period of sexual abstinence. There is usually no bacterial infection, but a degree of irritation. If possible, a woman should urinate before intercourse and soon afterward. One of the worst things we are encouraged to do as children is to hold our water. This habit sticks and often assists cystitis to develop. Urinate as frequently as you feel the need; that is the healthiest thing. Wash the vulva in warm soapy water, especially the clitoral hood and the urethral opening, rinse, and dry well.

Fibroid Tumors

These growths on or inside the uterus seem to occur more frequently in Black women than other racial groups. The cause for this is not yet known, although there is a definite correlation between the growth of fibroid tumors and hormone activity that can be stimulated by pregnancy and the taking of oral contraceptives. Although mostly benign, these tumors can grow as large as a nine-month gestation if unattended and can cause abdominal pain and bleeding. If the patient is over thirty-five, the tumor is usually removed with a hysterectomy and if she is younger a myoctemy is performed whereby only the tumor itself is removed.

Ovarian Cysts

When benign, these are simple capsulelike structures containing fluid that develop on the ovaries. They are only removed if they grow beyond a certain size, but regular examination is important.

Cancer

The word "cancer" applies to a family of diseases that is characterized by the abnormal and uncontrolled growth of cells whose spread destroys normal tissue. If this spread is not checked, the cells can travel in the blood to other parts of the body. Of cancer in general there has been an alarming rise in the mortality rate among the Black population of the United States. It has increased 20 per cent in as many years and, although in 1950 the rate was lower than for whites, it is now significantly higher. The reasons for this rise are varied but are socioeconomic, not physiological in nature. It really comes down to the fact that poverty denies us adequate health care and even in areas where it is available we do not avail ourselves of the opportunity to have the frequent examinations that will detect early signs of cancer. The female reproductive system is vulnerable to cancer of the cervix, cancer of the uterus, and cancer of the breast, each of which we will deal with separately. Uterine cancer among Black women is declining, but breast cancer is increasing and we have the highest rate of cervical cancer of any ethnic group in this country.

Cancer can strike at any age, but the woman past forty is more prone to it than a younger person. The causes are still largely unknown but it is quite definitely *curable if detected sufficiently early*. It is a very dangerous adversary, but once caught and treated in the early stages is effectively rid from the body forever. The billions of dollars being spent on cancer research throughout the world are bearing fruit. Once found, cancer can be treated by surgery, X-ray, radiation therapy, and chemotherapy. Cancer is not contagious, but it is very difficult to detect. There are no obvious symptoms that manifest themselves at an early stage. The only way for us to absolutely avoid the possibility of death from cancer is by having frequent, complete physical examinations combined with self-examination and an awareness of the following body changes that may indicate the presence of cancerous tissue:

Change in bowel or bladder habits.
A sore throat that does not heal.
Unusual bleeding or discharge.
Thickening, or lump, in breast or elsewhere.
Indigestion, loss of appetite, or difficulty swallowing.
Obvious change in a wart, mole, or birthmark.
Nagging cough or hoarseness.

Learn these signs, the first letters of each spell out C.A.U.T.I.O.N. Pain is not usually associated with the damaging stages of cancer and so the absence of pain is no indication that there is no cancer present in the body. The early detection of cancer among lower-income women is a prime target of two large organizations, the American Cancer Society and the National Cancer Institute. Both offer free examination to women over thirty-five, aimed at detecting breast cancer *before* the lump-forming stage. The cure rate when this happens is better than 90 per cent. Twelve state health departments recently received $10,000,000 from the National Cancer Institute for a three-year program to screen lower-income women for cancer of the cervix. In some parts of this country, "lower-income" is synonymous still with "Black," and we must seek out and take advantage of these programs. If you suspect you have cancer, do not let fear of knowing keep you from a physician because treatment is possible, and every day you delay you are shortening your chances of survival. Go to a doctor or the cancer clinic of a state or university-affiliated hospital. Up to the age of thirty-five, every woman must be examined once per year for uterine and cervical cancer (a Pap test), for breast cancer, for cancer of the colon (rectal examination). After the age of thirty-five, these examinations should be conducted *twice every year*.

UTERINE CANCER

Cancer of the uterus itself and the endometrium lining of the uterus often strikes mature women and usually occurs after menopause. The Pap test is very effective in determining uterine cancer and simply consists of painlessly taking a sample of fluid from the vagina and examining it under laboratory conditions. A new tool called a gravlee has recently been developed that washes the lining of the uterus and gathers cells for study. Once detected, uterine cancer is treated by removing all of the cancerous tissue by surgery or radiation, including surrounding healthy tissue to ensure that no cancerous cells remain.

CERVICAL CANCER

Cancer of the cervix, the neck of the uterus, is second only to breast cancer in frequency among all American women but is more prevalent among Black women than any other form of cancer. Many theories have been advanced to account for this startling and disturbing fact, and although none has been conclusively proved, we should examine some of the most important:

Physiological. That there are inherent physical characteristics of the cervical cells in Black women that predispose them to cancer. The evidence for this is weak and unsubstantiated.

Economic. That poverty inhibits substantial numbers of Black women from obtaining the kind of regular medical care that would reduce the possibility of this kind of cancer developing. If infections of the genital-urinary tract are untreated, the cervix will suffer and cancer cells can develop in any such weak area. This theory is supported by the fact that the poorest group measured, immigrant Puerto Rican women, have a rate of cervical cancer four times that of the national average.

Social. That frequent sexual intercourse in the teen-age years and childbearing in those years cause damage to the cervix that can encourage cancer. This might make sense if it could be proved that as a group our sexual mores are markedly different from other groups; since this cannot be so proved, this theory is most likely racist in origin.

Another theory that may have an equally shaky basis is that there is a correlation between lack of circumcision in the male and cervical cancer in the female, and that Black males tend to be uncircumcised. This idea is really based on the negative premise that Moslem and Jewish women (whose mates are circumcised) have a very low rate of cervical cancer.

Whether the answer is one of the above or a combination of factors does not alter our singular predisposition to this deadly disease. We are not helpless, though. The Pap test is 95 per cent effective in detecting cervical cancer and must be regularly and frequently taken by all of us Black women.

OVARIAN AND FALLOPIAN CANCER

Cancer of the Fallopian tubes is quite rare, but cancer of the ovaries is not unusual. It is quite insidious because there are rarely any symptoms and often by the time it is diagnosed it has reached the fatal stage. It can be detected before this but only by professional physical examination that may indicate a slight enlargement of the ovaries. Then they can be treated with radiation therapy or surgically removed before the cells have irrevocably spread to other parts of the body. This form of cancer has been noted in prepubescent girls but is most likely to occur in women over forty. This is the very important reason for semiannual complete checkups.

CANCER OF THE BREAST

Wide publicity regarding this in recent years has made a great number of women much more conscientious about the need for early diagnosis, which is immeasurably aided by establishing a regular program of self-examination. There is an X-ray procedure (mammography) that is used to detect breast cancer, but it is presently only available to those who may have a family history of such cancer or to confirm a diagnosis based on a physical examination. Thermography is also used to detect breast cancer by measuring the relative heat emanating from breast tissue. Malignant cells produce more heat. Both mammography and thermography are expensive and require skilled personnel to administer the tests and evaluate the results. At the present time there is really no substitute for self-examination and thorough examination by a physician on a regular basis. If a nodule or lump is found in the breast, a very tiny sample of the suspicious tissue is taken and examined microscopically to determine if the growth is malignant or benign. Three out of four such biopsies prove to be benign. There are three possible courses for the surgeon to choose to take if the lump is cancerous. The traditional, standard procedure is to perform a *radical mastectomy*. This is the removal of the breast as well as the lymph nodes under the armpit and part of the chest muscle. *Simple mastectomy* consists of the removal of the breast alone and *lumpectomy* or *partial mastectomy* is the removal of only the tumor mass itself and the surrounding tissue. There is considerable controversy over which is the best technique, but so far there is simply no alternative to surgery.

Postmastectomy Adjustment

Many women feel that breast removal is akin to castration and that they will never be "whole" again. The adjustments that must be made are emotional, psychological, social, and physical and cannot be made alone. Despite the fact that with the modern prostheses (artificial breasts) it is impossible to tell if a clothed woman has undergone mastectomy, it is probably this society's obsession with breasts as only sex objects that often makes it harder for a woman to adjust to a mastectomy than to a limb amputation. Society, she feels, accepts the latter but not the former. This is why the Reach to Recovery program is so important. It is a volunteer organization of former mastectomy patients who are available to counsel, reassure, and assist any mastectomy patient with help that begins immediately after the operation. She will train the patient how to use the prosthesis—which may be made of foam, plastic, or silicone—and advise her about recuperative exercises and marital adjustment. Most women find their mates more, not less, attentive after this operation. The only criticism I have of the current situation is that there are no breast forms manufactured in the wide range of colors that Black women require. Although the breast form is not seen, even when swimming, there are psychological factors that would make natural color breast forms for the Black woman most welcome. Both department stores and some smaller shops now have sections that cater exclusively to the woman who has undergone breast surgery. A sense of fashion does not have to be sacrificed by such women who find specially designed bathing suits and low-cut dresses still can be worn with assurance.

Breast Examination

There is no correlation between breast size and cancer, but you should be particularly wary if members of your family have suffered cancer.

Because of the emphasis placed upon the breasts as sources of sexual stimulation and gratification, some women may feel embarrassed or uncomfortable about feeling themselves. If this attitude prevails over common sense, you may not discover breast cancer until it is too late and not even a radical mastectomy can save your life. Ninety per cent of all breast cancer is first discovered (or at least, its possible symptoms are discovered) by the patient herself. Remember, you cannot tell if you have cancer or not, and you cannot treat yourself. What you must do, however, is search for a hard lump. Immediately inform your doctor; do not attempt to cure yourself. He will take steps to determine *if* it is serious, *if* a biopsy should be performed, and only then will

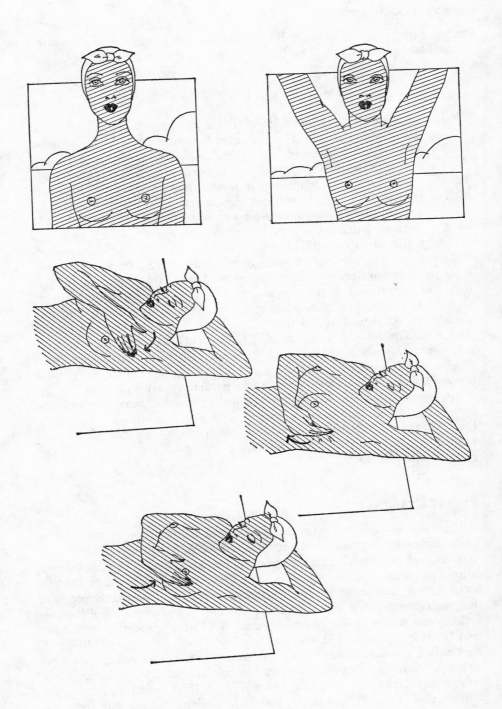

you know if it is cancerous. A lump does not mean cancer but it must be immediately reported.

Most doctors and the American Cancer Society advise us to examine our breasts at least once a month. The best time for doing this is the day after your menstrual bleeding has stopped. If you are on "the Pill," examine your breasts during that period you are not taking it. Just before menstruation the breasts tend to have a granular internal texture and this makes it difficult to detect a lump, but after menses the breasts should feel soft, jellylike, perhaps slightly ropy.

1) Strip to the waist. Stand or sit in front of a mirror with your arms relaxed at your sides. Look slowly for any changes in shape and size of the contours of your breasts and nipples. Raise arms above head and re-examine.

2) Lie on a firm bed or on the floor. With the left hand behind the head, place the tips of the fingers of the right hand on the outer edge of the left breast. Using a gentle, circular motion, feel around the perimeter of the breast and move in toward the nipple. Bring the left arm down and feel from the nipple out again.

3) Reverse the procedure; with your right hand behind your neck, examine the right breast with the left hand.

After a bath or shower, when still slightly wet, you may more readily detect a lump or thickening area. If you do, there is no reason for alarm; simply call your physician or clinic and make an appointment for as soon as possible.

Venereal Diseases (VD)

Gonorrhea and syphilis are the most common venereal diseases and although medical textbooks contain statistics purporting to indicate that Black women have a higher incidence than white of venereal disease, there are a number of reasons why this conclusion is wrong. My principal quarrel with such figures is that they are based on reported tabulations of the disease and although it is against the law to withhold reporting a case of VD to the local health authority, many doctors in private practice do not report their patients and these are mostly white women. Black women, being on the whole poorer, must be treated for VD at clinics that are bound to report the statistics. Consequently, one frequently finds male doctors, both white and Black, firmly believing that Black women are likely to have VD and sometimes diagnosing nonvenereal ailments of the reproductive system as VD simply because the patient is Black.

Venereal disease is communicated by intimate physical contact between one infected person and another, formerly noninfected, sexual partner. Contact may be of the mouth, sexual organs, or rectum. Prevention is virtually impossible unless the male wears a prophylactic condom at all times during the period of sexual contact.

GONORRHEA

This disease ranks number one among the most widespread communicative diseases in the United States. It is much more commonly identified as a male disease only because it is quite difficult to detect in the female. Gonorrhea may have few or no symptoms. Those that do appear are often increased vaginal discharge, abdominal pains, chills, fever. Such symptoms can often be misinterpreted by the patient and a physician not consulted until the infection is in the dangerous later stages. If untreated, gonorrhea causes pelvic inflammation that requires surgical sterilization. If gonorrhea is detected in good time, it can simply be treated with penicillin, a very effective, standard procedure.

SYPHILIS

Syphilis rarely shows and there are no symptoms in women in its initial stage. But from ten to ninety days after contact, a sore will form at the site of infection. This may be hidden in the labia or be on the mouth, fingers, or breast. The sore will often fade, but the disease is raging. Six weeks later a rash may be accompanied by headache and fever. These too can all but disappear, although the organism can remain in the body for up to twenty years, slowly destroying heart and brain tissue. All stages of syphilis can be effectively treated with penicillin, but obviously it is better thwarted right at the start of the cycle.

If you are alerted by a sexual partner that you may have VD, or you suspect the symptoms you have, there are VD clinics in almost every state where laboratory tests are given without charge. Your local hospital or physician can also help.

H. BIRTH CONTROL

Before I explain the advantages and drawbacks of the various different methods of birth control, I must state that as a Black woman and a Catholic I am opposed to a widespread, thoughtless, self-indulgent use of contraceptive methods. It is a matter for personal conscience, but that must be tempered by the needs of the family as a unit, the society as a whole, and our race as an expanding phenomenon. There is indeed serious consideration to be given to the question of whether or not it is right to bring Black children into a world if they cannot be fed or clothed or educated or employed; but on the other hand, we must be aware of the fact that the federal government, in the form of the Department of Health, Education and Welfare, is spending massive sums on population control and that control is strongly directed at the Black population—almost exclusively so. The goal of most population control groups is zero rate increase, a situation whereby the birth rate would equal the adult death rate. This may be a subtle form of genocide for us because our infant mortality rates and maternal mortality rates are higher than the rest of the population; our numbers would slowly decline at zero growth rate. This attitude is quite a reversal from that of the pre-Abolition years when we were encouraged and bribed by our white masters to breed many slaves. In a free society, as ours is supposed to be, the decision to practice birth control is a matter for the mother to decide, not the father or the government. It is she who bears and rears the child and it is a matter for her and her beliefs alone. We must not forget that contraceptive measures are not the only means of birth control. In the past and in the present, abortion, sterilization, and infanticide have been sanctioned in various civilizations.

Contraception

The woman who decides to take contraceptive measures must first be aware of her needs and then consult with a doctor. The effectiveness of any contraceptive device is related to the woman's mental and physical proclivities. You cannot determine these entirely yourself and you must take the advise of a physician. It is not simply a matter of the effectiveness of the method you wish to use, but whether or not it can cause temporary or permanent damage to your system, inhibit your childbearing capacity for the future, or have immediate unpleasant side effects. This chart of current contraceptive measures is not meant to substitute for a doctor's advice but to implement it and help you understand all the possibilities.

THE PILL

This is the most widely used method and if used correctly is almost 100 per cent effective. It prevents the release of the egg from the ovary but since this is accomplished by effecting hormonal change, there can be potentially dangerous side effects. Recently a minipill was approved that is less effective but much safer since it does not contain as much hormonal substances. Black women have a tendency to develop fibroid tumors in the uterus and the Pill can encourage such growth. Generally doctors will not prescribe the Pill for patients they know to be suffering from high blood pressure, sickle-cell anemia, kidney disease, or diabetes.

INTRAUTERINE DEVICE (IUD)

This very popular method of birth control is now being scrutinized more closely for defects. It consists of a small plastic or metal flexible device that is inserted into the uterus, and although it certainly inhibits conception, why it

Current Means of Contraception

Method	Theoretical effectiveness[a]	Limitations in usefulness	Associated reactions and side effects
Tubal ligation	Virtually 100 percent	Outpatient surgery or hospitalization required; reversibility difficult	Several days recuperation needed; risks associated with surgical procedures.
Vasectomy	Virtually 100 percent	Office or outpatient minor surgery; reversibility difficult	Temporary scrotal swelling, soreness, or discomfort in some cases; risks associated with minor surgical procedures.
Oral contraceptive ("the pill")	Almost 100 percent if taken as directed	Checkups required for supervision and complications; method not indicated for various medical reasons	Minor reactions such as headache, nausea, breast tenderness, irregular bleeding are common but tend to pass with continuing use and are readily tolerated by millions of users. Perhaps 15 percent of users will experience altered blood chemistry or sugar metabolism but without clinical manifestations. In some countries adverse effects on the liver are seen but not in others. About 5 percent of users will experience elevated blood pressure. Rare cases of blood clotting disease.
Oral contraceptive ("mini-pill")	Highly effective, but not as effective as "the pill"	Checkups required for supervision and complications; method not indicated for various medical reasons	Minor reactions such as headache and nausea less than "the pill." Irregular bleeding, spotting, and weight are common and continue with use. Changes in blood chemistry in some women, but less than "the pill." Generally considered to have less risk than "the pill" because of the absence of estrogen.
Injectable	Almost 100 percent, if schedule followed	Checkups required for supervision and complications, and return visits to clinic for periodic injections; method not indicated for various medical reasons	Minor reactions such as weight gain occur in some women. Most users experience menstrual cycle disruption starting with irregular bleeding and giving rise later, in many women, to amenorrhea. Delay in restoration of fertility after termination of use is frequent. Rare cases of excessive uterine bleeding.

Method	Effectiveness[a]	Requirements and problems	Side effects
Intrauterine devices (IUDs)	Highly effective but not as effective as "the pill"	Office or clinic visit required for insertion; checkups required for supervision and complications; method not indicated for some women	Minor reactions such as irregular bleeding, spotting, cramps, or discomfort are common initially but tend to pass with continuing use and are tolerated by millions of users. Rare cases of pelvic inflammatory disease (infection), perforation of uterus.
Diaphragm with jelly or cream	Highly effective if used correctly	Office or clinic visit required for fitting and for instruction on technique of insertion; method not indicated for medical reasons, in infrequent cases; requires insertion in anticipation of coitus	None but occasional complaints of discomfort.
Condoms	Highly effective if used correctly	Method requires interruption of sexual preparation and stimulation	None
Temperature rhythm	Highly effective if used correctly	Coitus limited to less than half of each menstrual cycle; careful instruction needed to learn interpretation of temperature chart; cannot be used if woman has grossly irregular menstruation	None
Calendar rhythm	Moderately effective if used correctly, but less than "temperature rhythm"	Coitus limited to less than half of each menstrual cycle; careful instruction needed to learn computation of safe days; cannot be used if woman has grossly irregular menstruation	None
Chemical contraceptives (foams, creams, jellies, suppositories and foam tablets)	Moderately effective; foams highest, foam tablets and suppositories lowest	Method requires interruption of sexual preparation and stimulation; insertion not more than one hour in advance	Rare minor, local allergic reactions or irritation.
Withdrawal	Moderately effective	Method requires interruption of intercourse; unsuitable if male partner cannot control ejaculation	None
Douche	Least effective	Method requires interruption immediately after ejaculation	None

[a] For all nonsurgical methods, effectiveness in actual use varies from significantly lower to much lower, depending on education and motivation.

Reprinted with the permission of the Population Council from "World Population: Status Report 1974," prepared by Bernard Berelson with the collaboration of staff members of the Population Council, *Reports on Population/Family Planning*, Number 15, January 1974, page 38.

does is not completely understood. One theory is that it inflames the wall of the uterus and makes the implanting of a fertilized egg impossible. Another theory is that the continual effort to expel the foreign object also forces the egg out of the Fallopian tube before it is developed enough to implant. It is now known that a number of women who have worn an IUD later had badly infected miscarriages, and health officials are asking for much stricter controls on the marketing of these devices. Because it is not a drug but a mechanical object, controls have formerly been lax. Many doctors will not prescribe it on the grounds that it is difficult to insert, often painful to wear, and tricky to remove.

RHYTHM METHODS

These are based upon determining exactly when ovulation occurs and avoiding intercourse during the fifteen to twenty most fertile days of the menstrual cycle. Although they are not infallible, if you have a very regular menstrual cycle and are willing to forgo intercourse on designated days, these are by far the safest methods.

MECHANICAL AND CHEMICAL METHODS

Spermicides are chemical substances introduced into the vagina in an attempt to kill the male sperm at the time of intercourse and thus prevent conception. They may be in the form of suppositories, creams, jellies, aerosol foams, and douches. Alone, they are less than effective but can be almost totally effective if combined with the use of a *diaphragm*. The latter is a rubber, saucer-shaped disc, about four inches wide, that is inserted sideways into the vagina, and when properly in place, covers the cervix, or entrance to the uterus. The most common artificial method of contraception is probably the *condom*, a rubber sheath that the male partner wears on the penis during intercourse which collects the sperm and prevents it from entering the vagina.

FUTURE METHODS

A drug known as Depo Provera has been approved for use in this country. It is administered by injection and apparently can prevent conception for up to three months at a time. It is not widely available, however, and has not been completely tested.

Sterilization

Many of us are aware of recent scandals that took place mainly in the South involving the involuntary sterilization of young Black women.

Sterilization laws became relaxed in recent years but are now being scrutinized more closely. Both men and women can be sterilized, the woman by tubal ligation or the covering and tying of the Fallopian tubes, and the man by vasectomy, or the cutting of the sperm-bearing tubes in the scrotum. Sterilization is not reversible, so it must be voluntary and it must be preceded by very careful consideration.

Vasectomy and the use of the condom are the only birth control measures that place part of the burden on the male. More research is now being done to investigate how the male reproductive system can be altered to inhibit conception. Even the most modern birth control methods for women have not been as safe, effective, reversible, acceptable, and inexpensive as had been hoped.

Abortion

Many doctors will refer to premature deliveries as well as miscarriages as abortions, but in daily use the word usually refers to an *induced abortion* whereby the pregnancy is deliberately terminated prematurely and the fetus does not survive. Induced abortion is legal in some parts of this country. As *therapeutic abortion*, it is justified, supposedly, by the adverse mental, physical, or economic condition of the mother. It is not possible to determine whether or not we, as a group, undergo more abortions than white women but we do know that unwed mothers do not make up the majority of women who seek abortions. Evidence suggests that as many as four out of every five abortions are performed on married women who have one or more children.

Never attempt to secure an illegal abortion. If you are seeking a legal abortion, you should first discuss the matter with some professional aware of local regulations. This person might be a minister, a nurse, a physician, or a social worker. If they cannot help you find a reputable facility, contact the local Planned Parenthood Office.

METHODS OF ABORTION

If the pregnancy is advanced by less than sixteen weeks, most doctors administer a D. and C., discussed earlier in this chapter. Sometimes a saline solution is injected into the uterus to induce contraction and expulsion of the fetus; this is sometimes called a *"salting out."* Other methods include the use of a plastic aspirator and suction pump, and a new method still being researched involves the injection into the uterus of a hormone solution that induces labor at any stage of pregnancy. There are risks attendant upon all these methods, and you must be under medical care not only immediately after the abortion but until you begin to menstruate regularly. Efforts to self-induce abortion by injuring the vagina or introducing implements into the uterus or taking unprescribed drugs often lead to sterility or death.

I. THE INTERNAL EXAMINATION

Most doctors recommend a complete internal examination at least once a year starting between the ages of eighteen and twenty. If a younger woman is indulging in sexual activity or notices any unusual condition in the genital area, then the first examination should take place at once. It is advisable that after the age of thirty-five we visit the doctor twice a year for this kind of checkup. The danger of cancer increases with age. There are four types of medical personnel who are authorized to examine you. If you suspect that the person you are seeing is not one of these, you have every right to know:

1) Gynaecologist—a doctor of medicine who specializes in women's diseases;

2) Obstetrician—a doctor of medicine primarily concerned with pregnancy and childbirth;

3) General practitioner or internist—also doctors of medicine;

4) A nurse or midwife certified by the American College of Obstetrics & Gynaecology.

The last category cannot diagnose or treat disorders, but may conduct examinations and report to a physician. It is important that you have a doctor with whom you can discuss your intimate parts candidly. In the past, women were "not supposed to know" about themselves, and this left all the responsibility for their internal health in the hands of a male doctor who was frequently unsympathetic to tales of "female complaints." With the advent of an outspoken women's movement we can expect a greater degree of awareness and sympathy from the medical profession, but it is still a profession 90 per cent of which is white and male. The chances for us to be examined by one of our own, a Black female doctor, are slim indeed, although their numbers are growing. The more we know about the way our body functions as Black and as female, the more prepared we are for any examination. Those of us not able to consult private practitioners may have to put up with the sometimes inhuman treatment meted out by health clinics where time is almost nonexistent for a full discussion of your problems. Although often overburdened and understaffed, these clinics are frequently run by talented and dedicated medical personnel working under the direction of a fully qualified supervisory physician. In such circumstances we must allow for some confusion and hurry, but it is well worth it if an early diagnosis saves you the anguish and cost of serious operations. I hope the following guidelines will suggest to you what MUST be done to constitute a thorough internal examination and what you can demand if it is absent.

Pre-examination

1) Make the appointment for a day following your period so that your breasts can easily be felt for lumps.

2) Avoid douching for twenty-four hours before examination.

3) A bowel movement the morning of your examination will minimize some discomfort.

4) Make a note of any questions you have or unusual conditions you remember since your last visit.

Examination

1) You should first be seen by the doctor in the office, fully clothed. If it is a first visit, the doctor should take down your case history. If they have your records, you should bring the doctor up to date regarding any ailments, however minor.

2) You should be asked to retire to a shielded area or bathroom to change into a clean smock and empty your bladder for a urine sample.

3) If a nurse is not present during the examination, you may request one.

4) First you should *sit* on a table in the examination room and the doctor will feel your breasts for any lumps and examine them for puckering of the skin or discharge. If the machinery is available, an X-ray of your breasts may be taken.

5) You will be asked to lie on the table while the doctor gently presses your abdomen for any indications of thickening in the uterus and ovaries.

6) You should be helped to place your feet in the stirrups on either side of the table. The smock should cover you from neck to knees. The doctor will stand or sit between your legs facing your vagina. First the doctor examines the outer genital area to make sure it is free from irritation and infection. Then a speculum is inserted. (This is a simple instrument that supports the walls of the vagina while the doctor takes a smear from the uterus with a swab or flat stick.) This is the Pap test and your secretions will be examined in the laboratory for any signs of abnormal conditions.

7) With a finger (the doctor is wearing sterilized rubber gloves) your rectum is probed to determine the presence of such conditions as hemorrhoids and cancer of the colon.

8) The doctor may make additional tests as your age and situation may warrant.

Postexamination

You will get dressed and return to the doctor's office for a brief diagnosis of your condition and to receive any prescriptions that may be necessary. Ask what the medication is for, how long you must take it, what side effects are possible.

J. EMERGENCY TREATMENT

Childbirth

The unborn child is protected by a bag of amnionic fluid, quite literally, water. In most cases the first indication of impending birth is the break of this water that will begin to leak or flow out of the vagina. Uterine contractions may occur before or after this; sometimes the birth does not happen until forty-eight hours after the water breaks, but once it does, the fetus is less protected and mother and child should receive tender care. The following rules should be observed if you or a friend should be surprised by a sudden birth without benefit of a doctor or midwife. Under normal circumstances, the hospital or doctor or clinic should be called as soon as the water breaks or uterine spasms begin.

1) Let nature take its course. Wash your hands and make sure the birth canal is clean. Support the emerging baby but do not let hands or tools enter the vagina.

2) Place the newborn baby between the mother's thighs, with the head slightly lowered; cover the baby to keep it warm.

3) If the infant is not breathing, gently employ mouth-to-mouth respiration.

4) Carefully massage the mother's abdomen to help the uterus contract.

5) Immerse scissors in boiling water or clean them with alcohol. Tie a clean tape or cloth in a square knot around the umbilical cord about four inches from the baby. Tie a second knot another four inches from the first, away from the baby. If no tapes are available, use shoestrings.

6) Do not be in a hurry to cut the cord; wait until the afterbirth has been expelled. Then cut the cord between the tapes with clean scissors.

7) Do not wash white substance off the baby; it protects the skin.

8) Don't touch the baby's eyes, ears, nose, or mouth. Keep baby and mother warm.

9) Call police, fire, or ambulance and transport mother and child to nearest hospital.

Rape

The National Commission on the Causes and Prevention of Violence reported in 1967 that in seventeen major U.S. cities, 60 per cent of all rapes were committed by Black men and the victims were Black women; 3 per cent were committed by white men against Black women; 27 per cent by white men against white women, and 10 per cent by Black men against white women. Most rapes occur in predominantly Black neighborhoods and in half the crimes the assailant is known by the victim. Most rapes are planned in advance and over half occur in the home in the daytime. Many rapists are married and lead ostensibly normal lives. In our society the judicial structure is such that often the rape victim herself bears the burden of proving her innocence from having enticed the rapist rather than enjoying the protection of the state and the prosecution of the criminal. For this reason many, many rapes are unreported: the victim fears the humiliation that a public trial might force her to endure. In recent years, however, the incidences of reported rape are increasing with startling rapidity. In 1973, 51,000 rapes were reported—an increase of 60 per cent over 1968. Statistics such as these and pressure from women's rights groups are slowly forcing some state legislatures to amend their rape laws so that the victim has at least the same protection as the accused. The other institution involved with rape—the hospital —is now on the whole more responsive and concerned about this emergency. For years many hospitals would be generally hostile to a rape victim. Rape can occur to any woman of any age regardless of position or wealth.

The Rape Crisis Center in Washington, D.C., presents the following suggestions for the prevention of rape and how to handle an attacker:

At Home

1) List only your initials and last name in the telephone directory and on your mailbox.

2) Keep your doors locked *at all times*.

3) When you move, have new locks installed *immediately*.

4) Never open the door automatically to a knock. If necessary, tell deliverymen to leave goods outside the door. Use a chain bolt to check identification of strangers.

5) Leave at least one light on when you go out, and make sure that your hall outside the door is well lit. If you return at night, have your key ready in your hand.

6) Protect ground-floor and rooftop apartments with bars or gates that are fire-code approved.

7) Never use a secluded basement laundry alone and be wary of unguarded underground parking lots.

8) If you return home and find a door or window has been forced, DO NOT ENTER. Leave silently and use a neighbor's telephone to call the police. Wait for their arrival.

9) Do not enter an elevator with a stranger. If someone who makes you uneasy gets on your elevator, leave at the next floor. Always stand near the control panel and if attacked, hit the alarm button as many times as possible. Press as many other buttons as you can.

On the Street

1) Avoid unlit areas.

2) Walk near the curb, away from doorways and alleyways where an attacker could hide.

3) Do not pass through groups of men but cross the street, or walk around them.

4) Listen for voices and footsteps and above all remain alert.

5) When you choose your clothes, bear in mind that certain items such as platform shoes, clogs, long necklaces, and scarves offer an attacker easy ways to render you helpless.

6) In the face of danger, always scream "FIRE!" This will bring out far more people than "Help" or "Rape."

Traveling

1) Take taxis, especially at night. Ask the driver to wait outside your building until you are safely in the door.

2) If the taxi is not licensed, look for identification and take a close look at the driver.

3) When traveling by bus, sit close to the driver. Ask only the driver for directions.

4) Avoid empty or near-empty subway cars. When possible, travel in a car that will deposit you close to the exit of your station so you avoid a long walk on the platform.

5) When driving, avoid unlit roads. Keep the windows and doors locked. Keep the car in gear at stop signs and traffic lights. Never leave your purse on the seat and check the back seat before entering the car.

6) If you are being followed by another car, drive to a well-populated, busy area for help. Do not ever leave your keys in the ignition. If you are attacked, lean on the horn.

Self-Defense

1) Unless you are trained in self-defense, do not resist an armed man. Tell him you are pregnant or have VD.

2) Do not carry a gun or a knife; not only are they illegal but they can be used by the attacker against you. If your attacker is unarmed, you can wield the following in order to get away:

a) *Perfume,* hair spray, or lemon juice that can be squirted into the attacker's eyes.

b) Lighted *cigarette* to smash into attacker's face.

c) Heavy *ring* worn with ornament inside the hand for a strong slap in the attacker's face.

d) An *umbrella* can be effective if held with both hands, one in the middle and one at the handle. Jab the neck and the stomach.

e) A *whistle* should be carried in the hand or at the wrist, never around the neck.

f) A *hatpin* held firmly in the hand should be aimed at the face and neck.

None of these are effective unless they are in your hand when attacked. They are useless in your purse.

3) Do not throw your hands out to strike the attacker; he can grab them and use them to push you down.

4) If he closes in on you, use your elbows and aim for his neck and stomach. His weakest points are his eyes, ears, nose, and mouth. If possible, strike these hard with your fists.

5) A loud scream into his ear may stun him; don't be afraid to use your teeth.

6) He may be aware that you will aim for his groin, so surprise him by kicking his knees and shins. If you aim too high, you risk losing your balance.

To Report a Rape

1) Immediately call the police; time is important.

2) Do not bathe, clean up, douche, or change clothes. Preserve as much evidence as possible.

3) Take a change of clothes and demand to go to the nearest hospital.

4) While waiting for police, write down as much as you can about the rapist and the circumstances of the attack.

5) Call a friend or local hotline for moral and professional support. Every woman should find out the number of her local rape-crisis office.

6) Six weeks after the attack, have an examination for venereal infection and a pregnancy test if your next period is missed.

The most important thing to remember when attacked is that you must save your life and, if possible, look for a chance to run. If you try to "win" the fight, you may only increase the danger to your life. The attacker may expect you to be cowed immediately and a ferocious counterassault may scare him off.

Chapter IX

MENTAL HEALTH

———◆———

Mental health and mental illness and the difference that lies between them are among the least understood facets of contemporary medical knowledge. The general public as well as writers for the press and television bandy about words and phrases such as "nervous breakdown," "psycho," "inferiority complex," and "crazy" to describe incidents and patterns of behavior that range from very mild peculiarities to chronic malfunctions of the brain. Even the doctors that specialize in psychiatry and psychology do not always agree on the definitions of such terms as "schizophrenia" or "neurosis," nor do they necessarily all subscribe to general principles of causes and cures for these disorders. This makes it very confusing for the woman who either has a healthy curiosity about mental illness or wishes to know more because she is concerned about herself or a friend or relative. I am going to try to outline broadly the practical aspects of mental hygiene. We may all have our personal biases concerning the efficacy of such things as psychoanalysis, drug therapy, and old-fashioned will power, but we must have a fairly clear picture of what it is we are discussing. As we shall see in a later section of this chapter, the Black woman is not subject to mental disorders that are markedly different from women in general, so we shall treat this outline without racial emphasis.

A. WHAT IS SANITY?

When we speak of the mind, in relationship to "sanity," we must incorporate into our thinking all that is conjured up by the words *intelligence, emotion, personality, nerves,* and *soul.* In the context of current language usage these albeit vague qualities constitute our "mind." Depending upon one's point of view, sanity is either conjectured as being a state in which the mind functions without overt or grave harm to oneself or others or, alternatively, *insanity* is considered as anything that deviates grossly from the norm in thought or behavior. Between these two extremes there lies the truth and, in fact, it consists of three parts: the normal, the neurotic, and the psychotic.

Normal

First of all, be assured that neither I nor you nor possibly anyone you know fits perfectly the clinical definition of what constitutes normality. The following qualities are generally considered to be desirable in a "normal" woman or man:

1) A realistic attitude to life, its joys and sorrows.
2) The ability to make long-range decisions and abide by them.
3) A willingness to be reasonably dependent on others, such as one's family, friends, and employers.
4) The ability to handle work and enjoy leisure without confusing the two.
5) The ability to express anger or annoyance without losing one's temper.
6) A love and tolerance for children.
7) Cultural, sexual, and racial understanding and compassion.

These are ideals, however, and most of us are lacking in one or more of these qualities. A recognition of their importance, though, is just as necessary as the ability to fulfill them. All of us, every day, are subject to tensions that sometimes seem insurmountable. A woman is by no means unbalanced if she occasionally succumbs to moments of despair, anger, or tears. In fact, these may be very "normal" ways of coping with the stresses and strains of life in twentieth-century America. If we can cope without creating excessive anxiety, then there is no reason to fear any kind of mental illness.

Neurotic

Sometimes we worry irrationally about problems and this can create disturbances that upset ourselves and those around us, and if they are not curbed, we can fall into patterns of abnormal behavior that by no means constitute insanity but make it hard for us to function properly and get the most out of life. One of the most common of these neuroses is a generalized fear or anxiety that appears to have no factual basis but is so strong that the individual develops the notion that insanity is just around the corner. This is never, in fact, the case. Insanity, or psychosis, as we shall see later, is far removed from neurotic tendencies which are really just uncontrollable exaggerations of normal methods of coping with stress. Shyness, timidity, hypochondria, neurasthenia (desire to sleep constantly), phobias, and depression are all possible products of deep-seated anxiety feelings that a woman may develop without knowing the underlying causes. Such causes may, in fact, be rooted in her daily life and revolve around work-related problems or a demanding spouse. In any event, the stress produces anxiety and the anxiety is expressed in any number of different ways such as obsessive-compulsive behavior (never being able to step on cracks in the street), conversion hysteria (partial paralysis), and many forms of psychosomatic illness in which the asthma, migraine, ulcer, or high blood pressure is quite real but finds its source in emotional rather than physical disorder. Neurosis is not the first step on the road to madness but encompasses many mild forms of mental disorder that are usually quite simple to overcome.

Psychotic

Although not always categorized in this way, I want to include in this section about the sick or diseased mind serious personality disorders that not only prevent the individual from functioning but infringe upon the rights of others. Chronic alcoholism, drug addiction, crimes involving sex and violence cannot be products of a normal mind nor simply the results of neuroses. Such behavior indicates personality disorders of the most serious type. As with other forms of psychosis, the individuals who practice these aberrations are out of touch with reality most of the time and completely incapable of functioning in a manner sympathetic to the needs of others, let alone conducive to their own health or welfare. A psychotic personality may be able to keep a job and raise a family but does not view the world with comprehension. The psychotic with a personality disorder generally believes that anyone who attempts to live honestly and maintain good relationships with others is stupid. In addition to this type of psychotic there is the individual suffering from either functional or organic psychoses who also cannot keep in touch with reality.

FUNCTIONAL PSYCHOSIS

There are three major categories of this type of disorder:

1) *Schizophrenia.* The truly schizophrenic personality withdraws so utterly from the world that comprehension of all but the simplest propositions is impossible. Acute attacks of confusion abound and quite baseless bouts of laughter and tears are not uncommon.

2) *Manic-Depressive.* The woman suffering from this condition often experiences regular periods of perfectly normal behavior interrupted by alternating moods of wild elation (accompanied by frenzied activity) and profound unhappiness and withdrawal.

3) *Paranoia.* We all have certain strong fears, and even though some may be exaggerated, real paranoia as a psychosis is total delusion of a world in which most individuals are plotting against, or out to harm, the patient. Perhaps I can use this to illustrate the three broad areas of mental health:

A *normal* woman approaches a busy intersection, is aware of the danger of a traffic accident, and takes suitable precautions while crossing the street.

A *neurotic* woman might walk several blocks out of her way to avoid that intersection, believing that it is inherently "wrong" for her ever to cross the street at that point.

A *psychotic* woman remains in the house because she is convinced that the driver of every car approaching that intersection will knowingly attempt to run her down.

ORGANIC PSYCHOSIS

Serious mental debility can be caused by damage to the brain as a result of certain types of poisoning, severe injury to the head, and, less often nowadays, birth complications. One of the most commonly held fears about mental illness is that it is easily inherited and that if there is a member of the family who is at all unbalanced, everyone should fear for the sanity of her children. Although, of course, babies are born with brain damage or congenital defects, only a very, very small fraction of mental cases is due to inheritance and there is no justification in fact for the widespread fear of "madness" running in the family. Anyone who has the slightest worry about this should seek out a physician and have her fears allayed.

B. MENTAL ILLNESS AND THE BLACK WOMAN

It is definitely true that proportionately far fewer Black women are treated for mental disorders than white women. From this we can conclude either that we are on the whole mentally healthy or that we suffer as much or more than whites and simply avoid treatment. I firmly believe that our common background does provide us inherently with greater strength to withstand serious mental illness. After all, the singularly shattering pressures that create so much mental grief to the middle-class-white population (such as family disunity, financial deprivation, and alienation from society as a whole) are pressures that many of us and our mothers and grandmothers before us have had to take for granted as part and parcel of this vale of tears. Even though more of us than care to admit it might need some form of mental help, we believe that we are unable to afford the luxury of such therapy as psychoanalysis and, moreover, that it is our responsibility to overcome our handicaps, material or spiritual, without the help of strangers. Thus we do see far too few Black women participating in mental health programs and far too many reliant upon the more anonymous but dangerous crutches of alcohol and drugs. In the recent past, and even to some extent today, the Black woman if brought up without the benefit of the family and social resources that most other women take for granted they can rely upon to counter mental illness. For many of us, our determination not to be felled by the vicissitudes of life helps us to develop healthy defenses against neuroses; all our lives we are very familiar with the social and economic problems that contribute to so much grief in this land. Out of these opinions and contradictions it is difficult to assess the current status of mental health in American Black women, and there is to date no complete study or reference work that can help us in a practical manner. My personal feeling is that although experience and heritage have made us mentally stronger than white women, there are still large numbers of mentally disturbed Black women who because of fear and ignorance shun any form of help. The big mistake that we (in common with most people) make about mental illness is that it is an unsavory subject that indicates personal weakness and is quite alien to physical health. In fact, our mental and physical beings are inextricably intertwined and no discussion of one is complete without strong reference to the other. To this day, researchers cannot define the invisible line between mental and physical pain because, really, there is no distinction. When we prick a finger, our mind registers the pain; when our mind is absorbed with worry, our stomach produces an ulcer. There cannot be a healthy mind in a diseased body and, conversely, it is not possible to sustain physical health if the intelligence is anxiety-ridden. Healing the body will strengthen the mind, and if your anxieties are under control and your mental outlook fairly stable, you will be subject to far fewer aches and pains and serious illness. As far as mental illness being a "taboo" subject, that attitude is in itself indicative of a narrow mind unwilling to face reality squarely and deal with any sickness, be it mental or physical, in an open, honest, precise, informed, and compassionate manner. This we must do if we are to progress as a race and a sex. In Chapter VII we have seen just how fatal hypertension (high blood pressure) can be for the Black woman. In order to reduce the incidence of this disease in our communities, we must recognize that, along with certain aspects of diet and behavior, mental stress is a key ingredient in the pattern of abuse to the body and mind that produces hypertension. We cannot treat most cases of hypertension unless the mental stress is isolated, realized, and combatted. In many such cases the appearance of some physical symptom will create such worry and distress that the body as a whole is weakened and disease can make further inroads into the system. Anxiety and stress are curable and even the most severe psychoses are treatable.

C. THE TREATMENT OF MENTAL ILLNESS

First of all, never try to diagnose yourself or someone else. The broad information I give in this chapter is not designed to allow the reader to become an amateur psychiatrist and "spot" tendencies in herself or her friends. That is an unhealthy and dangerous activity. Often the victim of mental disturbance is unwilling or incapable of realizing it. If we are beset by family problems or career difficulties, it is often very difficult for us to recognize the onset of what may be a mild but crippling depression. Because anxiety and depression are chiefly caused by an inability to cope with problems, it stands to reason that the afflicted woman cannot cure herself, cannot "pull herself together," cannot simply "face the issues squarely." The first and most important step of all is to realize that help is needed and to seek it. Even if your depression is vague or your anxieties very abstract (in fact, especially if they are of a diffused nature), you must admit to yourself that some kind of counseling is in order. Most mental afflictions can be dealt with far quicker, and cheaper, than the legendary ten years in psychoanalysis on the doctor's couch and, please, forget about padded cells and strait-jackets! Unfortunately, in our attempts to dispel the gloom of mental sickness with lighthearted humor, we have painted for ourselves a very false picture of the methods of modern psychiatric therapy. After deciding to seek help you should look for a professional counselor with a good listening ear. Do not assume in this regard that only a Black person can help. Black psychiatrists and psychologists do not have an exclusive understanding of Black problems, and it is even possible that some may be hardened to problems of the Black experience that a white counselor, with more distance from the situation, would have greater sensitivity about. Whomever you choose, it should be a stranger or semistranger, not someone part of your family or immediate circle who may also be part of your problems. Often it is easier to confide in a stranger and discuss personal matters with someone who is not privy to the particulars of your life. It does not matter who this first professional is, as long as you have confidence in his or her ability to render fair judgment and, if necessary, recommend further, more advanced therapy. Your personal physician is the most obvious first choice. All medical doctors are required to study mental illness and are quite qualified to help and, of course, their confidence must be trusted. If you do not have a personal doctor, get in touch with a local hospital and ask them to recommend a mental health agency or clinic. Simply state that you need to find someone with whom to discuss personal problems; do not be afraid that you will be thought of as mad or locked up. Few of us realize just how common such a request is and every day across the country thousands of people in distress are put in touch with counseling, and often it is enough just to be able to enumerate and analyze your problems. Even if you are not a regular church-goer, do not be afraid to seek help from a local minister. Most contemporary parishes are equipped to deal with troubled minds and can offer down-to-earth, sympathetic advice. Admirable though it is to bear misfortune stolidly, if you do not look for a cure and treatment of your mental distress, you are as foolish as the woman who disregards the symptoms of physical disease and allows the situation to deteriorate until it is almost irremediable. There is nothing cowardly about admitting to mental anguish. In fact, it is very brave of a woman to seek help so that she and her family and her friends can benefit.

It is one thing to admit to yourself that mental stress is changing your outlook and to seek help and quite another to decide that someone you know is similarly afflicted and needs help. If you suspect that a friend or loved one is mentally ill, do not try to diagnose or treat him or her yourself. First of all, examine your own reactions and make sure that they have in fact changed, not your attitude toward them. Maybe the change is in you. If you are convinced that they need help and if they are willing to admit to some anxiety, suggest a talk with a doctor or minister. If the person is very altered and possibly psychotic (if they are incoherent, highly suspicious, or totally uninterested in anything), do not discuss the matter with her or him unless your advice is asked for. Instead, try to persuade them to visit a doctor or clinic for a medical checkup and stress physical health, not mental. Never try to trick someone into going to a mental clinic or institution. If you yourself understand that no stigma should be attached to mental illness, it will be much easier to handle it should it appear in yourself or another. At the same time, realize that no matter how harmful or hostile a person's behavior, they may be suffering from acute mental problems and clearheaded understanding is necessary to control and cope with the situation.

Prevention

If it were possible to cure the social ills inherent in the way we live, most mental anguish would be eradicated. Unfortunately, we live in an imperfect world. The best protection that a woman can have against mental illness, other than, of course, a stable and enriching life, is a sound, healthy body. Here again I must emphasize my trio of necessities: a balanced diet, regular exercise, and adequate sleep.

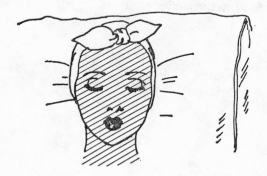

Charlatans

One must be very vigilant to avoid entanglement with the many dangerous, unethical, unlicensed, and unscrupulous individuals who promote themselves as "mind-healers" or therapists or even use, without authorization, titles such as "psychologist," "psychiatrist," and "doctor." Much damage can be done to the mind when it is disturbed if it is controlled by lay analysts and psychiatric practitioners who have no real medical knowledge and are not answerable to any code of medical ethics. Such therapy may involve elaborate mechanical gimmickry as well as subtle and insidious intimidation. On one thing you can be sure: Such quackery is not cheap and the cost, even though it might be cleverly disguised, will be considerable. Always, always, if in doubt, consult your state mental health association, give them the particulars of the alleged healer including her or his title and qualifications, and find out if they are a bona fide therapist of any kind. Above all, be wary of those who promote or advertise their services. Legitimate physicians cannot advertise as individuals. You may well see advertising in newspapers or in some cities on public transportation for crisis clinics. These may be quite legitimate, but inquire first if they are associated with, or authorized by, a city, state, or federal agency. In most parts of the country, free or low-cost mental health counseling by professionals is available to all.

D. EMERGENCY TREATMENT

If you are faced with a family member or friend whose behavior appears to be suddenly deranged, do not attempt to treat the individual yourself or advise her or him directly. Immediately call your doctor or local clinic and indicate that the person must have immediate attention and is not capable of arriving voluntarily at a doctor's office or hospital facility. Try to get a friend or neighbor to stay with you until help arrives, and remove any weapons, implements, or dangerous substances from the vicinity of the patient. She or he may attempt to harm themselves or others.

Chapter X

BEAUTY AND BEHAVIOR

For me, it is impossible to separate the concept of female beauty from a woman's patterns of behavior, speech, manners, and approach to life. I have met so many women renowned for their physical beauty who repulsed me with their ostentatious ignorance and vulgarity. Those experiences have more than been made up for by the many very fine women I have met who, although not blessed with a perfect figure or a radiant visage, have impressed me with their strength and grace and their ability to ignore superficial disadvantages. If you are gifted with good looks, you must not use them as an excuse to neglect the personal and social graces. If you are average or considerably less than average in physical beauty, you can stride ahead of the conventionally "pretty" woman if you follow the body-care advice in this book and develop your skills as a human being. Beauty is not skin-deep, but soul-deep!

We are all aware that, short of reconstructive surgery, little can be changed of the features one is born with, but the cleanliness and clearness of your skin, the set of your hair, and (within limits) your weight are all factors well within your control that add immeasurably to your appeal. Remember, you must first appeal to yourself in order to register the confidence that today's Black woman must have to compete. Your clothes do not have to be the most expensive nor do you need a closetful of cosmetics in order to be able to present yourself to other women and men with relaxed self-assurance. First, your face and body and your clothes must be clean and your appearance neat. The most beautiful pair of eyes in the world will fail to impress anybody if they are set above a nose (no matter how perfectly shaped) clustered with blackheads. Beauty is a composite of mental alertness, physical cleanliness, and a pleasing countenance. All of these are obtainable. So far we have dealt with cleanliness (health) and countenance. Now I would like to devote a few words to the well-finished personality, that all-pervasive force that can either make life an exciting, kind, and fruitful experience for oneself and others or, if it is incomplete or lacking, will eventually lead to tribulation. A distinctive, unique, and endearing personality is not arrived at by chance or luck of birth. It is the result of a mind that allows itself full freedom of expression, opinion, and emotion within a useful framework, a framework that is acknowledged by others as being the most pleasing. For want of a better word, I call this framework "manners."

Manners Make the Woman

It may be considered very old-fashioned among younger, political-minded Black women today to talk of manners. Perhaps they feel that manners are part of an alien, white heritage and have no place in today's "do your own thing" society that erupted in the last decade alongside the Civil Rights movement. I hold the opposite to be true, with reason and from some experience. All civilizations, and groups large and small within those civilizations, are based on agreed codes and symbols of mutual trust. Certain rituals are performed in all societies that make strangers into acquaintances and acquaintances into friends and sometimes friends into families. These rituals may be quite useless or meaningless in themselves: "Please," "Thank you," "Excuse me," "I'm sorry"; but, in fact, the more complex and potentially divisive the civilization becomes, the greater is the need for these "manners" to keep all the groups—small and local, large and national—structurally sound and healthy. Please, do not confuse manners with morals. I have no intention here to preach moral behavior; that is to be decided between the individual, her conscience, and her concept of God. Nonetheless, in reviewing what I know of the major religions, and especially the teachings of Christ, Mohammed, and Buddha, there is a persistent theme in all of them that courtesy must be practiced not only within the family group but, most importantly, extended toward the stranger, the foreigner, the individual of another faith, country, or race. I am well aware that poverty, lack of opportunity, and impatience have bred a deep streak of cynicism into a new generation of young Black women. The reasons for this attitude are very real, but the response is totally self-defeating. Adopting a permanent public stance of indifference or hostility, exaggerated by intentionally vulgar behavior, only exacerbates the alienation that exists and breeds tumultuous frustration. Unfortunately, many of our fine young Black women equate manners, poise, and, perhaps, charm with a Crow-Jane attitude signifying acceptance of white order. In fact, we have taught white America much over the years about correct and fitting behavior and it belittles our ancestors to assume that they were brainwashed to say "Please" and "Thank you." The brainwashing may have been more the other way around; it is far more likely that crude, pioneer plantation owners learned the meaning of the word *dignity* from their African slaves and not vice versa. Now, as we are approaching some semblance of at least legal equality in these United States, for us Black women to intentionally deprive ourselves of our natural grace and poise is a terrible thing to happen. I do believe most firmly that only by acknowledging the need for well-mannered behavior can we effectively achieve any kind of substantial progress. Unless we are, by and large, civil and graceful, how can our anger and our hurt, when it is shown, be in any way effective? The woman who cultivates her manners, her voice, and her charm (all attributes, incidentally, that a man should also cultivate; they are human, not feminine, qualities) can persuade, convince, love, hate, embrace, shun, and express her individuality honestly and to its fullest capacity in a way that a woman who is slovenly and coarse simply cannot. It is the woman who can only use obscenities to express her anger who is very weak; the woman with manners will stand proud, decisive, and firm and be, above all, strong. Think of a person, woman or man, whom you greatly admire—a politician, perhaps, or an entertainer. Can you imagine his or her being interested in or intrigued by a Black woman who flaunts her uncouthness in a shrill and ignorant manner? Of course not. The strong Black women in this country whom I admire, those who I believe are standing up for their sisters and brothers and all citizens in an intelligent, defiant manner, are women like Mamie Phipps Clark, Barbara Jordan, Shirley Chisholm, and Angela Davis. These are women of exceptional beauty. They are neither ill-mannered nor vulgar. In fact, despite their obvious anger at the gross inequities in our social system, they are surely teaching their fellow white and Black male political leaders of all persuasions much about the value of levelheaded, well-mannered behavior. There is nothing coy about good manners. Those men and women intelligent enough to grasp not only how useful manners are as a tool for ambition, but also how necessary for our survival as a civilization, are among the strongest leaders we have and the most decent human beings one wants to meet.

In order for a woman to be firm, she must be essentially polite, and both these qualities are important ingredients of the truly beautiful woman. We must understand that as Black women we share far more than a few physical characteristics. These, in fact, are the least common of our attributes: Some of us have ivory skin and others ebony; some have aquiline noses and others broad. We do indeed vary tremendously in looks, but we have a common past, a shared present, and, if we are unwilling to compromise, a great future in this country. We will not obtain that future if, as the eyes of the world turn upon us, we are unable to act with dignity. You and I know that the Black women who do not, or cannot, behave well constitute a very small part of our number, but they are, of course, the most noticed, being the loudest and most obvious. Because my definition of beauty includes the ability to know how to behave in any situation, I am going to enumerate some such situations and provide pointers for optimum behavior. No matter how well we think we do behave, everybody is ennobled by the occasional refresher course in manners.

The Home

THE FAMILY

We must not confuse politeness with stiff formality; in many cases the latter can be downright rude, especially in the bosom of the family. Warmth of spirit, mutual respect and consideration, generosity and elasticity regarding others' habits and foibles are mandatory for the happy functioning between all members of the family, wife and husband, siblings, children and parents. Mere correctness of form can wither affection whereas with genuine concern it will flourish. It is not enough that mutual likability and love be taken for granted within a family because every day each member is growing and changing and real, honest effort is required by all to constantly adapt.

One of the principal causes of divorce is selfishness. Women and men precipitate themselves hurriedly into marriage before they have had enough time to make an honest reckoning of their intended partners' likes and dislikes and habits—especially in matters of daily schedule and personal hygiene— and the result is that two virtual strangers get to know each other, even as they are starting a family, only to discover that there are deep-rooted incompatibilities. Couples, once married, will inevitably discover in each other practices that become annoying. My advice is to immediately let the other person know what you find wrong as soon as it happens. Do it in a very kind, straightforward way, without nagging. Be very firm about it. If you keep silent, your annoyance will increase until eventually in anger you will announce your distaste. You yourself must have habits that he dislikes; offer to "swap" evenly and each try to give something up together. Air your grievances before they become irreconcilable. Silence is the worst cause of incurable bitterness. Matters quite minor should be spoken of even on the honeymoon; in years to come they can assume gigantic proportions. If things are at a complete impasse, seek counseling; the least it can do is reopen doors of communication. A family must be structured with wife and husband sharing equally the burden of command, and the children, as they grow older, should be allowed to speak their minds but not make major decisions. Help your children understand responsibility by gradually sharing it with them; but also they must be made aware of the absolute necessity for respect for their parents and teachers and elders. As parents, we must provide our children with examples of behavior, compassion, and discipline that they can respect.

ROOMMATES

When two women decide to share a house or apartment, they should have prior acquaintance of each other. Personality conflicts between roommates can be every bit as emotionally destructive as between spouses. You must have some interests in common, not the least of which should be a work/play schedule that is mutually compatible. Generally speaking, you must want to retire and rise at the same time, and at the outset of the relationship, draw up a simple scheme for marketing, cleaning, and cooking. You and your roommate should be financial equals, sharing evenly the rent, telephone, and utility bills, and they should be settled together promptly. This is one situation that benefits from a written agreement of practices, no matter how casual, to which both can refer.

SERVICE PERSONNEL

Whatever the nature of your family unit, even if you are single, you must be in regular contact with a variety of women and men who perform services for you or your home. I am speaking of delivery persons, sanitation workers, superintendents, repair persons, housekeepers, domestic help, doormen, porters, and the like. I must admit that in the major cities one has almost come to expect antagonism and rudeness from this group as a way of life, but we must acknowledge that it is not a one-way street, and we must "do as you would be done by" and continue to treat each person as we would want to be treated. As Black women we are not unfamiliar with how demeaning and unpleasant service work can be, and when we are in a position to require it ourselves, we must make an extra effort to create a pleasant atmosphere of businesslike respect. Some women who find themselves rather suddenly in a position to afford household help, for instance, are rude to a point of bitterness and wish to consider any service worker a social inferior. Many such women simply do not know how to deal with others in a frank and open way and are perhaps slightly embarrassed by the situation. Every stranger deserves courtesy from you, no matter what his or her appearance or job. If that courtesy is not returned, you must retain communication with the person and try to achieve at least a working relationship without acrimony. The vast majority of people, even if they approach their service job with a chip on the shoulder, will let it drop if they are treated cordially and with respect. It is false, however, to suggest a tone of great familiarity to a service person simply because he or she also is Black. Do not lose sight of the fact that although you may be in your home (and not necessarily considering that a "job"), the service person is at work, earning a living, repairing, delivering, or cleaning, and for that situation a simple, kind, and disciplined employer-employee relationship must exist. If you work yourself, you may have an employer with whom you enjoy a good, cordial but not close relationship, and that is how it should be with helpers in the home.

THE TELEPHONE

I am going to make an observation that may anger many of you, will open me to charges of prejudice, and for which I have no exact statistics, but it is something about my sisters that I have constantly experienced throughout the four years of research on this book, something that many white people take so for granted that they no longer make racist jokes about, something for which there is no excuse: too many Black women cannot speak correctly on the telephone. I am criticizing both the housewife who answers her home phone with a grunt and the business receptionist who does exactly the same thing. In the course of my day I call many, many business offices. In the past few years, more and more such numbers are answered by Black secretaries or receptionists. There is often a reluctance on their part to say *anything* at first; a lack of comprehension concerning the nature of the call, the caller, or the person called; long, agonizing pauses; foggy, muffled speech; excessive gum-chewing and eating and a total lack of interest. I have no real objection to the use of colloquialisms and I am a great admirer of all genuine local and regional accents, but the telephone is an instrument of communication, as are a newspaper, a radio, a television, a camera, and a tape recorder. All such instruments require clarity and comprehension from the human element in order that they function correctly and efficiently.

When answering the telephone, always say "Hello" or identify yourself or your business. Do not eat, chew, drink, smoke, or listen to music at the same time; it can be very distressing to the listener. If the call is not for you, whether it is a personal or a business call, say, "Please hold on; I will see if —— is available." If you are placing a call, immediately identify yourself, even to a close friend; if the phone is not answered by the person to whom you wish to speak, say, "Please, may I speak to ——?" If it is not possible at that time, *do not insist*—the telephone is not a weapon with which to invade privacy; simply leave your name and number. Try not to drop the receiver or crash it down. One's manners on the telephone are very revealing of one's character, and friendly courtesy should be the hallmark of all telephone communication.

Business Behavior

The following advice applies to *all* kinds of work, including executive, secretarial, factory, store, and domestic positions.

APPEARANCE

Standards of what one is expected to wear to work are much more relaxed now than twenty years ago. This does not mean, however, that such license should be taken that your manner or type of dress disrupts your fellow employees or employers. Your working garments must be clean, neat, appropriate, and, above all, comfortable and well-suited to the job.

Punctuality

"CPT" (Colored People's Time) may be a tired old crudity, but all of us should make every effort daily to refute the cliché that Black folks are habitually tardy. If you are being paid to work for a certain number of hours per day, it is thievery to arrive late, leave early, or spend working hours primping in a restroom.

Giving and Taking Instructions

When you tell an employee to do a particular job, make your speech concise and clear and, if necessary, ask the instructions to be repeated back. Answer any pertinent questions and be firm but cordial. When receiving instructions, be attentive and immediately register any doubts you may have about the clarity of the instructions, but first listen carefully without interruption. If you object to the instructions or the manner in which they are given, say so then and there, calmly.

Coworkers

When you find yourself in a work situation with people of both sexes, various races, and different ages, it is normal for you to feel self-conscious at first, but do not hide behind a paranoid defense of hostility or aloofness. Let yourself unbend, allow others the benefit of the doubt, and be friendly and helpful. In most cases you will find that the more diverse the mixture of peoples gathered for a common purpose, the greater is their genuine desire to help and respect each other. You should, however, be wary of intimate relationships at work; politeness does not mean spontaneous affection. Avoid office gossip and petty jealousies.

Letter Writing

Never underestimate the power of the written word. The use of a letter to make your point to a relative, friend, or business person is almost always more effective than a telephone call and, if the circumstances are difficult, much easier than a confrontation. Few of my contemporaries seem to know how to write even the simplest letter, yet almost everyone I know of my parents' generation is very at home with pen and paper. There are really very few conventions that have to be adhered to in letter writing, although the idea itself is probably what many women find daunting. Simply assume a pleasant, conversational tone, avoid platitudes (especially about the weather!), and ask plenty of questions while trying to answer what you expect the reader will want to know about yourself. Try to get to the point quickly and stick to it. If you are not known to the reader, avoid being overly familiar and always try not to use slang expressions. For letters of a formal or business nature, "less is more," and the briefer you are, the more effective will be your message. Correct spelling is a must; no home should be without a dictionary, and if you get in the habit of using it, your spelling will improve quickly. Never guess with spelling.

Lay your page out neatly with your address and the date centered or in the upper right-hand corner. Always address your correspondent as "Dear ——" and start the letter on the next line. Clean, plain white paper makes a good impression, especially if it is without ruled lines. Use a pen, not a pencil, and start over if you have more than a couple of crossings-out. Every word must be legible; if you are writing to a stranger and your signature is undecipherable, print your name beneath it.

Table Manners

If you are presented with more than one service of cutlery per place setting, you proceed from the utensil farthest from your plate and work inward per course. Only children should tuck in a napkin, and after use, whether it is linen or paper, it is simply laid, unfolded, next to the used plate. Never remove "bad" food from your mouth in an obvious manner (screen your mouth with your napkin) and never spit food on your plate for any reason whatsoever. If it is very hot, take a sip of water. Put your hand to your mouth if you cough, but make no excuse. If you have a coughing or sneezing fit, leave the table. If you are unsure of how to eat a particular dish, no matter where you are, never be afraid to ask your hostess, your companion, or a waiter. There is never an absolutely *only* way to eat certain foods, but often there are more efficient, less messy ways, and no one will think less of you for asking; if you appear unsteady and embarrassed throughout the meal, that will ruin your own enjoyment. Eat the food as it comes and do not stir up or mash on your plate. You may reach across the table if it does not inconvenience your neighbor, but never so far that you have to rise from your seat. When serving dinner for your family or friends, the hostess is always served last. The women are served first, then the men, ending with the host, then the hostess. If the party is large, guests should be encouraged to start at once while the food is hot. At a table, keep relaxed; manners here are more common sense and comfort than convention.

Behavior in Public

As a group, we are judged by the rest of the world not according to our occupations or private lives but according to our public behavior. This may render a superficial judgment, but it is nevertheless how we, in turn, judge others. It should not be necessary for a Black woman to modify her public behavior in order to "make a good impression." Her public behavior should be as much a true reflection of her personality as her attitude toward her close friends and family. If you develop and practice the attributes of mutual concern and respect for all peoples, you will not be capable of behavior demeaning to yourself, your sex, or your race. If, on the other hand, you hold yourself in low esteem, you may easily be guilty of annoying or hostile public practices. Some of those that we are most prone to and should make the greatest effort to avoid are as follows:

Shouting. Never raise your voice for emphasis; you will only encourage others to do so and the level of noise pollution in our cities is high enough without adding the human factor.

Slang. Do not assume that strangers, even other Black women, understand your slang. Speak clearly and precisely.

Swearing. The use of profane, blasphemous, and obscene language is increasingly more common in our culture, seemingly condoned if not encouraged by popular literature, films, and television. Scatological language is openly used to express mild distaste and sexual epithets have become substitutes for more rational forms of emphasis. None of this makes it correct or particularly polite. In fact, the woman who stoops to the use of such language in anger or despair demeans herself utterly. There is nothing cool or strong about an ability to express yourself by using swear words. Neither do men have any greater excuse to swear than women; it is a petty, mean, and demeaning trait. If you are offended in public, summon your natural dignity and either ignore the offense or construct an imaginative riposte. Gutter language puts and keeps the user in the gutter and anyone using it in public deserves to be snubbed.

Spitting. I am shocked at the number of Black women I see who think nothing of spitting in the street. Needless to say, this is not only a filthy, lazy habit but very unsanitary. Always carry tissues.

Eating. Despite the growing number of fast-food emporiums that exist with adequate seating, it is increasingly common to see groups of young Black women eating in the street. All children eat candy and ice cream outside, but the repasts now consumed on the sidewalks are far more substantial —pies, hamburgers, pizzas, and french fries are gorged unremittingly. This is disgusting to witness and ruinous for the digestion.

Loud Music. Not everyone shares your taste in music and if you cannot get enough of the sounds you enjoy in your home, use earphones while enjoying it in the company of strangers. I doubt if anybody really plays very loud music outside unwittingly—it is usually in order to attract attention and willfully disturb the peace; both motives indicate a troubled mind.

Gum-Chewing. This alone is bad enough when done with open mouth and glazed expression, but should be considered a felony when loudly cracked repeatedly.

Demeanor. Give the public the benefit of the doubt and treat strangers, alone or in crowds, as you want to be treated. Be firm but polite. If you have problems of your own, do not foist them on others. It might be too much for me to ask you to whistle a happy tune (not too loud), but you might wipe the scowl off your face.

Appearance. Even if you are just going next door, never be seen outside in slippers, housecoat, or curlers. Always wear clean, mended clothes.

Dealing with Strangers

In shops, on the street, or in transit, men and women may try to scrape an acquaintance with you. If you are gregarious and enjoy such relationships, by all means go ahead, but be careful not to reveal too much about your personal life, your address, and your occupation, until you are sure that your new friend has innocent motives for wanting to meet you. If you do not, like me, enjoy being pestered in public, simply say so, very succinctly, right away. Always keep handy something you can read or be occupied with and just say, "I would rather not talk now, thank you." I have found this to deter almost everyone without giving offense except a certain species of Black malehood, God's gift to our race and our sex, who will not take no for an answer and will become increasingly hostile if rebuffed. This kind of man has the effrontery to take public liberties with a Black woman that he would not dare inflict on a white woman, which immediately says something about his personal values. I have even been treated in this manner by a number of very well-known Black male celebrities who have sent their managers or minions on crude errands of romance in airport lounges and are hostile almost to violence when I prefer not to swoon into their arms. When you are accosted in the street and seriously pestered in this manner, keep your mouth shut no matter what is being said and, if possible, seek a manager, an airport official, a security guard, or some such official and simply report that the man is a total stranger and is harassing you.

Traveling

Americans are the most chauvinistic travelers and Black Americans are no exception. We expect all nations to speak English, serve American food, and conform to our somewhat hysterical notions of sanitation. Thus we eliminate most of the reasons for traveling. To travel is to explore the differences between peoples, not to seek the similarities. Keep an open mind, travel light, and be prepared, within reason, to eat local food and adapt temporarily to local habits. Definitely do not assume just because your skin is the same color as your hosts' that they will necessarily share your views about anything. Even some African nations define a light-skinned American Black as a "European," not as a member of their race. Also, in certain African countries, women are far from liberated. Women alone or in groups, including visitors, have to expect slow and inferior service. Be careful how you criticize your host country, even if you think your suggestions helpful. Imagine how you would feel if a British- or French-educated Black African came here to ridicule your way of speaking, eating, and relaxing. Remember that we are all descended from "foreigners."

Parties and Dates

Black women do give the best parties with the best music and the best food and the best company—that I proudly acknowledge. Just as important sometimes as the party itself is the invitation and the thanks afterward. Always respond in the same manner as you have received the invitation—casually if it has been word-of-mouth or formally if it is written. If your letter, card, or note days "R.S.V.P." (Repondez, s'il vous plaît), then you must indicate to the sender if you are coming or not, and do not leave it to the final hour; that is very rude. If you have accepted and cannot go at the last minute, then a call or telegram briefly explaining the circumstances will suffice. After you have enjoyed yourself at someone's house or in their company at a restaurant or concert, it is quite correct and not at all forward to thank them with a simple, unostentatious gesture. Never make it expensive or elaborate, but send a wire with a few words, write a very brief note; one flower is very effective, or a candygram for fun. This habit should be extended to fill all those gaps we have about people and situations that require thanks in a simple way. Do it to thank someone for helping you in an emergency, for good advice, for an introduction. Just a note or a very inexpensive gift will do.

Parties and dates should be fun, relaxing times. Carry yourself with dignity, eat and drink in moderation, and do not be afraid to speak up if anyone's behavior offends you. If you find yourself in the company of a well-known person you would like to meet, neither ignore them (as often happens, paradoxically) nor push yourself upon them. If they appear friendly, introduce yourself, and if they are busy with other people, wait until you can be properly introduced. The art of introduction seems almost to be a lost art but it is very simple. Use the same name designation for both persons—just the first names or the full names—but never say, "Fred, this is Mary Wilkins"; say either, "Fred, this is Mary—Mary, please meet Fred" or "Fred Smith, this is Mary Wilkins." No matter how casual the affair, make sure everybody gets properly introduced.

Your Speaking Voice

American English has come into its own; you do not have to speak like Winston Churchill to be correct. American English is composed of many vernacular idioms and accents that have evolved over the past two hundred years, and our race has had much to do with enriching it. There is nothing particularly "white" about the way your television newscaster speaks (be he or she Black or white) and any woman who persists in illiterate patterns of speech, imagining such to be more "Black," is sadly to be pitied. Our varied accents and speech rhythms across this country constantly infuse and enrich the English language as a whole, but if we restrict our speech to catch phrases and fancy street talk, our particular language will simply die. Always enunciate your words, breathe while you speak, try to modulate the pitch of your voice so that it is not too high, and remember that it is better to speak slowly and pick your words than to garble fast and furiously. Everyone can achieve a good speaking voice; there are plenty of good public speakers to emulate, but if you do attempt to improve your voice, do a thorough job and do not just affect a clear, "classy" voice for special occasions or the telephone. Enunciate every vowel and consonant; do not rush your words together, and always choose a short, simple word in place of a long, complex one. If you train your ear to listen to the speech of others and try to correct in yourself what you object to about them, you will be on the way to perfecting a fully comprehensible, well-modulated voice.

Class Distinction

It is usually not very polite to remark that a particular woman "has class," but I think everyone knows what that means and every Black woman would like to feel that she also "has class." It may seem indefinable, but I would venture that it consists of items that every woman can achieve:

Poise
Posture
Dress
Self-discipline
and, most important of all, Manners.

Least necessary is a stunning face and gorgeous figure. In fact, with many women these attributes often obscure their real graces, their intelligence, and the ability to converse with all people as equals.

Chapter XI

FASHION: MYTH AND REALITY

A. THE MYTH

Cursory acquaintanceship with the fashion pages of newspapers and magazines often promulgates the entirely misleading concept that "fashion" is the exclusive property of High Society, the Jet Set, Beautiful People, or whatever one wishes to call what now passes for Society in our major cities. In fact, these people constitute the often-changing tip of a fashion pyramid, the broad base of which is made up by the hundreds of thousands of less celebrated women who spend billions of dollars per year on clothes that they simply consider smart and comfortable and which have very little to do with what the Paris or New York fashion world decrees season by season. In fact, the increasing trend among top designers is to be ultra-aware of this mass market and to avoid designing clothes that are so outrageous in design and cost that they can only appeal to the idle rich. Fashion, by definition, is the current style or custom or mode of dress and, by implication, that of the majority. Thus it is spurious, for instance, to state that knee-length skirts are "old-fashioned" when the majority of women in this country wear knee-length skirts; in fact, knee-length skirts are "the fashion" for these times. Also it is incorrect to propose either miniskirts or maxiskirts as being "new fashions" since neither style became popular enough to be enjoyed by the majority. It would be more appropriate to call such innovations "newfangled" than "new fashions."

The Black woman is often self-deluded that she has no heritage of fashionability and is often caught between choosing styles, which she may feel are too loud and brassy for her but express an ethnic bias, and simpler, plainer styles she may really prefer but because of their conservatism appear to her to be "white."

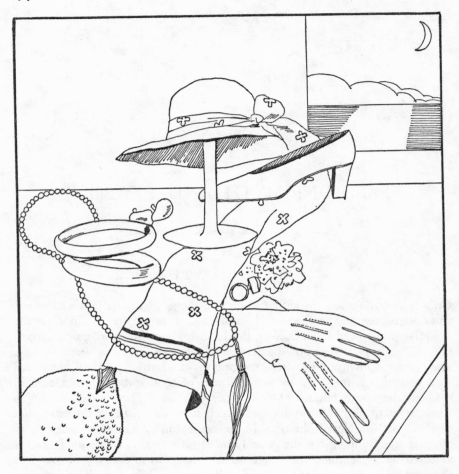

B. THE REALITY

Fashion has no color, but our color is wondrously suited to styles of all kinds. Consider our relatives across the ocean, the Masai, whose basic dress is a light cloak simply draped and hung from the shoulders, perfectly practical and tremendously dramatic, simple, elegant and, to our industrialized eyes, eminently "fashionable." Consider also the Nuba in the Democratic Republic of Sudan; over the centuries they have evolved a very complex, highly stylized, and visually stunning vocabularly of body painting whose dazzling but subtle geometrics could put many modern artists to shame. Our forebears in this country designed utility clothes that have become absolute standards in all parts of the world and, as our society gained affluence, very high standards of taste in fashion were set by the socially prominent "400s" in the early decades of this century whose imaginative but discreet styles were widely emulated by other Black women.

For the past few years, many of the leading new American designers have been Black, and although they are very highly regarded in the fashion world, not enough Black women have availed themselves of their talents. My personal favorites are Ed Austin, Scott Barrie, and Stephen Burrows.

Forget, please, that only the very wealthy can be fashionable. They are, in fact, as a group perhaps the worst dressed in the world since they do not have to budget and thus do not think hard about making choices. They can afford to indulge themselves in the most ludicrous caprices that are often presented tongue-in-cheek by the designers. The very rich woman does not necessarily consider the appropriateness of her clothes according to her figure, the occasion, or the season, but simply buys "the latest" as a vivid testament to her (or her husband's) ability to be able to afford the absurd prices of *haute couture*.

Most Black women can now buy a collection of clothes that is generous enough in quantity to cover the seasons and sufficiently versatile to enable the owner to present a fresh appearance several times a week by judicious manipulation of her basic garments and accessories—that is the key to being really well-dressed. Good taste in clothes is virtually undefinable, but I will venture that it is a combination of harmonious lines, seductive colors, ingenious ideas, and absolute tact. This is, of course, very subjective, and what one woman finds pleasing and in excellent taste another may consider quite abominable. There are, nevertheless, a few universals that I will enumerate in the course of this chapter to apply to the art of dressing well. The most frequent error made in our affluent society is to confuse luxury with taste. Often they are in inverse proportion to each other. To my eye, among the ugliest and most grotesque items in the fashion vocabulary are the endless lines of monstrously vulgar "initialed" garments and accessories that appeal to the basest instincts of ostentation and cost a small fortune. The woman is buying "a name." Well, she gets nothing else in most cases—not good workmanship, imaginative styling, or lasting fabric. She is even cheated on the "name" since in most instances all she gets are the initials, albeit repeated endlessly, in lieu of the designer's ability to create a pleasing print or solid. This kind of buying leads to a dreadful uniformity of dress that helps to dull the variety of daily life. You must first of all know yourself intimately in terms of your *real* figure and your *real* personal tastes. The joy of dressing is that it allows us to express our individuality and, in a perfectly legitimate way, display whatever flair we may have for co-ordination and design. Forget this season's color if you abhor it; think twice before you buy "fashionable" ankle-length dresses if you have good-looking legs and want to show them off. Your clothes must suit *you*, not the fashion-magazine editor. All women should dress with decorum, a word the Romans used to describe "that which is suitable." Your dress should be suitable to your age, your moods, your place of work, your style of relaxation, and in harmony with your character. It is worthwhile to plan your dress carefully and from then on be free to enjoy your day and evening without constantly worrying about the appropriateness of your clothes. Avoid the radically new; if you chase after the latest "in" styles, you will be a follower of fashion. If you exercise your own judgment and train your taste, you will be a fashion leader. Fashion is not a one-way street with the designer dictating to you. Many designers that I know look to the average women in the street for clues to incorporate into their new collections. There are no absolutely "new" styles. We invent new fabrics, new methods of manufacture and, perhaps, new colors, but fashion is an endless cycle of basic forms that revolve through the centuries. From the draped, loose look from Hellenic times to the simple tailoring of the Middle Ages, we have not really produced much that is new other than an infinite array of juxtapositioning. Perhaps the greatest revolution that has occurred in our time has not been the emergence of any one new, typical style, but the liberation of women from specific, regimented, universal fashions. With this freedom to wear just about what we want, we must exercise great care, however, and develop the very real responsibility of being each her own designer. Clothes do not make or remake a woman, so do not expect a dress to compensate for untidy hair or a dirty skin. Your basic wardrobe must have a theme which you can carry through from year to year, a marked bias in terms of color or style that reflects your personal desires and which will suit you in all seasons.

First, you must be aware of the archetypal shapes of fashion and learn to be able to differentiate between a look that is flattering to you and one that simply makes you "feel" contemporary. For this you must use the mirror, full-length and often, and be very critical about how you actually look—not just how you think you look. Secondly, you must know the difference between clothing and costume. Clothing evolved anthropologically first as protection, then incorporated elements of ornamentation. Costume involves symbolic communication such as black "widow's weeds" to announce mourning and multicolored, fanciful garb to indicate festive revelry. We frequently wear costumes such as a particular uniform if we are policewomen, and without crashing the boundaries of good taste we can safely consider some of our evening "party" dresses as coming under the category of costume. Too many of us, however, negate the whole joy and meaning of costume as a method of communication by "dressing up" each and every day for every occasion instead of creating a wardrobe diverse enough to render service appropriate to the needs of the occasion and our individual moods. Sometimes elements of costume become absorbed into the everyday garments of a group or society, and recently Black women have been largely responsible for incorporating African-derived ceremonial wear into items of standard elegance such as capes, turbans, and caftans, as well as such allied fashions as braided hair. In many ways we seem to be creating a new sense of fashion that has very much to do with our political and social emergence but which is in many cases the opposite of the garb worn by the white would-be liberals who on occasion express empathy for our causes. While they on the one hand delight in blue-jean, work-shirt wrappings of the cotton fields, we prefer to celebrate whatever freedoms we have won by indulging in fashion adventures. To me, even the most bizarre style of dress is preferable to the self-consciously drab attire of the white middle-class drop-out. One of our sisters, Flo Kennedy, the attorney for, and founder of, the Feminist Party, spoke recently of antiestablishment groups making inroads into the world of fashion: "Many of these women have had to wear shapeless hand-me-downs all their life and to them wearing nail polish and gold lamé may be a declaration of independence." Personally, I am not so keen on gold lamé, but the point is very well made that since diversity is the hallmark of our social revolution, no Black woman should be criticized for a desire to dress elegantly. Just because some white woman finds blue jeans a liberating garment (after years of being forced into a tailored image) does not indicate that as Black women we consider such attire as anything but symbolic of hard work and in fact we may express our liberation by way of a hand-stitched, tailor-made suit. In my thoughts that follow, I am going to assume that the reader does not have a fortune but can afford, from time to time, to spend some money on quality garments. Since all taste is very subjective, you will have to forgive me for imposing my own opinions on these judgments; my personal taste tends to the conservative. I am a believer in the dictum "less is more," particularly when applied to extravagance of dress. I believe that the cut, the material, the lines and the tones and the fit make a much stronger, glamorous, personal statement than vivid colors or elaborate frills and bows.

C. A BASIC WARDROBE

The Color Scheme

The color of our skin is not only the most immediately noticed facet of our appearance but our great asset in terms of fashion. Our hues work better, from a visual standpoint, with all colors of the spectrum, than those of any other race. Many Black women are ultrasensitive about their color and the color of their clothes. This self-consciousness is usually based on a belief in such vague generalizations as "never wear yellow if your skin tone is at all yellowish." This sounds as if it could be correct, but it is in fact a gross exaggeration and no such dictum can have a universal application. In fact, I often purposefully search for clothes that have brown tones that exactly match my own, and such matching can be very flattering indeed. The colors that in my opinion best dramatize our natural tones are black, blue, brown, gray, and white. If that sounds dull, consider all the delicate variations such as aquamarine, tan, toast, beige, and ivory. My wardrobe is entirely based on these colors, the only departure being very pale pastel shades of pink or light green, and I accent my appearance with Chinese lacquer red, a very hot color, on my nails or perhaps a belt. I sternly advise all of us to restrict the use of bright oranges, reds, yellows, and purples to make-up and accessories. Not only is it very difficult to create a multipurpose wardrobe with a variety of garments in very strong, loud colors, but they dominate our complexions, which should be allowed to come first and foremost. Your favorite color may not be the one that actually looks best on your person. Once you are wearing a dress, you see less of it than everybody else, so you should choose the color very carefully with your eyes, not your heart. Try the garment on in front of a full-length, well-lighted mirror, and ask yourself very honestly if the color flatters your complexion, your hair color, and your eyes. If the color stands up well on you when you are wearing little or no make-up, you have made a wise choice. Keep in mind that the color of a coat or a dress will appear quite different in daylight than in the artificial light of a store, and, if you tan in the summer, you may be able to wear some colors that are not possible for you in the winter. Not only can a carefully and well-chosen color add a glow to your own skin tones, but it can vary the appearance of your figure. Dark and neutral solid colors have a slenderizing effect; bright colors and busy prints add bulk. I have no enthusiasm for wild prints and strong plaids, and a woman should have no more than a couple of such items. Your wardrobe should not look like a theatrical costumer's storeroom. Keep the vibrating patterns and fluorescent hues for a few items such as belts and scarves.

If you plan your wardrobe according to a predetermined color scheme, after critically examining what really best suits your appearance, you will get much greater and more imaginative use out of your clothes because you will be able to circulate and rotate your garments, mix sets, suits, and skirts without wasting precious minutes every morning worrying if things "go together." If there is no color consistency to your clothes-buying, and you choose according to your whim or someone else's advice, you end up with a dizzy array of items none of which perhaps can be suitably worn with each other.

Accessories

These are the items in which to indulge yourself if you so desire. With judicious and imaginative purchase of accessories, you can increase times ten the excitement and variety of any wardrobe. The accessory should never be necessary to save the total look, and if ever a salesperson attempts to talk you into making a purchase of a major item such as a dress or coat by indicating how well it will look with the right belt or buckle or pin, you would be well advised to look at something else. The accessory should just enhance the rest of your appearance, create a focal point, and express your individuality. I consider all jewelry, scarves, handbags, belts, gloves, hats, and shoes to be potential accessories. They can transform an otherwise forgettable dress into something special if the dress is basically simple and well made. "Restraint" should be your password when shopping for any item of apparel, and this is true also of accessories. They do not have to be flashy to be dramatic. If they are too large, too small, too gimmicky, too vivid, or too many, you can destroy the balance that must always exist between your body height, shape, color, and your clothes. Your accessories must not overpower the appearance. Avoid the temptation to dress up black with glitter, for instance. Red shoes are enough of an accent. (You do not need also a red scarf and a red blouse.) If a little is good, more is worse, not better. Our best accessory is our color; do not upstage it. Always keep the size of your handbags, belts, and scarves in direct proportion to your own scale. If you are petite, you cannot wear large shoulder bags, chunky jewelry, and six-inch platform heels. If you are tall or large-boned, delicate jewelry and dainty purses are out; carry tote bags and choose dramatic jewelry with flair. Accessories can help your body as well as your clothes. For a short neck, wear a few long chains or a graded string of beads; if you try to disguise it with a choker, you will simply emphasize its deficiency. If your legs are heavy, wear dark stockings; if they are sticklike, choose light shades of hose. A big ring on a small finger is ludicrous—petite hands should be qualified with thin, delicate rings. I have hands in proportion to my figure; they are large and long and I never draw attention to them by wearing anything on them except my wedding band. Bracelets can be a great help. If you have heavy arms and wrists, wear big, loose bracelets to minimize them.

Keep your accessories as casual or as formal as the rest of your clothes and according to the occasion. Diamonds in the day, no matter how expensive, look cheap; on the other hand, it might seem like a fun idea to go to a formal dinner party wearing a gay plastic brooch, but please resist the temptation. Accessories that depend on a fad for their appeal are very quickly dated; they are toys only and should be treated as such.

It is worthwhile to spend a little extra on your accessories if the better quality belt costs more. It will endorse and enrich the rest of your outfit and add a real touch of distinction.

Coats

In my climate it is much wiser to invest in a really good winter coat ($90–$200) than in a summer dress for the same price. The former I may have to wear again and again in the fall, winter, and early spring. If only one good cloth or fur coat is possible on your budget, avoid high-fashion styles and choose a basic dress coat, three-quarter or full-length. It should have a classic cut with pockets, buttons, and a roll collar—not a cape, shawl, or bolero style. Among furs, of course, mink is the most expensive to buy but in the long run the cheapest; it loses its value hardly at all and lasts forever. Persian lamb is also very good and slightly less expensive. Muskrat in mink tones, seal, and beaver are all very hardy and should last at least seven years. Rabbit and fox shed quickly; the skins tear easily and are less durable than a cloth coat. If you want to help protect our endangered wildlife, by all means choose a good man-made fake-fur coat, but be sure of its quality; the less expensive ones barely last one season.

An often overlooked solution for the one-winter-coat woman is a well-tailored fabric raincoat with a removable lining. This can be very smart and also double as a year-round raincoat.

Spring is a short season and I avoid buying spring coats altogether; they are too high-styled and expensive for the little wear they get. For spring and summer I suggest a white, black, gray, brown, or camel-colored loose-fitting lightweight coat (not a "tent" shape) in classic lines that can be worn over a heavy sweater if the weather gets cool or a very light summer dress for formal evenings. In between seasons I just toss on a shawl, a cape, or an extra large scarf.

Hats

I regret that in the past decade Black women seemed to wear hats less than ever before. I enjoy hats and wear them frequently and hope to see a return of the hat as a basic fashion item. My faith no longer requires me to wear a hat in church and I do not mourn the loss of the hat as a symbol of propriety, but I simply think that a well-chosen hat can add great chic and elegance to any woman. We have been very hat-conscious in the past and very talented in creating and adapting styles from simple scarves and turbans to highly elaborate brims and crowns. As a practical notion also, hats can provide a healthful rest from complicated hairstyles.

When buying a hat, first measure your head and take the measure of the hat; it must fit well. Its size and ornateness must be in proportion to your body scale and do not try to make yourself a lot taller by wearing a very high hat; it will be very obvious what you are trying to do. Just avoid saucer styles if you are rather short. For the winter, buy a very good fur hat ($50–$100) with a fairly straightforward style. It will last forever and, if it is well made, can be restyled again and again by an adroit milliner. It should protect your head, stay on in a high wind, and keep your ears warm as well as look good.

A solid-color straw is best for the summer. Again, my favorite colors would be black, navy blue, beige, natural, or white. The body must be the best you can buy; the trimming you can always change from season to season. If you want to own only a couple of hats, get good ones that you can alter. Cheap hats look tawdry and fall apart.

Suits

Every Black woman's wardrobe should contain at least one good tailored suit of a year-round fabric such as gabardine, crepe, or tissue-thin, 100 per cent wool. Neither the jacket nor the skirt should be too short so that there is enough material to make minor alterations in length from year to year if you wish. The best buys are often three-piece suits, consisting of jacket, pants, and skirt, and should cost from $80 to $150. A cheap suit with a highly stylized cut is a sheer waste of money and is, moreover, quite tasteless. Your suit should be unremarkable for everything except its simplicity. The lines, like those of a Chanel suit, must be perfectly clean and clear; the fabric and color should be neutral and conservative. With a change of accessories, a good suit can be worn anywhere, on almost any occasion and look stunning.

For my honeymoon I invested in an ivory gabardine suit with a tailored jacket and pleated skirt. It cost $300. I have worn that suit every month of the year with numerous different colors and types of blouses, sweaters, and accessories, different shoes (brown leather in the day, ivory satin at night) and, especially when traveling across the country for business and press interviews, I have worn it for the working day and at casual evening occasions. I have never received so many compliments about an item of apparel, and I never before felt so comfortable traveling, working, and meeting people. With a change of shoes or blouse it becomes a different suit.

Sweaters and Blouses

I shy away from flashy, printed batwing shirts with enormous flyaway collars and most of my blouses are tailored with a round or turnover collar in soft, solid pastels. Sweaters can be very inexpensive and very smart and can be bought in a very wide variety of styles; use your imagination when buying and wearing them. Choose complimentary colors and in warmer weather use them as accessories draped over your shoulders or with the arms knotted around your neck. My only advice about sweaters and body shape is that tight-fitting tops are not for the heavy-breasted woman.

Dresses

I do not care if maxi lengths have been "in fashion" for six years. If you or I look better showing our knees, then by all means we should show them. If "body" dresses are considered in style and you look better in more formal, tailored dresses, do not change. If baggy, tentlike chemises simply make you look pregnant, give them a miss. Always think of yourself, your body, your very subjective, personal likes and dislikes when choosing a dress. You make the fashion to be worn and emulated, so make it your way—the way in which you are comfortable and best able to express yourself. On the premise that we can only have one dress, it should be of a durable fabric, a solid color (rich, but not jazzy), and with a continuity and fluidity of line. Spend not less than $50 in order to get solid workmanship; prices can be as high as $110 for even a fairly workaday dress. Only buy clingy, matte jersey dresses if you already have a serviceable day dress or two. These body huggers can be very pretty, but they lose their shape on hangers and get stretched when cleaned; some have a marked propensity for opening at the seams also.

Pants

Trousers for women are now so widely accepted that many of us even wear them to work, as do our grandmothers. The prime pants problem is fit. They must fit well, otherwise they will destroy any affection anyone might have for your legs, thighs, and behind. Our derrières are not the same as those of most American women, and mass-produced pants simply do not fit off the rack. If you have a large behind, potbelly, thigh bulge, wide hips, or a high crotch, only wear pants if they can be altered and tailored to you individually. Otherwise avoid them. Even if you feel you can wear pants straight out of the store, make sure they are not too short (they should "break" on your shoe) or too long. (They should never bag over the shoe.) When trying on pants, wear the shoes and the undergarments you most expect to be wearing with them. My preferences are straight lines, solid colors, and substantial fabrics. Pants may cost from $30 to $60 and, unless you have money to burn, avoid very exaggerated bell-bottoms, enormous cuffs, and hip-huggers.

Underwear

The lingerie manufacturers are among the most innovative in the industry, and they have responded to the consumers' demand for undergarments to match every kind of fashion and figure. Good lingerie must be simple in style, well made, and washable. This does not mean it necessarily has to be handmade because many mass-produced items are sturdy. You should avoid knits and cheap rayon garments; although they appear neat and strong at first, they very quickly lose their finish and in the wash become torn and limp. Cotton is by far the best material for *panties*. Your *girdle* must not be expected to create an instant body beautiful. At the most, it should hold in your stomach slightly, give a smooth line to your hips, and hold up your stockings. If it does more than that, it is simply moving bulges from one place to another. The most comfortable type of girdle is the two-way-stretch girdle that allows free body movement and it should have a fairly loose weave to permit perspiration to evaporate. After a few hours of wearing a new girdle, you should be completely unaware of its presence, otherwise it is wrong for you. There is no point in torturing your body (and risking an irritated countenance) just to squeeze into something you consider fashionable.

Brassieres should be worn regularly by all women with a bust measurement of 34B or larger. This is as much for the sake of your health as your appearance. Elsewhere in this book I discuss the dangers of unsupported, pendulous breasts. If your brassiere is framed with wire, make sure none is pressing on soft tissue. No woman today should have to look droopy or flat-chested, but be realistic when choosing a brassiere to emphasize your chest. Nature tends to create in proportion and your lines are probably better left as they are.

Make sure that your underwear fits properly. If your weight fluctuates, measure yourself frequently and always buy the correct size. If your underwear is good, not only will your clothes fit better, but they will last longer too.

Evening Wear

Standards of evening wear have relaxed a lot in recent years. It is only a few distaff members of European royal families that still wear full evening dress with trains, sashes, bustles, and elaborate trimmings and then only on ceremonial occasions. A good evening dress today should cost from $50 to $120 and, again, it is wise to choose something fairly plain but striking that has a solid color or a pattern so simple you can effortlessly renew its appearance with accessories of various colors. You should be able to add a chiffon scarf or a fresh flower or a satin or grosgrain ribbon of almost any color. Never throw away an evening dress that is still in good shape, no matter how tired of it you become. In a year or two it may be perfect for a simple summer's day or a spare outfit for a vacation.

Many lingerie companies are producing "At Home" wear based on long lingerie items that sell quite reasonably ($20–$100) and that are often surprisingly suitable for evening wear.

Even though few people are shocked these days to see pants, minidresses, and elaborate jumpsuits being worn on formal evening occasions, to my eye the woman who is wearing an appropriate, well-cut evening dress always takes top honors.

Shoes

In "Our Feet and Legs" I have admonished you only to wear "sensible" shoes for the sake of your feet. I know, however, that we will keep buying smart shoes that are not the best for our feet, but we should always avoid the very faddish, outlandishly high or embellished shoe that is downright unsafe and an eyesore. Ideally you should have a sound pair of oxford walking shoes ($20–$50), a pair of brown, black, or tan classic leather pumps with a minimum of decoration (one buckle or strap; these should have a medium heel and can be lace-up), and a pair of low-vamped black silk, peau-de-soie grosgrain or satin classic pump also with a medium heel. The day shoes may cost from $18 to $40 and the evening shoes from $18 to $50. Avoid patent leathers and very bright colors; they are difficult to co-ordinate with any clothes and impossible to keep clean. I accept and enjoy colorful fabric sandals for evening wear if the rest of the outfit is appropriate.

Sports Clothes

When participating in specific sports, tennis for instance, always dress according to the accepted code. It is not only polite to your fellow players, but there are good reasons for the styles of certain sporting outfits. For simple relaxing at home, save your good clothes and just wear old but clean garments, blue-jeans, comfortable shirts, or whatever. I often just wind and tie large pieces of fabric Indian- or African-style around my body. This gives me maximum comfort, I am suitably covered, and I am not wrinkling or getting dirty my good suits and dresses.

How Many Clothes Must You Have?

To be really well dressed all you need are five daytime outfits (some of which should be mixable), two evening dresses, three pairs of shoes and one pair of boots, one solid warm coat and one light raincoat and many, many scarves. If you can spend the time now to plan your wardrobe and begin to build up a consistent collection of clothes and accessories, you will save much time in the future by not having to worry about your clothes every morning and evening, and, moreover, you will have a basic confidence that you will never be caught without the proper item.

D. MAKING YOUR OWN CLOTHES

Our dollar earnings vainly try to keep up with the upwardly spiraling prices of manufactured goods. Nowhere is it more true than in the fashion industry (often less grandly referred to as the garment business). The manufacturers on Seventh Avenue in New York City, fashion capital of the country, find their costs increasing so much that a recent study concentrating on the price analysis of a perfectly plain, simple, but well-made dress found that the wholesaler required $59.75 to pay for fabric, labor, rent, overhead, and taxes, and it cost the retail store $57.75 in salaries, advertising, and overhead to carry the product. It sold at a loss for $110. This is a dress that you might easily think you yourself could make for fifteen or twenty dollars! Perhaps you are quite right. I have the misfortune to be the only female member of my family who is not a talented seamstress. Despite my proximity to the fashion scene and close friendships with many leading designers, my sister Doris living in Pittsburgh gives me pretty stiff competition when it comes to being well dressed. I would be very surprised if she spent one quarter the amount I have to spend for clothes because she is a wizard with the sewing machine and has a great flair for adapting styles. Pattern books and sewing magazines are readily available everywhere and as the price of manufactured garments rises, patterns for every type of apparel in all sizes and styles are becoming available. All of us should be able to handle a sewing machine. There is little that is more satisfying than really making a very smart skirt for yourself, becoming your own designer. Always try to make preliminary adjustments in size and style to the pattern itself before you cut and sew. Search in the Yellow Pages for manufacturers' fabric houses and purchase your material at these outlets. Never throw away buttons or zippers from old clothes but recycle them. If you spray an old zipper with spray starch, it will be refortified. Sewing and tailoring classes for raw beginners and advanced practitioners are open to all ages at many community colleges, recreation centers, and YWCAs. The allied crafts of crocheting and knitting are not only very fulfilling hobbies but really slice the bills for sweaters, vests, socks, and apparel for every member of the family as well as for gifts. Even the most modest ability with a needle and thread should be put to use when purchasing inexpensive clothing. Often quite cheap dresses can become very elegant if you are able to remove the flashy "extras," replace the loud buttons with your own choice, remove belt loops, and alter collars and cuffs.

E. DRESS YOUR AGE

"These fashions are all for young women!" bemoans the older woman over and over again. Frustrated in her desire to be up-to-date, she finds the fashion press promoting styles that to her seem entirely geared to a younger generation. Often she is perfectly right and it is something she should accept. I agree with the pre-eminent doyen of tastemakers and the fashion press, Diana Vreeland who, although herself no longer young, consistently defends the role of seasonal and annual fashion changes as the exclusive prerogative of those whose bodies are young enough to be tastefully exposed. The older woman who seeks to regain her lost youth by assuming the trappings of the young simply makes herself look much older and very foolish. The wise woman realizes as she is aging that there is a very wide range of styles of dress not in the least old-fashioned that will flatter her maturing figure and face and help her remain graceful and attractive if not become more so as she ages. She will have to settle for a look that is perhaps overall more conservative than that worn by the beautiful girls on "Soul Train," but that does not make her out of fashion. A teen-ager can make an outrageous fad look like fun; on a mature woman the same pair of tight purple hotpants is only embarrassing. To recognize this does not consign the older woman to despair but should elevate her and encourage her to new levels of simplicity and dignity in dress. I have been horrified and appalled in the not-so-subtle changes that have occurred in the fashion choices of the mature Black woman over the past ten years. Some of my own acquaintances, women whose chic taste and elegance I not only applauded but as a child wished to emulate, did, in the past decade, follow the so-called "youth explosion" to absurd levels. They abandoned the well-tailored suit and classic pumps, simple hairstyle, and just a touch of flattering make-up to embrace a "look" that relied upon gargantuan Afro wigs, skin-tight pants, pop jewelry, and make-up more appropriate for the circus than the dinner table. The fault is not with these older women but our society that so neglects the middle-aged and the mature person that many feel they have to mimic the antics of the young and foolish in order to obtain any kind of social recognition.

I urge all mature Black women to exploit their natural dignity and grace, intimidate the young with simple and elegant hats, handbags, shoes, hairstyles, dresses, and coats, and as the eternal fashion carousel is moving faster, I predict that soon the tables will be turned and the grandchildren will be trying to recreate the single-strand-of-pearls elegance of their grandmothers.

F. DRESS YOUR SHAPE

Curb your impulse to buy a dress because it looked great in the advertisement. What you may be really wanting to buy is the model's figure, not the dress. Certain clothes can flatter any figure and play down the negative points, but before you try to buy this way, you must take a very hard look at yourself and first recognize what kind of figure you have. Few styles are suited to all figures. There are many kinds of clothes that I would not wear simply because I feel they are best suited to women smaller than I am, or wider than I am. The following guidelines are very broad and will not be effective unless you are prepared to be realistic about your clothes-buying and not attempt to create a vision of yourself that will exist only in your mind's eye.

Tall and Thin

Your clothes should have a rounded, softly tailored look. Avoid vertical lines that will emphasize your height. Wide belts are useful for interrupting the vertical bias. Round necklines and natural or low waistlines should be favored. Wear contrasting tops and skirts and experiment with pleated, full, and straight skirts, as well as double-breasted jackets, long sweaters, and bulky coats. Choose fabrics that have body and texture. If you wish to appear slightly heavier, lean toward the lighter colors. Avoid the short-waisted silhouette and severe, angular details. Frills and "cute" detailing are not for your figure.

Tall and Slender

No tight, clinging styles for you. Favor bloused tops, slightly flared skirts, jackets and suits with pockets set high on the bodice, rounded shoulder lines, and full sleeves. Big, bulky coats will look especially good on you; try belting them at the waist. You can wear all those fabrics that make other women look heavy—satins, bulky knits, and furs. You can afford to wear prints and plaids and light, pastel colors. Your best swimsuit is probably a one-piece tank top.

Tall and Full-Figured

Tailored styles in low-key colors and lines that are vertical or diagonal will flatter your height and girth. Avoid trimming; it will always look too small and ridiculous. Collarless dresses, especially V-necklines, are excellent for you. Straight, easy-fitting skirts with center stitching or a center pleat will slenderize your hips. Choose narrow or medium-width belts and avoid either very long or very short jackets. Semifitted A-line styles will suit you very well since both body-hugging or loose tent styles are quite wrong for your fuller figure. Try medium-weight fabrics in well-spaced but regular patterns. Steer clear of bulky, shiny, or sheer fabrics and sharp, one-color costumes. Dolman sleeves, round necklines, and large pockets will only exaggerate your size. For choice of swimsuit, a one-piece is better than a bikini.

Short and Thin

Everything you buy must be geared to your scale, not only in actual size but appearance. Vertical tucks and patterns are flattering; big splashy prints are not. Whatever you choose should be quite soft, such as a chiffon dress with floating panels, or draped matte jersey outfits. White and pale colors are best and fabrics with body, such as tweeds, are ideal. Your wardrobe should have plenty of blouses, slacks, and short jackets.

Short and Slender

Keep your clothes simple and favor vertical lines for height. Choose round or shallow necklines and short-waisted dresses. Try to match your tops and skirts so your color balance is uniform. Avoid fussy details, low necklines, heavy fabrics, and loud patterns. Crisp, flat fabrics and small-patterned materials in soft colors are much more flattering. Keep away from very short skirts and clunky high heels. If you want to increase your height with heels, the shoe and heel must be petite.

Short and Plump

Always look for a strong vertical line. Straight, full-length coats are good and dresses should include a clear line from shoulder to hem. Skirts should be slightly flared or straight with a center closing or pleat. Your sweaters and blouses should close in the center also. Modified V-necklines flatter, as do thin or medium-weight fabrics with flat finishes, not shiny or sheer. One-color dark or muted outfits are best. Wear a dark, well-fitted, one-piece bathing suit.

Fat

My guidelines for the short and plump are also for you. You will be doomed to failure if you try to buy clothes that have a close fit. A classic tent dress well tailored to the shoulders with enough room to give comfort to the bust can be very elegant. Let it flare out as large as you wish. The neckline should be ultrasimple—no collars. Long sleeves help, but with no cuffs. Mid-knee is the very best length. Your colors should be rich, not light, and never very mixed. Wine, dark brown, bottle green, black, and navy blue are very flattering. Your stockings should be dark and match your shoes, classic pumps with just a medium heel. You will be best served by just a few excellent accessories. Invest in a gold neck ring, a very good bracelet, and a tasteful ring. Never wear pants, and wear sweaters only if they are very full and loose. No swimsuit can make you look thin.

If you are small-bosomed with very full hips, place the emphasis above your waist. Jackets and sweaters must reach no lower than the hipbone. Avoid any tight-fitting clothes, especially pants.

If you are large-breasted with small hips, wear two-tone combinations with the darker color on top.

If you are large-breasted with full hips, de-emphasize your waist by wearing narrow belts and keep the accents below the waist—for instance, a dark jacket with lighter (but not pale) pants.

If you have wide shoulders, wear simple tops and full skirts. Narrow shoulders look best in set-in sleeves.

Vertical and Horizontal Lines

Most of us know that wide women should avoid horizontal lines and tall women vertical lines, but most of us tend only to think of bold stripes in this regard. A "line" in this context can be one of many different things such as a seam itself, a bodice dart, a stitch pattern or a design that tilts to the vertical or to the horizontal. A solid-color dress without any discernible pattern can still have a strong line bias up or across, depending on the weave of the fabric and the way the article has been constructed.

The Art of Buying Clothes

I have given you some pointers about how to choose your clothes and I have to stress, above all, that you do not spend one penny on a single stitch until you have a realistic idea of the good points and limitations of your figure and be prepared to buy accordingly.

Although you should create a budget and stick to it, that does not mean you have to avoid fashion magazines. In step with contemporary mores, most allegedly high-fashion magazines now cater more and more to the average working woman, not just the society queen. Both in terms of articles and fashion layouts there is a long overdue breath of realism and practicality abounding in these pages. Even the models they use no longer represent an ethereal, other-worldly type of beauty, and many may seem no more attractive than yourself. When you see an item that catches your eye in a magazine or newspaper, cut it out and keep it for your next shopping day. You may want to wear a fifty-cent scarf the same way as the picture demonstrates a fifty-dollar one, or your eye may be attracted by an unusual fabric you want to try.

The mark of quality is not absent from inexpensive clothes any more than it is automatically present in expensive ones. If you are well informed and develop a sharp eye about not only what is available but what suits you personally, you can build a great wardrobe. We, the consumers, must keep pressuring for high quality at reasonable cost and also support those manufacturers who do produce (even mass-produce) merchandise that is solidly well made and lasting rather than the slick bargain producers who are only interested in a one-shot profit at your expense. Is it not better to pay $50 once for a really splendid beige cashmere sweater that can last and look wonderful for fifteen years than to pay $20 every third Saturday for a puce knit item that is not colorfast, immediately shrinks and mats on the first washing, and which you discard after one wearing? Quality is not hard to spot and it is not always necessarily at the most expensive counter.

Sizing is one of the first clues to quality. Styles and fabrics can alter the exact fit of a particular size, but if you regularly wear size-8 pants comfortably and the pair you are trying on are size 8 but feel very snug and skimpy, the manufacturer has saved on fabric and the item is shoddy.

Look at the seams of a garment very carefully. If they are open, avoid it, but if they are overcast at the edges with machine stitching or seam binding, then the article is solidly made and will last. Open seams ravel, rip, and split. The seams of a knit or any stretch fabric should give just as much as the fabric itself when you tug gently. If the seams remain stiff and in place, they will split with the first real strain. When an article is on a hanger, the back and side seams must fall straight with no puckers. Often salespersons have told me that uneven seams will iron out flat. Do not be fooled: If they could be made flat, the manufacturer would have done so. Avoid them.

For preventing wear and tear and sustaining good lines, all skirts should be lined, at least enough to cover the hips. The state of the buttonhole is often indicative of the care that has gone into making the whole garment. Make sure there are no loose threads and that the stitching is generous and tight.

Plaid, striped, and print garments should match at all the seams except the inside leg above the knee. Sleeves and jacket fronts should keep the pattern continuous.

Check the linings of your jackets and coats. If they are stiff, they will crack and split. If the garment is unlined, there should be no unfinished seams or loose threads; it should be as neat inside as out (a very good rule of thumb about any kind of clothing purchase).

Hard-finish fabrics like tweeds, gabardines, and many synthetics give better wear than softer cottons, silks, and matte jersey.

Crumple a small piece of the fabric in your hand; it should bounce back fairly easily without many discernible creases.

Always, always try on clothes. The store should provide you with a three-way mirror and a good light if they expect you to buy quality clothes. Unless you are a professional seamstress, you should not imagine that you can correct major deficiencies of fit. If the bodice stands out at the back, you may be able to take it in if there is a center seam and a simple neckline, but shoulders, sleeves, and side seams are very difficult to handle and you are better off searching for a good fit in the store. Examine yourself carefully from all angles. Does the skirt dip at the back or the front? Are the sleeves flat on the inside and full on the outside (like a man's shirt) as they should be? Do you have to tighten belts or move buttons? Take your time and listen to your eyes. A dress too small will make you look large, not petite. That very short skirt may make you look older, not younger.

If you are making an important, expensive purchase, wear the shoes, stockings, and underwear you expect to wear with the item. Go home and change, if necessary, before making your decision. The carfare may be worth the hundred dollars you save or spend well. The fall of the dress or coat may depend upon a particular heel height and your best silk underwear. Always bear in mind what is already in your wardrobe that you can wear with the outfit and expand your purchases logically so that they flatter your older clothes as well as you. Before letting the sale be finalized, ask about care and cleaning instructions. If the salesperson is vague or impatient, think twice. Also, ask yourself if you have been unduly influenced by an overanxious sales staff.

How to Know If It Fits

1) The collar or neckline should lie perfectly flat and even without gaping.

2) The tip of your shoulder bone should be aligned with the set of the shoulder seams.

3) Sleeveless garments must be comfortable and neat at the arms and shoulders.

4) Full-length sleeves must be not too long and not too short.

5) Bodice darts should be at the fullest point of your bustline.

6) The waist, if natural, should really match your own.

7) The side seams of the skirt should be perpendicular to the floor.

8) On a slim skirt, the darts should end at the fullest part of your hips.

Before you buy, not only stand in the garment but walk, sit, and bend; none of these motions should be in the least uncomfortable.

G. CARE AND MAINTENANCE OF YOUR CLOTHES

Start with your closets and drawers. All of us lack enough space, so we must organize. No matter how limited your space, always keep it neat and tidy and you will find what you want quickly and your garments will stay unwrinkled. Your closet or section of the closet must be ONLY for clothes, not for records or books or toys as well. If your closets and drawers are a mess, the odds are your appearance also leaves a lot to be desired. Rearrange your clothes frequently; they will get out of shape if you do not. If they are always put away on hangers or folded neatly and are clean, you never need to hurriedly press or iron a garment. Clothes that you simply never use anymore should be given away or stored in suitcases elsewhere in the house, in the attic or basement or even just under the bed. Do not mix your old, tired, worn clothes with your neat, new ones, or the latter will pick up bad habits from the former. Sweaters and shoes should be kept in plastic bags so you avoid cleaning, dusting, and lint-picking when you pull items out to wear. Keep out-of-season clothes neatly folded in storage areas. You may be surprised at how much space you actually have for hooks in your closet. A few well-placed hooks can hold all your hats, scarves, belts, and bracelets and necklaces that otherwise get tangled and shifted from shelf to shelf or drawer to drawer and cannot be viewed all at once when you want to make a choice. Never let your clothes get mixed with the garments of other members of your family, and separate your own indoor wear from your outdoor wear. Hang as much as you can on hangers—coats, dresses, skirts, suits, and slacks; this takes up the least space. Please throw away or give back to the cleaners those awful wire hangers; for a few cents, buy large strong plastic or wooden hangers with natural shoulders that will keep the shape of your clothes. Divide your drawers and keep your underwear items and all lingerie in individual spaces. I keep all my accessories in partitioned plastic boxes in my drawers.

Never put away dirty clothes; even if you cannot have them cleaned or laundered at once, keep them in tied linen laundry bags. Maintain a good sewing box and even if (like me) you are no expert, sew on your buttons and mend split seams as soon as possible. If you leave these little things, the item will quickly deteriorate.

Manufacturers do not print fabric-care instruction cards for their own amusement. Keep a box just for these tags and when you remove one from a garment, mark down on the tag what garment it came from; you may forget. Follow the instructions and you will have the dress or skirt or suit or sweater much longer. Do not assume everything can be tumbled into the washing machine nor, alternatively, that all your clothes must be dry-cleaned. Take time to familiarize yourself with the instructions; buy the recommended washing product and follow the steps as outlined on the container.

Chapter XII

HOSPITALS AND HEALTH AGENCIES

As I have tried to repeat throughout this book, the best form of medical care is prevention. It is not exactly pleasant to think of serious illness when one is sound in mind and body, but if you spend a small amount of time organizing your preventive-care possibilities, including health insurance, any disorder that you may sustain can either be diagnosed and treated very early or at least contained and cured in a way that does not cause social and financial catastrophe to you or your family.

The health-care picture in this country varies from region to region, and although it can be very favorably compared in scope and opportunity to that of many other nations, we are still behind a few European countries that despite being far less wealthy than the United States can virtually assure every citizen of adequate medical care. Elsewhere in this book I have discussed doctors and clinics. In the event that you are required to enter a hospital either in an emergency or for a routine examination, you or your family should determine which of three possible types of hospital it is:

PRIVATE

Private hospitals are run in order to make money and are usually owned by groups of businessmen and doctors. In general they offer surgery and nursing care to the wealthy, but rarely do they have any emergency-care units or facilities to treat ambulatory outpatients.

MUNICIPAL

Municipal hospitals are run for the benefit of the community and are supported by the tax dollars you pay to either the city, state, or federal government.

Volunteer

A volunteer hospital is a private, nonprofit institution that may be affiliated with a university or a church and is funded by nongovernment subsidy.

Municipal and volunteer hospitals cater to the general public and in most cases offer emergency-treatment facilities and outpatient care. If you do not have any form of health insurance and you are admitted to a municipal or volunteer hospital, you will be required to pay for your treatment according to your ability and in most cases a sliding scale of fees is used to match the cost of such care to your income. Even so, such care can be a great burden financially and I urge all Black women to investigate the possibilities of joining a health insurance group or plan.

Health Insurance

Before signing any health insurance policy, you should contact one or more of the following consumer-oriented organizations that will help you plan a personal or family or group policy to obtain the most benefits for the lowest premium. It is also possible that health insurance is available on a group plan at your place of work, or at your husband's. This often supplies very adequate protection.

Group Health Association of America
1717 Massachusetts Avenue, N.W.
Washington, D.C. 20036
(202) 483-4012

National Association of Blue Shield Plans
211 East Chicago Avenue
Chicago, Illinois 60611
(312) 943-8181

Health Insurance Association of America
1701 K Street, N.W.
Washington, D.C. 20006
(202) 638-3336

Health Insurance Council
750 Third Avenue
New York, New York 10017
(212) 986-8866

Health Insurance Institute
277 Park Avenue
New York, New York 10017
(212) 922-3000

Medical Care Problems

Any question or complaint that you may have concerning any aspect of medical care (such as a physician's qualifications or a clinic's fees) that you cannot obtain satisfaction about on a state or city level you should forward to:

Patient's Aid Society
509 Fifth Avenue
New York, New York 10017
(212) 687-0890

This society is dedicated to protecting the health of the public and improving medical practices.

Medical Care Outside the United States

If you are planning to live or travel abroad, the following organizations can provide information regarding English-speaking medical personnel almost anywhere in the world:

International Association for
Medical Assistance to Travelers
350 Fifth Avenue
New York, New York 10022
(212) 279-6465
American Women's Hospital Service
225 West 34th Street
New York, New York 10019
(212) 947-1721

The American Medical Association

This association, commonly referred to as the AMA, serves both the medical profession as a fraternal organization and the public as a disseminator of information regarding current trends and legislation in all medical fields, including drug therapy, nutritional requirements, cosmetic ingredients, surgical procedures, and the AMA also acts as a watchdog agency against medical chicanery and charlatans.

American Medical Association
535 North Dearborn Street
Chicago, Illinois 60610
(312) 751-6000

Another such watchdog agency that aims to promote and protect both personal and environmental health is:

American Public Health Association
1015 18th Street, N.W.
Washington, D.C. 20036
(202) 467-5000

Black Physicians

If you are seeking a bona fide physician in your community area who is Black or you wish information regarding clinics or hospitals serving the Black community, there is an excellent and very worthy professional society of Black physicians that will give you the necessary assistance:

National Medical Association
2109 E Street, N.W.
Washington, D.C. 20037
(202) 338-8266

The National Medical Association publishes a bimonthly newsletter covering their services and news to which you may subscribe.

For families or groups that would like to receive material about current educational programs in the area of medical care, I advise applying to:

American Social Health Association
1740 Broadway
New York, New York 10019
(212) 582-3553

Health Agencies

I have compiled the following list of national organizations dedicated to combatting specific disorders. Do not be afraid to contact them regarding any problems or questions you have; they exist to serve and educate the public and relieve suffering.

ALLERGIES

Allergy Foundation of America
801 Second Avenue
New York, New York 10017
(212) 684-7875

ALCOHOLISM

National Committee for Prevention of Alcoholism
6830 Laurel Street
Washington, D.C. 20012
(202) 723-0800

National Council on Alcoholism
2 Park Avenue
New York, New York 10016
(212) 889-3160

Alcoholics Anonymous
24 East 22nd Street
New York, New York 10010
(212) GR3-6200

ARTHRITIS

Arthritis Foundation
475 Riverside Drive
New York, New York 10025
(212) 678-6363

CANCER

American Cancer Society
219 East 42nd Street
New York, New York 10017
(212) 867-3700

National Cancer Institute
U. S. Public Health Service
9000 Rockville Pike
Bethesda, Maryland 20014
(301) 656-4000

CEREBRAL PALSY

United Cerebral Palsy Associations, Inc.
122 East 23rd Street
New York, New York 10010
(212) 677-7400

CYSTIC FIBROSIS

National Cystic Fibrosis Research Foundation
3379 Peachtree Road N.E.
Atlanta, Georgia 30326

DENTAL CARE

American Dental Association
211 East Chicago Avenue
Chicago, Illinois 60611
(312) 944-6730

DERMATOLOGY

American Academy of Dermatology
2250 N.W. Flanders Street
Portland, Oregon 97210
(503) 224-0320
American Dermatological Association
17 East Grace Street
Richmond, Virginia 23219
(504) 895-8687

DIABETES

American Diabetes Association, Inc.
600 Fifth Avenue
New York, New York 10020
(212) 541-4310

DRUG ADDICTION

International Federation for Narcotic Education
144 Constitution Avenue N.E.
Washington, D.C. 20002
(202) 543-0839
National Family Council on Drug Addiction
401 West End Avenue
New York, New York 10024
(212) 787-7202

Odyssey House
309 East 6th Street
New York, New York 10003
(212) 674-9160
Synanon Foundation
1910 Ocean Front
Santa Monica, California 90406

EPILEPSY

National Epilepsy League, Inc.
116 South Michigan
Chicago, Illinois 60603
(312) 332-6888
Epilepsy Foundation of America
225 Park Avenue
New York, New York 10017
(212) 677-8550

HEART AND HYPERTENSION

American Health Foundation
1370 Avenue of the Americas
New York, New York 10019
(212) 489-8700
American Heart Association
44 East 23rd Street
New York, New York 10010
(212) 533-1100

KIDNEY DISEASE

National Kidney Foundation, Inc.
116 East 27th Street
New York, New York 10016
(212) 889-2210

LEUKEMIA

Leukemia Society of America, Inc.
211 East 43rd Street
New York, New York 10017
(212) 573-8484

MENTAL HEALTH

National Institute of Mental Health
U. S. Public Health Service
9000 Rockville Pike
Bethesda, Maryland 20014
(301) 656-4000
American Mental Health Foundation
2 East 86th Street
New York, New York 10028
(212) RE7-9027
Federation of Mental Health Centers
241 Central Park West
New York, New York 10024
(212) SU7-1913
Social Psychiatry Research, Inc.
150 East 69th Street
New York, New York 10021
(212) 249-6829

MUSCULAR DYSTROPHY

Muscular Dystrophy Association, Inc.
810 Seventh Avenue
New York, New York 10019
(212) 828-3355

MULTIPLE SCLEROSIS

National Multiple Sclerosis Society
257 Park Avenue South
New York, New York 10010
(212) 674-4100

NUTRITION

American Nutrition Society
P. O. Box 158-C
Pasadena, California 91104
(213) 839-7231
American Board of Nutrition
Department of Medicine

University of California
Davis, California 95616
(916) 752-2723

PREGNANCY AND CHILDBIRTH

American Association for Maternal & Child Health
116 South Michigan Avenue, Suite 806
Chicago, Illinois 60603
(312) 782-3618
Maternity Center Association
48 East 92nd Street
New York, New York 10028
(212) 369-7300
Childbirth Without Pain Education Association
20134 Snowden
Detroit, Michigan 48235
(313) 341-3816

SICKLE-CELL ANEMIA

Sickle-Cell Disease Foundation
144 West 125th Street
New York, New York 10027
(212) 850-1920
Association for Sickle-Cell Anemia
521 Fifth Avenue
New York, New York 10036
(212) 682-5844

SIGHT

American Foundation for the Blind
15 West 16th Street
New York, New York 10011
(212) 924-0420

American Association of Ophthalmology
1100 17th Street N.W.
Washington, D.C. 20036
(202) 833-3447

Speech and Hearing

American Speech & Hearing Association
Old Georgetown Road
Bethesda, Maryland 20014
(301) 530-3400
National Association of Hearing & Speech Agencies
919 18th Street N.W.
Washington, D.C. 20006
(202) 296-3844
Alexander Graham Bell Association for the Deaf
1537 35th Street N.W.
Washington, D.C. 20007
(202) 337-5220

Smoking

National Inter Agency Council on Smoking & Health
419 Park Avenue
New York, New York 10016
(212) 532-6035
Action on Smoking & Health
2000 H. Street N.W.
Washington, D.C. 20006
(202) 659-4310

Tuberculosis

Tuberculosis Welfare League
155 West 72nd Street
New York, New York 10023
(212) TR3-5861
American Lung Association
1740 Broadway
New York, New York 10019
(212) 245-8000

Venereal Disease

American Venereal Disease Association
State Department of Health, Room 416H
47 Trinity Avenue S.W.
Atlanta, Georgia 30334

Committee to Eradicate Syphilis
P. O. Box 92941
Los Angeles, California 90009

The following organizations are concerned with the treatment and rehabilitation of the permanently disabled:

Institute for Crippled & Disabled
340 East 24th Street
New York, New York 10010
(212) 679-0100

National Amputation Foundation
12–45 150th Street
Whitestone, New York 11357

Shut-In Society, Inc.
225 West 99th Street
New York, New York 10025
(212) AC2-7699

Appendix

FURTHER READING

ANGELOGLOU, MAGGIE, *A History of Make-Up*. Macmillan, 1970.

ARCHER, ELSIE, *Let's Face It*. J. B. Lippincott Co., 1968.

BALSAM, *Cosmetics, Science and Technology*. Vols. I and II. Wiley Interscience, 1972.

BAUER, WILLIAM, and SCHALLER, WARREN, *Your Health Today*. Harper & Row, 1965.

BERNE, ERIC. *A Layman's Guide to Psychiatry and Psychoanalysis*. Grove Press, 1957.

BOUCHER, FRANÇOIS, *20,000 Years of Fashion*. Abrams, 1972.

COHEN, SIDNEY, *The Drug Dilemma*. McGraw-Hill, 1969.

CLARK, KENNETH B., *Pathos of Power*. Harper & Row, 1974.

DAVIDSON, BASIL, *The African Past*. Grosset & Dunlap, 1964.

DRAKE, RUTH, *Redbook's Complete Guide to Beauty*. Grosset & Dunlap, 1973.

ELLWOOD, CATHRYN, *Feel Like A Million*. Pocket Books, 1970.

FARIS, JAMES C., *Nuba Personal Art*. University of Toronto Press, 1972.

FREESE, ARTHUR S., *Managing Your Doctor*. Briar Books, 1974.

HALL, ROBERT E., *Nine Months' Reading*. Bantam Books, 1973.

HARRIS, JOSEPH, *Africans and Their History*. Signet Books, 1972.

HARRIS, MIDDLETON, *The Black Book*. Random House, 1974.

HENSLEY, MILLIE, *The Art of Make-Up, Skin and Hair Care*. Milady Pub. Co., 1960.

HILLIARD, MARION, *Women and Fatigue*. Pocket Books, 1962.

HUGHES, LANGSTON, *A Pictorial History of the Negro in America*. Crown Publishers, 1968.

HYMAN, REBECCA, *The Complete Guide to Synthetic Hairpieces and Wigs*. Bantam Mini-Books, 1970.

HYMAN, REBECCA, *The Brand Name Wig Book*. Bantam Mini-Books, 1974.

JANTZEN, INC., *What You Should Know about Your Breasts*. Jantzen, Inc., 1974.

JONES, JOHN HENRY, *All About the Natural*. Clairol Inc., 1971.

KRANE, JESSICA, *How to Use Your Hands to Save Your Face*. Avon, 1969.

LA BARRE, HARRIET, *Plastic Surgery: Beauty You Can Buy*. Holt, Rinehart, Winston, 1970.

LAWRENCE, SEYMOUR, *Pregnancy, Birth and the Newborn Baby*. Delacorte Press, 1973.

LOUIS, M., *Six Thousand Years of Hairstyling*. Louis, 1939.

MATTHEWS, LESLIE, *The Antiques of Perfume*. Bell & Sons, 1973.

MIDDLETON, JOHN, *Gods and Rituals*. Natural History Press, 1967.

MILLER, BENJAMIN, *The Complete Medical Guide*. Simon & Schuster, 1967.

MORINI, SIMONA, *Body Sculpture: Plastic Surgery from Head to Toe*. Delacorte Press, 1972.

MORROW, WILLIE, *Curly Hair and Black Skin*. Black Publishers of San Diego, 1973.

NULL, GARY, *The Complete Question and Answer Book of General Nutrition*. Dell Pub. Co., 1972.

ORENTREICH, NORMAN, "Hair Transplantation in Blacks." *Journal of the National Medical Association*, November 1973.

PATTERSON, BELLE, *Belle on Beauty*. Popular Library, 1973.

PAULME, DENISE, *Women of Tropical Africa*. University of California Press, 1963.

PECKEN, MARY BROOKS, *Dressmakers of France*. Harper & Bros., 1956.

PERUTZ, KATHRIN, *Beyond the Looking Glass*. William Morrow, Inc., 1970.

POWITT, A. H., *Hair Structure and Chemistry Simplified*. Milady Pub. Co., 1972.

PLOSKI and KAISER, *The Negro Almanac*. Bellwether, 1971.

RICCIARDI, MIRELLA, *Vanishing Africa*. Reynal & Co., 1971.

RIEFENSTAHL, LENI, *The Last of the Nuba*. Harper & Row, 1973.

ROBBINS, SIDNEY, *1001 Questions to Your Skin Problems*. Dell Pub. Co., 1964.

ROSENBAUM, HELEN, *Afro Make-Up and Hairstyling Secrets*. Signet Books, 1972.

ROTH, BEULAH, *Organic Beauty Secrets*. Paperback Library, 1970.

SEAMAN, BARBARA, *Free and Female*. Coward, McCann & Geoghegan, Inc., 1972.

SCHOENER, ALLON, *Harlem on My Mind*. Random House, 1968.

SPENCER, GERALD, *Your Hair and You*. Milady Pub. Corp., 1957.

THOMAS, VALERIE, *Accent African*. Col-Bob Associates, 1973.

THOMSON, JAMES C., *Healthy Hair*. ARC Books Inc., 1969.

TRAHEY, JANE, *100 Years of the American Female*. Random House, 1967.

TRAVEN, BEATRICE, *Here's Egg On Your Face*. Pocket Books, 1971.

WALKER, MORTON, *Your Foot Health*. Arco Pub. Co., 1972.

WENIG, STEFFAN, *Women in Egyptian Art*. McGraw-Hill, 1969.

WRIGHT, LAWRENCE, *Clean and Decent*. Viking Press, 1960.

ZAX, MELVIN, *The Study of Abnormal Behavior*. Macmillan, 1964.

INDEX

Abortion, 203, 225, 281
Acne, 3, 140
Action on Smoking & Health, 282
Acupuncture, 174
Adolescence, 190, 192–93
Afro hairstyle, 69–70
Age, dressing to suit, 265–66
Aging
  facial skin, 18
  and menopause, 209–10
  skin, 9–11
Alcohol. *See* Drinking
Alcoholics Anonymous, 277
Alcoholism, 165, 167, 277
Aldomet (drug), 175
Alexander, Rowland, 54
Alexander Graham Bell Association for
  the Deaf, 282
Allergies, 4, 276
Allergy Foundation of America, 276
Alopecia (hair loss), 83
Aluminum chloride deodorant, 147
American Academy of Dermatology, 278
American Association for Maternal and
  Child Health, 281
American Association of Ophthalmology,
  282
American Board of Nutrition, 280–81
American Board of Plastic Surgeons, 139
American Cancer Society, 186, 214, 219,
  277
American College of Obstetrics &
  Gynaecology, 226
American College of Surgeons, 139
American Dental Association, 278
American Dermatological Association, 278
American Diabetes Association, Inc., 278
American Foundation for the Blind, 281
American Health Foundation, 279
American Heart Association, 279
American Lung Association, 282

American Medical Association (AMA),
  25, 275
American Mental Health Foundation,
  280
American Nutrition Society, 280
American Public Health Association, 276
American Social Health Association, 276
American Speech & Hearing Association,
  282
American Venereal Disease Association,
  283
American Women's Hospital Service, 275
Amphetamines, 168
Antiperspirants, 146, 147
Anxiety, 234
Appearance, 246–47, 250
Arm-pull exercise, 128
Arteriosclerosis, 175
Arthritis Foundation, 176, 277
Association for Sickle-Cell Anemia, 281
Astringents, 15
Athlete's foot, 118
Austin, Ed, 255

Backache, 172–73, 198
Bad breath, 49
Barbiturates, 168
Barrie, Scott, 255
Basic wardrobe, 257–72
  accessories, 258–59
  art of buying clothes, 269–71
  blouses, 261
  brassieres, 263
  care and maintenance, 271–72
  coats, 259–60, 264
  color scheme, 257–58
  daytime outfits, 264
  dresses, 261–62
  dress your age, 265–66
  dress your shape, 266–69
  evening wear, 263, 264

girdle, 262–63
hats, 260
how to know if clothes fit, 271
making your own clothes, 264–65
pants, 262
shoes, 113–15, 263–64
sports clothes, 264
suits, 261
sweaters, 261
underwear, 188, 262
Bathing, 7–9
  during menstruation, 146
  during pregnancy, 146
  personal hygiene, 187–88, 189–90
Beauty
  and behavior, 241–52
  and health, 149
Behavior, 233
  and appearance, 246–47, 250
  beauty and, 241–52
  business, 246–47
  class distinction, 252
  and coworkers, 247
  dealing with strangers, 250
  family, 244
  giving and taking instructions, 247
  language, 252
  letter writing, 247–48
  and loud music, 249–50
  manners, 242–43
  neurotic, 234–35, 236
  normal, 234, 235
  parties and dates, 251
  psychotic, 235–36
  public, 249–50
  punctuality, 247
  roommates, 244–45
  service personnel, 245
  table manners, 248
  telephone, 246
  voice, 252
Benson, Stella, "Story Coldly Told" by,
  146
Benzedrine, 168
"Best Slaves Got Drunk, The"
  (Douglass), 166
Biofeedback, 174
Birth control, 220–25
Birth-control pills, 4, 5
Birthmarks, 137
Blackheads, 23
Bladder, 184
Blood poisoning (toxemia), 199–200
Board-certified surgeons, 139, 140
Body, 123–48, 148–81
  annual checkup, 177, 178–80, 206–07,
    215, 226–28
  common complaints, 171–74
  and drinking, 165–67

and drugs, 167–71
excessive hair, 140–45
and exercise, 19, 123–33
internal disorders, emergency treatment,
  180–81
major diseases, 174–77
and nutrition, 150–51, 156–57
odor, 145–48
posture, 133–35, 252
and smoking, 163–65
surface appearance, 123–48
temperature, 1, 146
weight (see Weight gain, Weight loss)
See also Menopause; Menstruation;
  Pregnancy
Body hair, 140–45
  breast, 145
  ingrown, 144
  legs, 142
  pubic, 145
  removal of excessive, 141–45
  underarm, 141, 142
Body odor, 145–48
  antiperspirants for, 146
  deodorants for, 146
  foot, 118
  genital, 189–90
  racial scents, 146
Body surgery, 135–40
  before-surgery considerations, 139–40
  congenital defects, 137
  corrective, 137, 139
  cosmetic, 135, 136–37, 137–40
  reconstructive, 135, 136, 139
  reductive, 137
Brassiere, 194, 205, 263
Breast cancer, 214, 216–17
  mastectomy for, 216–17
  postmastectomy adjustment, 217
  self-examination for, 216, 217–18
Breasts, 185–86
  artificial (prostheses), 217
  and menopause, 207
  and menstruation, 192
  and pregnancy, 199
  self-examination, 216, 217–18
  surgery, 138–39, 216
Breast-shaping surgery (mammaplasty),
  138–39
Bunions, 117
Burns, 11
Burrows, Stephen, 255

Callous, 98, 118
Cancer, 213–19, 277
  breast, 214
  cervical, 214, 215
  of colon, 215
  and drinking, 167

Fallopian tube, 216
  ovarian, 216
  and smoking, 163
  uterine, 214, 215
Carbohydrates, 151
Cellulite, 132–33
Cereal food group, 152, 154, 160
Cerebral palsy, 277
Cervical cancer, 214, 215
  Pap test for, 215, 216, 227
Cervix, 183, 184, 211, 214, 215
Cesarean section, 200, 204
Chafing (intertrigo), 137
Change of life. See Menopause
Charm, 242, 243
Cheeks, make-up for, 42–43
Chemosurgery, 140
Childbirth, 281
  Cesarean section, 200, 204
  emergency treatment, 228
  episiotomy, 200
  premature, 203, 225
  stillbirth, 203
  and women athletes, 204
Childbirth Without Pain Education
    Association, 281
Chiropodist, 119
Chisholm, Shirley, 243
Chloasma (melasma), 4, 5, 176, 198
Choking, emergency treatment for, 180
Cholesterol, 150–51
Churchill, Winston, 252
Circumcision, 216
Civil Rights movement, 242
Clark, Mamie Phipps, 243
Class distinction, 252
Cleft-palate surgery, 137
Clinics, 178, 276
Clitoris, 183, 184
Clothes, 256
  and menstruation, 194
  and pregnancy, 205–06
  See also Basic wardrobe
Cocaine, 170
Collagen, 10, 21
Cologne, 147–48
Colon, cancer of, 215
Committee to Eradicate Syphilis, 283
Conception, 195–96
Condom, 224, 225
Congenital-defect surgery, 137
Contact lenses, 41
Contraception, 221–25
  abortion, 203, 225, 281
  condom, 224, 225
  current-methods chart, 222–23
  diaphragm, 224
  future methods, 224
  intrauterine device (IUD), 221, 224

mechanical and chemical methods, 224
  minipill, 221
  the Pill, 197, 219, 221
  rhythm methods, 224
  spermicides, 224
  sterilization, 224–25
  tubal ligation, 225
  vasectomy, 225
Cooking, 154, 156–57
Corn-row hairstyle, 69, 70
Corns, 117
Corrective surgery, 137, 139
Cortin (hormone), 197
Cosmetic surgery, 135, 136, 137–40
  breast shaping (mammaplasty), 138–39
  eye shaping (blepharoplasty), 138
  face lifting (meloplasty, rhytidectomy),
    138
  lip thinning (cheilotomy), 138
  lower-body shaping, 139
  nose shaping (rhinoplasty), 137
Cosmetics. See Make-up, Make-up base
Cosmetologists, 25
Courtesy, 242
Coworkers, and manners, 247
CPT (Colored People's Time), 247
Creams and lotions
  bleaching, 30
  cleansing, 15
  lip care, 43
  protein-enriched, 21–22
  vitamin-enriched, 21–22
Crisis clinics, 240
Cup-ear surgery, 137
Curlers, 250
Cuts, 11
Cystic fibrosis, 278
Cystitis, 213

Dairy-food group, 152, 154
Dandruff (seborrhea), 81–83
Davis, Angela, 243
Deafness, 282
Delivery. See Childbirth
Dental diseases, 50
Dental examination, 50
Dental plaque, 48
Dental surgery, 51
Deodorants, 146, 147, 189
Department of Health, Education and
    Welfare, 220–21
Department of Labor, Women's Bureau,
    113
Depilatories, 141, 143
Depo Provera (contraceptive drug), 224
Dermabrasion, 140
Dermatitis, 24
Dermatologists, 11, 19, 24–25, 93, 94–95,
    106

Dermatology, 278
Dermis, 1
Dexedrine, 168
Diabetes, 199–200, 221, 278
Diaphragm (contraceptive device), 224
Diet, 19, 31, 80, 100, 159
  balanced, 80, 150, 152, 158
  and menopause, 208
  and menstruation, 192–93
  and pregnancy, 200–01
Dietetic food, 161
Diet pills, 161, 203
Dilation and curettage (D. and C.), 192,
  207, 225
Discoid lupus (pigment loss), 24
Diuretics, 161, 193
Doctors, 178–79
  Black, 178, 276
  female, 178
  for internal examination, 226
  and mental illness, 238, 240
Douching, 187–88
Douglass, Frederick, "The Best Slaves
  Got Drunk" by, 166
Drinking, 165–67
  and drugs, 171
  and menopause, 208
  and pregnancy, 203
  and smoking, 170
Drugs, 167–71, 278–79
  and menopause, 208
  and menstruation, 193
  and pregnancy, 203

Earrings, 47
Ears, 46, 137
Eating habits, 151–52, 161–62
  and menstruation, 192–93
  in public, 249
  table manners, 248
Electric rollers, 75
Electrolysis, 143–44
Embryo, 195, 196
Epidermis, 1
Epilepsy Foundation of America, 279
Episiotomy (childbirth surgery), 200
Estrogen, 10, 21, 184, 192, 206, 207, 211
Exercise, 19, 123–33
  arm pull, 128
  for backache, 173
  and cellulite, 132–33
  "correct," 125–27
  facial, 132
  for the feet, 112–13
  gross motor activity, 126, 127, 133, 204
  head nod, 129
  head rotation, 128–29
  jogging, 126, 127, 130–31
  and menopause, 209

and menstruation, 193–94
  postnatal, 204–05
  and pregnancy, 204
  prone body raise and stretch, 129–30
  seated forward press, 129
  standing back press, 129
  and weight control, 124–25
Exfoliation (skin peeling), 22, 140
Eyebrow pencil, 40
Eyebrows, 38–40
  make-up, 39–40
  shaping, 38–39
Eye drops, 31–32
Eyelashes
  curling, 37–38
  false, 36–37
Eye liner, 35–36
Eye make-up, 33–42
  color selection, 34
  and contact lenses, 41
  and eyebrows, 40–41
  and glasses, 41
  removal of, 41–42
  tools for, 34
Eyes, 31–42
  blindness, 281
  circles under, 41
  close-set, 40
  examination, 32
  protruding, 41
  puffy eyelids, 41
  wide-set, 40
Eye shadow, 35
Eye-shaping surgery (blepharoplasty), 138
Eye tumor (melanoma), 31
Eyewash, 31

Face, 13–51, 132, 140
  cheeks, 42–43
  ears, 46–47
  eyes, 31–42
  lips, 43–46
  skin, 13–31
  teeth, 50–51
Face lifting (rhytidectomy, meloplasty),
  138
Facial mask, 20–21, 98
Facial sauna, 20
Facial skin, 13–31, 140
  cosmetics for disorders, 25
  dry, 13, 16–17
  oily, 13, 17
  problems, 23–24
Facial treatments, 18–19
FACS (Fellow American College of
  Surgeons), 139, 140
Fallen arches, 118–19
Fallopian tubes, 184, 195–96, 216, 225
Falls (hairpieces), 92

Family manners, 244
Fashion, 253–72
Fatigue, 171–72
Fats, 150, 151
Federation of Mental Health Centers, 280
Feet, 107–20
  ailments, 116–19
  care of, 108–09, 111–12, 119–20
  exercise, 112–13
  pedicure, 109–11
  and pregnancy, 205
  structure, 107–08
Feminist Party, 257
Fibroid tumors, 207, 213, 221
  and the Pill, 221
  and pregnancy, 200
Fingernails, 99–106
  and diet, 100
  injuries and diseases, 105–06
  manicure, 100–04, 106
  patching, 104–05
  after pregnancy, 105
  rate of growth, 100
  structure, 99
Fish, 153, 156
Flat feet, 118–19
Flesh moles, 24
Fluoride, 49
Food, 149–62
  basic groups, 152–53, 157
  basic nutrition, 150–51
  dietetic, 161
  eating habits, 151–52
  health, 158
  natural, 158
  organic, 158
  shopping for, 153–56
  soul, 152
  supplements, 157–58
  vegetarianism, 158
Food and Drug Administration (FDA), 21, 157
Foot odor (bromodrosis), 118
Footwear, 113–16
  how to buy shoes, 114–15
  ideal working shoe, 114
  pantyhose, 116, 188
  stockings, 116
Fragrances, 147–48
Fruit, 153, 155

Genital odor, 189–90
Genital-urinary tract infections, 215
German measles, and pregnancy, 200
Gingivitis, 50
Glaucoma, 31
Gonorrhea, 219, 220
Gravlee (cancer research tool), 215

Gross motor activity exercise, 126, 127, 133, 204
Group Health Association of America, 274
Gum-chewing, 250
Gums, 49, 50
Gynaecologist, 226

Hair, 1, 53–95
  anatomy, 55–57
  basic care, 63–68, 92–95
  basic hygiene, 57–61, 94
  body (see Body hair)
  conditioners, 60
  dry, 63–64
  drying, 61
  emergency treatment, 95
  fine (thin), 65–66
  function, 53–55
  gray, 67, 77
  grooming, 61–63, 79–80
  health, 80–81
  loss, 83–86, 176
  lubricants, 62
  and menopause, 208
  oily, 64–65, 81
  pigmentation, 75
  and pregnancy, 198
  problems and their treatment, 81–86
  professional care, 92–95
  rinses, 59–60, 76–77, 82
  shampooing, 58–59
  sprays, 77, 79
  styling (see Hair styling)
  thick, 66
  thinning (physiological), 67–68
Hair brushes, 61–62
Hair combs, 61
Hair cutting, 77–79
Hair styling, 69–71
  Afro, 69–70
  chemical straightening, 70, 72–74
  coloring, 75–77
  corn row, 69, 70
  curling and waving, 74–75
  cutting, 77–79
  hairpieces, 87, 91–92
  hot-comb straightening, 70, 71–72
  shaping, 78
  thinning, 78
  trimming, 78
  wigs, 86–92
Hairdresser, 93–95
Hairnets, 79–80
Hairpieces, 87, 91–92
  braids, 92
  cascades (clusters), 92
  demiwigs, 92
  long falls, 92

mini falls, 92
wig falls, 92
wiglets, 92
Hairpins, 79
Halitosis, 49
Hammertoe, 117
Hand care, 97–98, 106
  callouses, 98
  manicure, 100–04
  perspiration, 98
  prominent veins, 98
Hangnails, 105
Headache, 173–74
Head-nod exercise, 129
Head-rotation exercise, 128–29
Health
  and beauty, 149
  and nutrition, 149
  See also Health care; Mental health
Health agencies, 276–83
Heath care, 178, 179, 180, 206, 215
  clinics, 178, 276
  government health departments, 214
  hospitals, 178, 179, 214
  insurance, 274
  internal examination, 226–28
  medical checkup, 177, 178–80
  national agencies, 276–83
Health Insurance Association of America,
  274
Health Insurance Council, 274
Health Insurance Institute, 274
Hearing, 282
Heart, 279
Heart attacks, 175, 180
Henna, 60, 76
Heroin, 170
High blood pressure. See Hypertension
Hormones, 10, 21, 80, 184, 207
Hospitals, 178, 179, 276
  municipal, 273, 274
  private, 273
  university-affiliated, 179, 214
  volunteer, 274
Hymen, 184
Hyperpigmentation, 2
Hypertension, 174–76, 235, 237, 279
  and the Pill, 221
  and pregnancy, 199–200
Hypodermis, 1
Hypopigmentation, 2
Hysterectomies, 173, 207–08, 213

Insanity, 233–34
International Association for Medical
  Assistance to Travelers, 275
International Federation for Narcotic
  Education, 278
Institute for Crippled & Disabled, 283

Instructions, giving and taking, 247
Internal disorders, emergency treatment
  for, 180–81
Internal examination, 226–28
Internist, 226
Intradermal suturing, 136
Intrauterine device (IUD), 221, 224
Introductions, 251
Invitations, 251
Iron, 192–93
Ismelin (drug), 175

Jogging, 126, 127, 204
  in place, 130–31
Jordan, Barbara, 243

Kanekalon Preselle fiber, 87
Karp, Laurence E., 145–46
Keloids, 3, 46, 47
  and cosmetic surgery, 136, 137, 138,
    139, 140
Kennedy, Flo, 257
Kidney diseases, 175, 279
  and the Pill, 221
  and pregnancy, 199–200

Labia, 183, 184
Language, 249, 252
Laxatives, 161, 193
Legs, 120–21, 142
Letter writing, 248–49, 251
Leukemia Society of America, 279
Librium, 168
Life expectancy, 174
Lips, 43–46
Lipstick, 44–45
Lip-thinning surgery (cheilotomy), 138
Lobeline (stop-smoking aid), 165

Make-up
  cheeks, 42–43
  eyebrows, 39–40
  eyes, 33–42
  face, 25–31
  lips, 43–46
Make-up base, 26–31
  application, 28–29
  color, 27–28
  dry skin, 29
  light intensity effect on, 30
  natural look, 29–30
  oily skin, 29
Manic-depression, 235
Manicure, 100–04
Manners, 242–43
  table, 248
Marcel wave, 74
Marijuana, 169–70
Mascara, 36, 38

Massage, 133
  scalp, 81, 94
Mastectomy (breast-cancer surgery), 216
Maternity Center Association, 281
Matzeliger, Jan Ernst, 113
Meat and fish food group, 153, 155–56
Medical-care problems, 275, 276
Medical checkup, 177, 178–80
  after age thirty-five, 206, 215
  for cancer, 215
  complete physical examination, 179
  eye examination, 32
  internal examination, 226–28
  laboratory studies, 179
  medical history, 178–79
  and menopause, 206–07
  preventive, 50, 179
Melanin, 2, 10
Melanocytes, 2
Melasma. See Chloasma
Menopause, 186, 190, 206–10
  abnormalities of, 207
  and aging, 209–10
  and bathing, 146
  and body odor, 146
  and breasts, 207
  and cholesterol build-up, 150
  and diet, 208
  and exercise, 209
  and excessive body hair, 141
  and hair, 208
  signs of, 206
  and skin, 208
  and surgery, 207–08
  treatment of, 206–07
Menstrual cycle, 184, 190
Menstruation, 190–94, 206
  abnormalities of, 191–92
  amenorrhea, 191
  and the breasts, 192
  and clothes, 194
  and diet, 192–93
  dilation and curettage (D. and C.),
    192
  and douching, 188
  and drinking, 193
  and drugs, 193
  dysmenorrhea, 191
  and elimination, 193
  endometriosis, 191
  and exercise, 193–94
  and genital odor, 190
  irregular bleeding, 191
  and posture, 194
  and pregnancy, 195, 196
  prolonged, 192
  shortened cycles, 192
Mental health, 233–36, 280
  functional psychosis, 235–36

  manic-depressive, 235
  neurotic, 234–35, 236
  normal, 234–35
  organic psychosis, 236
  paranoia, 235
  sanity, 233–34
  schizophrenia, 235
Mental illness, 236–40, 280
  and the Black woman, 236–37
  emergency treatment, 240
  prevention, 239–40
  treatment, 237–39
Methadone, 170
Methysergide (drug), 174
Midwife, 226
Migraine, 235
Minerals, 151, 156
Miscarriage, 200, 225
Moisturizers, 10, 15, 21, 97–98
Moles, 24
Mouth-to-mouth resuscitation, 181
Multiple sclerosis, 280
Muscular Dystrophy Association, Inc.,
  280
Myoctemy (tumor surgery), 213

Naomi Sims wig collection, 86–87, 91
National Amputation Foundation, 283
National Association of Blue Shield Plans,
  274
National Association of Hearing & Speech
  Agencies, 282
National Cancer Institute, 214, 277
National Commission on the Causes and
  Prevention of Violence, 228
National Committee for Prevention of
  Alcoholism, 277
National Council on Alcoholism, 277
National Cystic Fibrosis Research
  Foundation, 278
National Epilepsy League, Inc., 279
National Family Council on Drug
  Addiction, 278
National Institute of Mental Health, 280
National Kidney Foundation, Inc., 279
National Inter Agency Council on
  Smoking & Health, 282
National Medical Association, 276
National Multiple Sclerosis Society, 280
Nembutal, 168
Neurosis, 234–35
New York Times, 145–46
Nikoban (stop-smoking aid), 165
Normality, 234
Nose blowing, 46
Nose-shaping surgery (rhinoplasty), 137
Nurse, 226
Nutrients, 151

Nutrition, 150–51, 280–81
  and cooking, 156–57
  and health, 149
  and menstruation, 192–93
  for pregnant and nursing women, 202

Obstetrician, 226
Odyssey House, 279
O'Leary, Lydia, 25
Olympic games, 193, 204
Onycholysis (nail disease), 105
Ophthalmologist, 32
Ophthalmology, 282
Optician, 32
Optometrist, 32
Oral contraceptives, 141, 191, 213
Orthodontist, 51
Otosclerosis (middle-ear disease), 46
Ovarian cysts, 213
Ovaries, 184, 216

Panties, 188
Pantyhose, 116, 188
Pap test, 179, 215, 216, 227
Paranoia, 235
Paronychia (nail disease), 105
Parties and dates, 251
Patient's Aid Society, 275
Pedicure, 109–11, 120
Pedicurist, 119
Perfume, 147–48
Permanent disability, 283
Permanent waving, 74
Personal hygiene, 187–90
Perspiration
  and body-temperature regulation, 1, 146
  foot, 108–09
  hand, 98
  and racial scents, 146
  underarm, 141, 146
pH factor, 22–23, 58
Physical examination, 179
Pigmentation, 1, 2, 31, 75, 136, 140, 198
  loss of, 24, 30
The Pill, 197, 219, 221
Pimples, 23–24, 30
Placenta, 196, 197
Planned Parenthood, 225
Plastic surgeons, 139–40
Podiatrist, 119
Poise, 242, 243, 252
Poisoning, emergency treatment for, 180
Population control, 195, 220–21
Posture, 133–35, 252
  and menstruation, 194
  and pregnancy, 205
Pregnancy, 186, 190, 194–206, 281
  and basic nutrition, 202
  bathing, 146

body change, 197–99
body hair, 141
body odor, 146
breasts, 199
clothes, 205–06
diabetes, 199–200
diet, 200–01
douching, 188
drugs, 203
embryo, 195–96
exercise, 204–05
fibroid tumors, 200, 207, 213
fingernails, 105
genital odor, 190
German measles, 200
hair, 198
hypertension, 199–200
kidney diseases, 199–200
mask of, 4, 198
menstruation, 195, 196
miscarriage, 200
ovulation and conception, 195–96
posture, 205
and race, 196–97
signs of, 196
and skin, 197–98
smoking, 203
stretch marks, 4, 198
symptoms of, 196
teeth, 50, 198–99
toxemia, 199–200
urinary infection, 197
varicose veins, 197
weight control, 202–03
Progesterone, 184, 192
Prone body raise and stretch exercise,
  129–30
Propalol (drug), 174
Protein, 10, 21–22, 151
Protorace, 1
Psychiatry, 233, 238, 240, 280
Psychoanalysis, 233, 236, 238
Psychology, 233, 238, 240
Psychosis, 235–36
  functional, 235
  manic-depressive, 235
  organic, 236
  paranoiac, 235
  schizophrenic, 235
Psychosomatic illness, 235
Puberty, 186, 190
Public behavior, 249–50
Pulmonary anemia, 168
Punctuality, 247

Racial scents, 146
Rape, 228–31
Rape Crisis Center suggestions, 229–31
Reach to Recovery program, 217

Reconstructive surgery, 135, 136, 139
Rectum, 185, 215
Reproductive organs, 183–86
    breasts, 185–86, 214, 216–17
    cancer of, 213–19
    cervix, 183, 184, 211, 214, 215
    clitoris, 183, 184
    Fallopian tubes, 184, 195–96, 216, 225
    and genital odor, 189–90
    hymen, 184
    and hysterectomies, 173, 207–08, 213
    internal examination, 226–28
    labia, 183, 184
    ovaries, 184, 213, 216
    personal hygiene, 187–90
    self-examination, 186–87
    and sterilization, 224–25
    and urinary diseases, 213
    uterus, 183, 184, 207, 213, 214, 215
    vagina, 183, 184, 189
    vaginal diseases, 210–12
    venereal diseases (VD), 176, 219–20
    vulva, 183
    womb, 184
    See also Menopause; Menstruation;
        Pregnancy
Rhythm contraceptive methods, 224
Ringworm, 117
Roommates, and manners, 244–45
Rouge, 42–43

Salting out (abortion induction), 225
Sanity, 233–34
Sarcoidosis, 176
Sauna, 133
    facial, 20
Schizophrenia, 235
Seated forward press exercise, 129
Sebaceous glands, 7, 8, 10, 18, 56
Seborrhea (dandruff), 82
Seconal, 168
Service personnel, 245
Shampoo, 58–59, 94
Shaving, 141–42, 144
Shoes, 113–15, 263–64
Shut-In Society, Inc., 283
Sickle-cell anemia, 31, 49, 167, 177, 221,
    281
Sickle-Cell Disease Foundation, 281
Sight, 281
    eye examination, 32
Silicone, 138
Sitting posture, 135
Skin, 1–10
    advantages of Black, 4
    ashiness, 2
    and chemosurgery, 140
    cleansing, 7–9
    color, 1–2

dark patches, 2
effect on of protein and hormone
    deficiency, 10
facial. See Facial skin
light patches, 2
and menopause, 208
normal-to-dry, 6, 8–9
normal-to-oily, 6, 7
and pregnancy, 197–98
special conditions, 2–3
special problems, 3–4
Skin specialists, 11
Slang, 249
Sleep, 19, 124, 126
Sleeping posture, 135
Smoking, 163–65, 282
    and drinking, 170
    and drugs, 171
    and menopause, 208
    and pregnancy, 203
    to stop, 164–65
Soap, 8, 16, 22–23, 146
Social Psychiatry Research, Inc., 280
Soul food, 152
Speech, 252, 282
Spermicides, 224
Spitting, 249
Spot reducing, 125, 133
Standing back press exercise, 129
Standing posture, 134–35
State Board of Cosmetology, 25
State health departments, cervical cancer
    program, 214
Sterilization, 224–25
Stockings, 116
Stomach pain, emergency treatment for,
    180
"Story Coldly Told" (Benson), 146
Strangers, dealing with, 250
Stress, 126, 234
Stretch marks, 4, 198
Strokes, 175
Sunglasses, 32
Sunlight
    effects of on eyes, 32
    effects of on skin, 5, 9–10, 18
Surgeons
    board certified, 139
    plastic, 139–40
Surgery
    childbirth, 200
    D. and C., 192, 207, 225
    dental, 51
    spinal, 173
    unnecessary, 173
    See also Body surgery; Cosmetic
        surgery; Hysterectomies;
        Reconstructive surgery
Swearing, 249

Swimming, 126, 127
   and menstruation, 193–94
   and pregnancy, 204
Synanon Foundation, 170, 279
Syphilis, 176, 219, 220, 283
Systemic lupus erythematosis (SLE), 176

Table manners, 248
Teeth, 47–51
   care, 48–49, 50, 51, 278
   diseases, 50
   examination, 50
   extractions, 50–51
   and pregnancy, 50, 198–99
   surgery, 51
   whitening, 49
   yellowing, 51
Telephone behavior, 246
Thalidomide, 203
Toenail ailments, 116–17
   club nails, 117
   fungus toenail, 117
   ingrown toenails, 116
   raised toenails, 116
Toilet water, 147–48
Tooth sticks, 48–49
Toxemia (blood poisoning), 199–200
Tranquilizers, 168
Traveling behavior, 250–51
Tubal ligation, 225
Tuberculosis Welfare League, 282
Tumors. *See* Fibroid tumors

Ultraviolet rays, 5, 9–10
Underarm shaving, 141, 142
Underwear, 188, 262
United Cerebral Palsy Associations, Inc.,
   277
University of Washington, 146
Urethra, 184
Urinary-digestive tract, 184
Urinary diseases, 213
Urinary infection, 197
Uterine cancer, 214, 215
   Pap test for, 215, 227
Uterus, 183, 194, 214, 215
   and menopause, 207
   tumors of, 207, 213, 221

Vagina, 183, 184, 210–12
   deodorants, 189
Vaginal diseases, 210–12
   atrophis vaginalis, 211
   cervicitis, 211
   discharge, 210
   moniliasis (candidiasis), 211
   treatment for, 212
   trichomoniasis, 211
   vaginitis, 210–11
Valium, 168
Vasectomy, 225

Vegetable cooking, 156–57
Vegetable and fruit food group, 153, 155,
   160
Vegetarianism, 158
Veins
   of hands, 98
   varicose, 120–21, 197
Venereal diseases (VD), 176, 219–20,
   283
   gonorrhea, 219, 220
   syphilis, 219, 220, 283
Virginity, 184
Vitamins, 21–22, 151, 156, 158–59, 203
   A, 21, 31, 151, 153, 159
   B, 151
   B-12, 168
   C, 153, 159
   D, 151, 157, 159
   E, 21, 151
   K, 151
Vitiligo, 24
Voice, 243, 249, 252
Vomiting, and pregnancy, 198
Vreeland, Diana, 265
Vulva, 183, 211

Walker, Madame C. J., 57, 71
Walking, 126, 135, 204
Water waving, 74
Waxing, body-hair removal, 142–43
Weight gain, 162
   and breast size, 185
   and exercise, 124
   and smoking, 164
Weight loss, 159–62
   and backache, 172
   and breast size, 185
   and exercise, 124
   and face lifting, 138
   and massage, 133
   and menstruation, 191
   and pregnancy, 202–03
Wella Kolestral Concentrate hair
   conditioner, 60
Whiteheads, 23
Wiglets, 92
Wigs, 86–92
   color, 87
   fit, 88
   hairline, 89
   human hair, 86
   Naomi Sims collection, 86–87, 91
   style, 87
   synthetic, 86, 90
   texture, 87
   and your own hair, 88, 89, 90–91
Woman's Liberation Movement, 195
Womb, 184
Wrinkles, 140, 164

X-rays, 143, 179